Evidence-based medical monitoring

From principles to practice

Evidence-based medical monitoring

From principles to practice

Edited by

Paul P. Glasziou
Professor of Evidence-Based Medicine
University of Oxford
Centre for Evidence-Based Medicine
Oxford, UK

Les Irwig
Professor of Epidemiology
Screening and Test Evaluation Program
School of Public Health
University of Sydney
Sydney, Australia

Jeffrey K. Aronson
Reader in Clinical Pharmacology
University of Oxford
Department of Primary Health Care
Oxford, UK

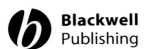
Blackwell
Publishing

BMJ | Books

BMJ Books is an imprint of the BMJ Publishing Group Limited, used under licence

Blackwell Publishing, Inc., 350 Main Street, Malden, Massachusetts 02148-5020, USA
Blackwell Publishing Ltd, 9600 Garsington Road, Oxford OX4 2DQ, UK
Blackwell Publishing Asia Pty Ltd, 550 Swanston Street, Carlton, Victoria 3053, Australia

First published 2008

1   2008

Library of Congress Cataloging-in-Publication Data

Evidence-based medical monitoring : from principles to practice / edited by Paul Glasziou,
Jeffrey Aronson, Les Irwig.
     p. ; cm.
   ISBN 978-1-4051-5399-7 (pbk. : alk. paper)   1. Patient monitoring.   2. Chronic
diseases–Treatment.   3. Evidence-based medicine.   I. Glasziou, Paul, 1954–
II. Aronson, J. K.   III. Irwig, Les.
   [DNLM: 1. Chronic Disease–therapy.   2. Aftercare–methods.   3. Aftercare–trends.
4. Evidence-Based Medicine–methods.   5. Evidence–Based Medicine–trends. WT 500
E93 2007]

RT48.55.E95 2007
616.07′5–dc22

                                                                              2007032639

ISBN: 978-1-4051-5399-7

A catalogue record for this title is available from the British Library

Set in 9.5/12pt Meridien by Aptara Inc., New Delhi, India
Printed and bound in Singapore by COS Printers Pte Ltd

Commissioning Editor: Mary Banks
Editorial Assistant: Victoria Pittman
Development Editor: Simone Dudziak
Production Controller: Rachel Edwards

For further information on Blackwell Publishing, visit our website:
http://www.blackwellpublishing.com

The publisher's policy is to use permanent paper from mills that operate a sustainable
forestry policy, and which has been manufactured from pulp processed using acid-free
and elementary chlorine-free practices. Furthermore, the publisher ensures that the text
paper and cover board used have met acceptable environmental accreditation standards.

Contents

Contributors

Jeffrey K. Aronson, MA, MBChB, DPhil, FRCP, FBPharmacolS
Reader in Clinical Pharmacology
Department of Primary Health Care
University of Oxford
Oxford, UK

John Bedson, MD MRCGP
GP Research Fellow
Primary Care Musculoskeletal Research Centre
Keele University
Keele, UK

Katy Bell, MBChB, MMed(Clin Epi)
Screening and Test Evaluation Program
School of Public Health
University of Sydney
Australia

Jan M. Binnekade, RN, PhD
Researcher
Department of Intensive Care
Academic Medical Center
University of Amsterdam
Amsterdam, The Netherlands

Patrick M.M. Bossuyt, PhD
Professor of Clinical Epidemiology
Department of Clinical Epidemiology
Biostatistics and Bioinformatics
Academic Medical Center
University of Amsterdam
Amsterdam, The Netherlands

Jamie J. Coleman, MBChB, MRCP (UK)
Lecturer in Clinical Pharmacology
Department of Clinical Pharmacology
Queen Elizabeth Hospital
Birmingham, UK

Jonathan Craig, MBChB, FRACP, MMed (Clin Epi) PhD
Senior Staff Specialist
Department of Nephrology
Children's Hospital at Westmead
Subdean, Clinical Epidemiology
Screening and Test Evaluation Program
School of Public Health
University of Sydney
Australia

Nicholas B. Cross, MBChB, FRACP
Centre for Kidney Research
Children's Hospital at Westmead
Screening and Test Evaluation Program
School of Public Health
University of Sydney
Australia

Jefferson D'Assunção, BEc
Research Officer
Screening and Test Evaluation Program
School of Public Health
University of Sydney
Australia

Andrew J. Farmer, DM, FRCGP
University Lecturer in General Practice
Department of Primary Health Care
University of Oxford
Oxford, UK

Robin E. Ferner, MSc, MD, FRCP
Director
West Midlands Centre for Adverse Drug Reactions
City Hospital
Birmingham, UK

Paul Glasziou, MBBS, FRACGP, PhD
Professor of Evidence-based Medicine
Department of Primary Health Care
University of Oxford
Oxford, UK

Paul R. Healey, MBBS(Hons), B(Med)Sc,
MMed, FRANZCO, PhD
Clinical Senior Lecturer
Centre for Vision Research
University of Sydney
Australia

Carl Heneghan, MA, MRCGP
Senior Clinical Research Fellow
Department of Primary Health Care
University of Oxford
Oxford, UK

Stephane Heritier
Head of Statistical Methodology
The George Institute, Sydney
Senior Lecturer in Biostatistics
University of Sydney
Australia

Andrea Rita Horvath, MD, PhD,
FRCPath, EurClinChem
Head of Clinical Chemistry
Albert Szent-Györgyi Medical and
    Pharmacological Centre
University of Szeged
Szeged, Hungary

Les M. Irwig, MBBCh, PhD, FFPHM
Professor of Epidemiology
Screening and Test Evaluation
    Program
School of Public Health
University of Sydney
Australia

Malinee Laopaiboon, PhD
Associate Professor
Department of Biostatistics and
    Demography
Faculty of Public Health
Khon Kaen University
Khon Kaen, Thailand

Pisake Lumbiganon, MD, MS
Professor in Obstetrics and Gynaecology
Department of Obstetrics and
    Gynaecology
Faculty of Medicine
Khon Kaen University
Khon Kaen, Thailand

Petra Macaskill, BA, MappStat, PhD
Associate Professor in Biostatistics
Screening and Test Evaluation Program
School of Public Health
University of Sydney
Australia

Kirsten McCaffery, BSc, PhD, MBPsS
Senior Research Fellow
Screening and Test Evaluation
    Program
School of Public Health
University of Sydney
Australia

David Mant, FRCP, FRCGP, FMedSci
Professor of General Practice
Department of Primary Health Care
University of Oxford
Oxford, UK

Susan Michie, BA, MPhil, DPhil,
CPsychol, FBPsS
Professor of Health Psychology
Department of Psychology
University College London
London, UK

George Peat, PhD, MCSP
Senior Lecturer in Clinical Epidemiology
Primary Care Musculoskeletal Research
    Centre
Keele University
Keele, UK

Rafael Perera, DPhil
Lecturer in Medical Statistics
Department of Primary Health Care
University of Oxford
Oxford, UK

Mark Porcheret, MBBS, FRCGP
GP Research Fellow
Primary Care Musculoskeletal
  Research Centre
Keele University
Keele, UK

Christopher P. Price, PhD, FRSC,
FRCPath, FACB
Visiting Professor in Clinical
  Biochemistry
Department of Clinical Biochemistry
University of Oxford
Oxford, UK

W. Stuart A. Smellie
Consultant Chemical Pathologist
Clinical Laboratory
Bishop Auckland Hospital
County Durham, UK

Alison M. Ward, BPsych, PhD
Research Support Director
Department of Primary Health Care
University of Oxford
Oxford, UK

PART 1
The Theory of Monitoring

CHAPTER 1

An introduction to monitoring therapeutic interventions in clinical practice

Paul P. Glasziou, Jeffrey K. Aronson

'Know which abnormality you are going to follow during treatment. Pick something you can measure.'

—CLIFTON MEADOR, *A Little Book of Doctors' Rules*

1.1. Introduction

Monitoring is repeated testing aimed at guiding and adjusting the management of a chronic or recurrent condition [1]. As the opening quote suggests, monitoring is a central activity in the management of patients and a major part of the ritual of routine visits for most chronic diseases. Measuring the patient's current state and responses to treatment is central to managing hypertension, diabetes mellitus, thyroid disease, asthma, depression, chronic pain and a host of other long-term conditions. Although managing acute diseases may begin with diagnostic testing, the focus should soon shift to monitoring. For example, much of the activity of intensive therapy or high-dependency units is monitoring, such as the repeated measurement of blood gases and electrolytes in a patient with trauma, or the tracking of glucose and other variables in diabetic ketoacidosis. The principles of monitoring are similar in both cases.

Although neglected as an area of research, monitoring is a substantial part of the clinical workload. Chronic conditions account for 80% of consultations by general practitioners (GPs, primary-care physicians), and such visits usually involve interpreting a set of monitoring tests and perhaps ordering some more. In the UK, the use of monitoring has accelerated as many of the quality indicators for GPs have involved monitoring, for example the targets and

Evidence-based Medical Monitoring: from Principles to Practice. Edited by Paul Glasziou, Les Irwig and Jeffrey K. Aronson. © 2008 Blackwell Publishing, ISBN: 978-1-4051-5399-7.

intervals of blood pressure, Hb_{A1c} (Chapter 16), cholesterol (Chapter 18), TSH (Chapter 19), FEV_1 and drugs such as lithium, aminoglycosides and digoxin [2]. The costs of such monitoring are substantial and not all of them are clearly worthwhile. Despite weak evidence for the effectiveness of self-monitoring in type 2 diabetes [3], the costs of blood glucose monitoring strips alone in 2002 in the UK was £118m—larger than the expenditure on oral hypoglycaemic agents [4]. However, despite financial and emotional investment in monitoring, many patients are poorly controlled. For example, in a UK study before the new GP contract was introduced in 2006, only 14% of 21,024 patients with newly diagnosed hypertension had met the target blood pressure after 12 months [5], and among treated patients about 40% of INR measurements are outside target ranges, compared with the ideal of 5% [6].

Intuitively, monitoring should obviously be beneficial. Nevertheless, clinicians forgo monitoring in many areas; for example, aspirin is used for preventing stroke without assessing aspirin responsiveness by measuring platelet aggregation. Deciding whether and how to monitor is clearly of central interest to both good clinical care and to the wise use of resources. In this book, we outline the principles needed to guide better monitoring and then illustrate those principles with examples. In doing so, we have built on what is known, but have also found many unexplored areas in which we have attempted to outline the problems and suggest directions for both clinical practice and research. In this chapter, I shall review the problems involved in monitoring and provide a guide to how these are dealt with in the other chapters in this book.

1.2. Is monitoring always helpful?

To be useful, a monitoring test must pass criteria similar to those for a good screening test:
- it should be accurate and simple;
- it should guide a strategy for achieving a target;
- achieving the target should improve patient outcomes.

The question of whether monitoring is helpful can be rephrased: Is a specific monitoring regimen better than no testing? Actually, there is never 'no testing', as a patient's symptoms and signs provide a default monitoring strategy. For some interventions this may be adequate; for example, phenytoin and digoxin toxicity both cause symptoms that may be sufficient for monitoring, and additional testing is required only for clarification. For other conditions, such as diabetes or thyroid disease, there may be a long silent phase, and hence some specific monitoring is desirable.

Figure 1.1 illustrates some of the possibilities. The arrows at the bottom indicate three monitoring tests that are done at regular intervals. The test at (i) does not detect the abnormal state in any of the four scenarios, but the tests at (ii) and (iii) do, at least in some of them.

In scenario (a) a test may detect the abnormal state before the event, and it may never have been detected by symptoms; for example, an abnormal

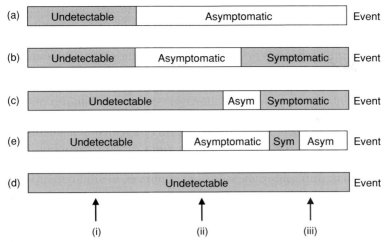

Figure 1.1 Four different scenarios that affect the frequency and timing of monitoring (see text for discussion).

prothrombin time (INR) in someone taking warfarin may be asymptomatic until a major bleed (the event).

In scenario (b) a test may detect an abnormal state, but symptoms would also detect it, albeit a little later. Hence, the question is whether early detection is clinically advantageous; for example, monitoring peak expiratory flow rate may detect a pending exacerbation of asthma a little early, but not early enough to make a difference to alterations in therapy.

In scenario (c) the asymptomatic period is too short to be feasibly detectable; for example, patients taking stable carbimazole treatment can suddenly develop neutropenia and soon afterwards develop symptoms such as a sore throat, but this happens too rapidly to be feasibly detectable by routine haematological monitoring.

In scenario (d) the asymptomatic period is too short to be detectable and does not occur at times of routine monitoring; for example, with stable lithium treatment, changes that alter lithium excretion (e.g. a fever or diarrhoea) can lead too rapidly to toxicity to be detectable by routine screening of serum lithium concentrations; routine monitoring misses the critical periods, which can only be detected by monitoring at times when the risk of toxicity is identifiably increased.

In scenario (e) the abnormal state is never detectable—that is, the current measurements do not provide a warning before the event; for example, we currently have no feasible means of detecting a period before the occurrence of ventricular fibrillation (implantable defibrillators detect this when it occurs and respond by defibrillation).

Proving that there is clear benefit, particularly in the prevention of long-term outcomes, often requires a randomized trial. Unfortunately, there are few of these. However, in the few good monitoring studies that have been done there have been surprises. For example, Swan–Ganz catheters for monitoring pulmonary artery pressure have been standard in intensive-care monitoring for decades, but a pooled analysis of over 5000 patients in randomized trials showed no impact on either mortality or length of stay [7]. On the other hand, B-type natriuretic peptide (BNP), which has become important in the diagnosis of heart failure, may also be useful for monitoring. Two randomized trials have shown reductions in hospitalizations from heart failure with BNP monitoring [8, 9]. And a meta-analysis of comparisons of self-monitoring of INR with usual care showed not only that it was safe, but also that it led to a greater reduction in all-cause mortality [10]. Table 1.1 lists some examples of monitoring strategies that have been subjected to randomized trials. One lesson from these trials is that it is not easy to predict whether monitoring will provide benefit.

Monitoring can optimize the benefits of therapy, by tracking a surrogate marker for benefit (e.g. adequate blood pressure control). It can also detect adverse effects (e.g. the toxic effects of methotrexate); the principles are similar to those outlined above, but there are some important differences, as discussed in Chapter 15.

1.3. The five phases of monitoring

To help with thinking about the elements of monitoring, it is helpful to break monitoring down into five phases as shown in Table 1.2. The central phase of monitoring is maintenance in stable control (phase 3), but this must be preceded by the establishment of a baseline—and the diagnosis—followed by a titration phase. Chapters 6–9 focus on elements of these phases. Titration requires assessment of the initial response to treatment, but detecting that response within the 'noise' of our usual unreliable measurements can prove a challenge. Sometimes checking for an adequate response is crucial and sometimes it is completely unnecessary, depending on the predictability of the response and our ability to detect important individual deviations from the average. The maintenance phase involves setting up a schedule of regular measurements (Chapter 8), and there are guidelines for deciding when a measurement or sequence of measurements suggests that a patient has drifted too far from the target range (Chapter 7). Some methods borrowed from industrial process control are worthy of further development here. Finally, when we have detected a deviation, we need to consider the options for adjusting treatment (Chapter 9).

1.4. Development and evaluation of monitoring

The final decision to monitor must take into account the balance of the benefits against the harms, such as inconvenience and cost, and the impact of false-positive results and false-negative results, which can lead to inappropriate or

Table 1.1 Examples of monitoring strategies subjected to randomized trials

Clinical area	Evidence	Results
Monitoring appears to be helpful		
Anticoagulation: INR self-monitoring for patients taking warfarin	Systematic review of eight randomized trials [9]	Self-monitoring reduces all-cause mortality compared with usual clinical care
Intensive follow-up of colorectal cancer after curative surgery	Systematic review of five randomized trials [11]	A one-third reduction in mortality
BNP and monitoring of heart failure	Two randomized trials [7, 8]	BNP monitoring reduces hospitalizations in severe heart failure
Temperature monitoring for diabetic foot ulcers	Randomized trial of 173 patients [12]	Temperature monitoring led to an 80% reduction in ulcers
Nitric oxide monitoring for asthma	Systematic review of three randomized trials [13, 14]	Nitric oxide monitoring improves control, with less use of medications
Monitoring not helpful or equivocal		
Pulmonary artery pressure in intensive care	Systematic review of randomized trials [7]	No impact of monitoring on length of stay or mortality
Peak expiratory flow rate (PEFR) monitoring in asthma	Systematic review of six randomized trials, and one later trial [15, 16]	Self-management based on PEFR was equivalent to self-management using symptoms
Urine or blood sugar monitoring for non-insulin dependent (type 2) diabetes	Systematic review of randomized trials [2]	Neither blood or urine self-monitoring affected Hb_{A1c}
Foetal heart rate monitoring during labour	Systematic review of randomized trials [17]	Equivocal results, with a reduction in seizures, but no difference in foetal mortality, and an increase in caesarean and forceps deliveries

delayed actions. Hence, establishing patient's benefit is important, but evaluation must be preceded by the development of a good monitoring strategy.

A monitoring test may be simple, but a monitoring strategy is a complex intervention, involving multiple components and adaptive decision-making on the part of the clinician and patient. The UK's Medical Research Council has proposed a framework for the development and evaluation of such complex interventions [18]. Chapter 2 considers the processes and elements needed

Table 1.2 The objectives of the five phases of monitoring*

Phase	Monitoring objectives	Optimal monitoring interval
1. Pre-treatment	• Check need for treatment • Establish a baseline for determining the response and change	Short; based on the within-person variability and analytical variation
2. Initial titration	• Assess the individual response to treatment • Detect immediate adverse drug reactions • Achieve control	Medium; based on both pharmacokinetics (for example, drug half-life) and the pharmacodynamics (physiological impact time)
3. Maintenance	• Detect drift from control limits • Detect long-term harms	Long; based on rate of random and systematic 'drift'
4. Re-establish control	• Bring value back within control limits	Medium; as for phase 2
5. Cessation	• Check safety of cessation	Medium; as for phase 2

Note: *Modified from [1].

to develop an optimal testing regimen and to evaluate it. These elements are expanded in subsequent chapters.

1.5. A few general principles

In this chapter I shall not attempt to give a complete overview of monitoring, but it is useful to draw together some of the pitfalls and lessons that emerge from the discussion in the succeeding chapters. These will necessarily be briefly mentioned here—the detailed background to these lessons will be covered in the chapters themselves.

1.5.1. Avoid the 'ping-pong' effect

Chasing random fluctuations can be dangerous. A common error when adjusting treatment is over-adjustment—changes in treatment that are too large can increase the variation in the monitored variable. A sequence of false alarms and inappropriate changes leads to increasing fluctuation and instability. This type of 'ping-pong' effect with subsequent overshoot (see Figure 9.1) has been observed in clinicians' adjustment of INR [1]. A typical sequence might be as follows:

• the INR is above the target range, but is in fact not significantly so;
• the clinician misunderstands this and reduces the dose of warfarin;
• the adjustment is too large;
• the INR falls below the target range;
• the clinician re-adjusts the dose, etc.

It is generally best to be cautious in making changes and when making changes to make small ones. Chapter 7 discusses some methods of more accurately sorting out real from spurious changes, and Chapter 9 gives details on the options for appropriate adjustment.

1.5.2. Do not remeasure until there is a chance of a real change

This follows from the principle of the ping-pong effect. If a patient is in a relatively stable condition, measuring too frequently can be misleading. There will have been little chance for the condition to change, but the random fluctuations in many clinical measurements may mislead us into changing therapy. Chapter 8 discusses the problems of developing an appropriate monitoring schedule and Chapter 18 looks at the specific example of cholesterol concentration monitoring. In the latter, it is suggested that we currently monitor cholesterol far too often, and would be better to shift to monitoring only every 3–5 years. This seems counter to clinical experience, since changes in cholesterol concentration occur in a short time, but most of this apparent change is due to short-term biological variation and analytical variation. The true underlying cholesterol changes only very slowly, unless there is a dramatic change in diet or drug therapy. However, other conditions fluctuate more, and earlier detection in the asymptomatic phase can be useful; for example, exhaled nitric oxide appears to be a good marker of airways inflammation in asthma and can signal a need for increased treatment [19, 20].

1.5.3. Sometimes we can 'hit and run'

Usually, we need to check whether the patient has had a sufficient response to treatment. However, if there is little or no individual variation in response, we can assume the average response instead. In fact, when there is no individual variation and the measure has considerable variation, trying to monitoring for a response can be misleading. In this case we can use a 'hit and run' strategy, i.e. measure once and not again. Of course, the patient's symptoms are a form of monitoring, and the hit and run strategy may rely on them for the trigger to change treatment. Chapter 6 discusses how we can decide when to hit and run, when we need to check repeatedly, and how to interpret the resulting checks.

1.5.4. There are several ways of adjusting therapy

If a patient's condition is not sufficiently well controlled, there are three basic strategies for improving the outcome:

1 *Intensify* treatment; for example, increase the dose or increase the frequency of administration.
2 *Switch* treatments; for example, to another similar agent or a different class of therapy.
3 *Add* a different therapy; for example, a low dose of an additional drug or another form of adjuvant therapy.

Different disease areas seem to concentrate on different options. For example, treatment of hypertension has been dominated by stepped care (option 1), but others have suggested using a switching option (option 2), and still others have suggested a 'Polypill' approach (option 3, with low doses of multiple agents) [19]. It is helpful to be aware of these generic options to avoid being trapped by a local paradigm.

In the case of over-treatment, with adverse effects, the opposite strategies apply:

1 *Reduce* treatment. For example, reduce the dose or decrease the frequency of administration; temporary withdrawal of treatment may be necessary before restarting at a lower total dose.

2 *Switch* treatments.

3 *Withdraw* the treatment altogether.

1.5.5. Understand the relation between dose and effect

When titrating and adjusting treatment, it is helpful to understand how the effect varies with the dosage. For drugs, this is an understanding of the pharmacological (pharmacokinetic and pharmacodynamic) properties of a drug, which are more fully discussed in Chapter 3.

1.5.5.1. Pharmacokinetics: the processing of the drug by the body

Detailed discussion of pharmacokinetics [20] is beyond the scope of this book. However, there are a few simple principles that are relevant. After the start of therapy with a regular dose of a drug, it takes about four half-lives for a steady state to be reached. The same is true after a change in dose (both an increase and a reduction); a new steady state takes about four half-lives to achieve. Knowing the half-life of a drug therefore helps to predict how long it will take before a change can be expected and whether to use a loading dose to produce the change more quickly. Knowing whether the drug is eliminated by the kidneys or the liver helps to predict the effects of renal or hepatic disease. Knowing the mechanisms of hepatic elimination helps in understanding drug interactions that involve inhibition of drug metabolism.

1.5.5.2. Pharmacodynamics: the dose–response curves for benefit and harms

The pharmacodynamic effect of a drug is summed up in its dose–response curve (or concentration–effect curve), which is the central dogma of pharmacology, as important, for example, as the central limit theorem is to statistics. If you choose to titrate the dose of a drug, an understanding of the dose–response curves of its benefits and harms is vital to predicting the impact of different doses, which will depend in part on the slopes and maximal efficacies of each curve. Chapters 3, 4 and 9 explore these concepts, but a few simple ideas are worth remembering:

- Once the peak response is reached, further dose increases only cause harm.
- There is a law of diminishing returns—increasing the dose does not produce a proportional increase in benefit unless the dose is within the short segment of the dose–response curve that is approximately linear. This is because the sigmoid curve of the beneficial response is log-linearly related to dosage only for the short central segment portion.
- The dose–response curves for benefits and harms are usually different. We can take advantage of this. If a drug has toxic effects (see Chapter 15, Figure 15.4) we can generally gain benefit at low doses, while harms tend to occur at high doses, and we can select medicines with this in mind. On the other hand, if a drug has adverse effects that are due to hypersusceptibility or collateral effects, avoiding adverse reactions may be impossible (in the former case, Figure 15.2) or at least difficult (in the latter, Figure 15.3).

1.5.6. Involve the patient in monitoring

Patients are often more capable than some health-care providers think. And they are often more motivated to manage their condition. The first pregnant woman with diabetes to monitor her blood glucose at home needed to be considerably persuaded, but her success led to a change in our paradigm of monitoring. However, we should remember that patients vary considerably in their ability to self-monitor effectively for chronic conditions. Some patients are very capable at both self-testing and self-management, whereas others are poor at self-monitoring, and still others may not agree or may be incapable.

Chapter 17 looks at the specific example of INR self-monitoring for patients taking warfarin. The systematic review of trials discussed there shows that self-monitoring was more effective than conventional clinical monitoring and equally safe. However, it appeared to be most effective when patients both self-tested and self-adjusted treatment rather than merely self-testing. Clearly, self-adjustment of therapy requires more skill and training, but it is more motivating.

1.5.7. Monitoring can adjust the mind as well as the treatment

While a key aim of monitoring is to detect clinically important changes and adjust treatment in response, it is also a learning and motivational tool. Indeed, simply monitoring weight by keeping a diary, hand written or electronic, can lead patients to lose weight without any specific intervention [21]. Hence, we need to be aware that monitoring has influences beyond the clinician's adjustment of treatment. Patients can learn what causes their condition to become worse, such as dietary changes or exercise in diabetes and other conditions, or can become more motivated by seeing progress, which in turn may improve adherence. Chapters 10 and 11 explore these issues further.

1.5.8. Do not read single measurements in isolation

Because of random fluctuation in monitoring measurements, it is helpful to think of a moving average of measurements. Some statistical rules have been

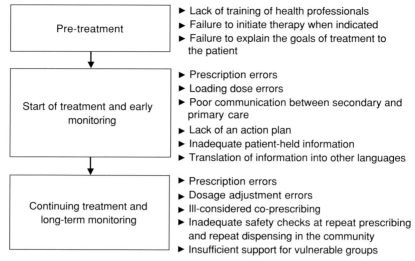

Figure 1.2 Some problems that can arise during monitoring at different stages.

developed to help interpret multiple tests. For example, one rule suggests that we can conclude that there is a real change if there is

1 a single measure 3 or more standard deviations from target, or
2 two of the last three measurements were at least 2 standard deviations from the target, or
3 four of the last five measurements were at least 1 standard deviation from the mean.

These are known as the WECO (Western Electric Company) rules. They are useful, but may not be sufficiently sensitive in some medical settings. However, the concept of using the combine deviation of several measurements is useful in clinical monitoring. Chapter 7, on control charts, discusses the various approaches to interpreting a sequence of test results.

1.6. Problems in monitoring

Some problems that can arise during monitoring at different phases are shown in Figure 1.2. The problems can be system failures, such as prescription errors or availability of translations of materials, or errors from the clinician, patient or laboratory, or the communication between these. These are discussed in Chapters 6–15.

1.7. Conclusions

Monitoring is a large and rapidly rising area of laboratory testing. However, unlike diagnostic testing there has been little interest in and development of methods for assessing the value of monitoring tests. These methods need further development. Nevertheless, there are some simple principles, such as the eight outlined above, that can be applied to the development and evaluation of optimal monitoring strategies.

References

1 Glasziou P, Irwig L, Mant D. Monitoring in chronic disease: a rational approach. *BMJ* 2005; **330**: 644–8.

2 Aronson JK, Hardman M, Reynolds DJM. *ABC of Monitoring Drug Therapy*. London: BMJ Publishing Group, 1993.

3 Coster S, Gulliford MC, Seed PT, Powrie JK, Swaminatham R. Self-monitoring in type 2 diabetes mellitus: a meta-analysis. *Diabet Med* 2000; **17**: 755–61.

4 Farmer A, Neil A. Letter in response to "Variations in glucose self-monitoring during oral hypoglycaemic therapy in primary care." *Diabet Med* 2005; **22**: 511–2.

5 Walley T, Duggan AK, Haycox AR, Niziol CJ. Treatment for newly diagnosed hypertension: patterns of prescribing and antihypertensive effectiveness in the UK. *J R Soc Med* 2003; **96**: 525–31.

6 Oden A, Fahlen M. Oral anticoagulation and risk of death: a medical record linkage study. *BMJ* 2002; **325**: 1073–5.

7 Shah MR, Hasselblad V, Stevenson LW, et al. Impact of the pulmonary artery catheter in critically ill patients: meta-analysis of randomized clinical trials. *JAMA* 2005; **294**: 1664–70.

8 Troughton RW, Frampton CM, Yandle TG, Espiner EA, Nicholls MG, Richards AM. Treatment of heart failure guided by plasma aminoterminal brain natriuretic peptide (N-BNP) concentrations. *Lancet* 2000; **355**: 1126–30.

9 Jourdain P, Jondeau G, Funck F, et al. Plasma brain natriuretic peptide-guided therapy to improve outcome in heart failure: the STARS-BNP Multicenter Study. *J Am Coll Cardiol* 2007; **49**: 1733–9.

10 Heneghan C, Alonso-Coello P, Garcia JM, Perera R, Meats E, Glasziou P. Self-monitoring of oral anticoagulation: a systematic review and meta-analysis. *Lancet* 2006; **367**: 404–11.

11 Powell H, Gibson PG. Options for self-management education for adults with asthma. *Cochrane Database Syst Rev* 2003; (1): CD004107.

12 Buist AS, Vollmer WM, Wilson SR, Frazier EA, Hayward AD. A randomized clinical trial of peak flow versus symptom monitoring in older adults with asthma. *Am J Respir Crit Care Med* 2006; **174**: 1077–87.

13 Graham EM, Petersen SM, Christo DK, Fox HE. Intrapartum electronic fetal heart rate monitoring and the prevention of perinatal brain injury. *Obstet Gynecol* 2006; **108**(3 Pt 1): 656–66.

14 Campbell M, Fitzpatrick R, Haines A, et al. Framework for design and evaluation of complex interventions to improve health. *BMJ* 2000; **321**: 694–6.

15 Wald NJ, Law MR. A strategy to reduce cardiovascular disease by more than 80%. *BMJ* 2003; **326**: 1419.

16 Grahame-Smith DG, Aronson JK. The pharmacokinetic process. In: *The Oxford Textbook of Clinical Pharmacology and Drug Therapy*. Oxford: Oxford University Press, 2002, Chapter 3.

17 Yon BA, Johnson RK, Harvey-Berino J, Gold BC, Howard AB. Personal digital assistants are comparable to traditional diaries for dietary self-monitoring during a weight loss program. *J Behav Med* 2007; **30**: 165–75.

18 Jeffery GM, Hickey BE, Hider P. Follow-up strategies for patients treated for non-metastatic colorectal cancer. *Cochrane Database Syst Rev* 2002; (1): CD002200.

19 Lavery LA, Higgins KR, Lanctot DR, et al. Preventing diabetic foot ulcer recurrence in high-risk patients: use of temperature monitoring as a self-assessment tool. *Diabetes Care* 2007; **30**: 14–20.

20 Smith AD, Cowan JO, Brassett KP, Herbison GP, Taylor DR. Use of exhaled nitric oxide measurements to guide treatment in chronic asthma. *N Engl J Med* 2005; **352**: 2163–73.

21 Petsky H, Kynaston J, Turner C, et al. Tailored interventions based on sputum eosinophils versus clinical symptoms for asthma in children and adults. *Cochrane Database Syst Rev* 2007; (2): CD005603.

CHAPTER 2

A framework for developing and evaluating a monitoring strategy

David Mant

About 20 years ago the *Lancet* published an editorial about cervical cancer screening in the UK, subtitled 'death by incompetence' [1]. The fatal error that it described was the introduction of a new screening test (the Papanicolaou or 'Pap' smear) in the absence of the development and evaluation of a screening strategy. The same error is now being made with monitoring. Clinicians are too often concerned only with an individual monitoring test. The purpose of this chapter is to demonstrate the importance of developing and evaluating a monitoring strategy.

A clinical example that will be widely recognized is the measurement of serum electrolyte concentrations in patients taking a number of commonly used drugs, such as thiazide and loop diuretics and angiotensin converting enzyme (ACE) inhibitors. The test is simple and reliable, but the timing and frequency of testing are usually haphazard, as often is the action taken on the basis of the test result. This does not imply that it is difficult to know what action to take if the test result shows life-threatening hyperkalaemia, for example, but the purpose of monitoring is to avoid extreme results with life-threatening implications. We currently know much more about what to do when monitoring goes wrong than what to do to stop it going wrong.

The defining characteristic of monitoring is that it involves a series of tests over time. A monitoring strategy therefore needs to consider the frequency and timing of tests and the appropriate clinical response to a test result, not in isolation but in the context of a series of sequential results. Once developed, the effectiveness of the strategy in attaining monitoring objectives needs to be formally evaluated. And once shown to be effective in principle, its implementation must itself be monitored to ensure that it continues to be effective in clinical practice.

Evidence-based Medical Monitoring: from Principles to Practice. Edited by Paul Glasziou, Les Irwig and Jeffrey K. Aronson. © 2008 Blackwell Publishing, ISBN: 978-1-4051-5399-7.

2.1. Considering the strategic options

It is important to be clear about what you are trying to achieve by monitoring—the clinical outcome you want to attain or avoid. This decision will determine who should be monitored (i.e. only those at risk of the outcome). However, it will not determine the best monitoring target, the best test, the optimal frequency of monitoring, nor who should do the monitoring. Nor will it determine the clinical action that should be taken on the monitoring test result. Table 2.1 illustrates the necessary process of options appraisal and decision-making by listing strategic options for monitoring a common condition (asthma) in relation to six key strategic questions.

Simply drawing up an 'options appraisal' list of this kind for the condition you are interested in monitoring will usually make clear that:

- It is unlikely to be cost-effective to monitor all possible outcomes—a strategic choice must be made.
- It may not be necessary to monitor everyone with the condition—the population to be monitored should be restricted to those at risk of the outcome

Table 2.1 The process of options appraisal and decision-making in monitoring, illustrated for the case of asthma

Question	Options
What outcome should be monitored?	Premature deaths; hospital admissions; episodes requiring emergency care; lung function; limitations on normal activity; growth or bone problems
Who should be monitored?	All patients with asthma; those at risk of adverse outcomes because of age or co-morbidity; those with frequent acute exacerbations; those with recurrent hospital admissions; those taking high-dose glucocorticoids
What test should be used?	Symptoms; frequency of use of beta-agonists; peak expiratory flow rate; emergency visits; hospital admissions; growth charts (children); markers of bone density (e.g. densitometry); home humidity/allergen concentrations
When, and at what interval, should it be monitored?	Scheduled (everyday to 5 yearly, depending on monitoring test); triggered by risk indicators
Who should do the monitoring?	Self; carer; doctor; nurse; pharmacist; other health professionals
What action will be taken on the monitoring result?	Education; aids to adherence (e.g. drug packaging aids); aids to drug delivery (e.g. spacer devices); changes in medication (e.g. increase or decrease glucocorticoid doses); environmental changes

(for example, there is no point in monitoring markers of bone growth or bone density except in those at risk of delayed growth or osteoporosis because they use glucocorticoids).
- When you have made a choice of outcome, you are likely to be faced with more than one strategy for best achieving that outcome—what to measure, at what interval, and who should do the test.
- There are usually further choices to be made on what action to take on the monitoring test result.

However, listing the options is insufficient. The rest of this chapter explains how to set about choosing between them. Although the process is straightforward, it cannot be done quickly on the back of an envelope. The process of moving from a list of monitoring options to an optimized monitoring strategy that precisely defines the test, the test interval, and the clinical action to take on the test result is a time-consuming task. However, it can be short-circuited by asking a single question: Can monitoring be justified? If it cannot be justified on the three simple criteria outline below, there is no point in expending further energy.

2.2. When is monitoring justified?

The comparison between monitoring an intervention and screening for a disease, such as cervical cancer, is relevant, because they both involve the repeated application of a diagnostic test to an individual over a period of time. We can learn much about monitoring from the experience of screening. For example, in deciding whether a screening strategy is justifiable, we have learned to apply three criteria [2]:

1 The clinical condition that screening identifies must be important.
2 There must be a screening test (or combination of tests) that reliably and cost-effectively distinguishes between people with and without the condition.
3 Effective treatment must be available for the condition at the stage at which it is identified by screening.

Monitoring needs to meet very similar criteria, modified only to reflect the key objective of detecting change over time. The suggested minimum criteria for monitoring are shown in Table 2.2.

The clinically significant change required by the first criterion may be in the condition (e.g. altered mood in bipolar affective disorder), the treatment (e.g.

Table 2.2 Suggested minimum criteria for monitoring

1 Clinically significant changes in the condition or effect of treatment occur over time
2 There is an available monitoring test that reliably detects clinically significant changes when they occur
3 Cost-effective action can be taken on the basis of the test result

a change in the serum concentration of a drug, such as lithium, used to treat the disorder), or an adverse effect caused by either the condition (neuropathy in diabetes) or the treatment (potassium depletion due to a diuretic). It may also be the clinical recurrence of an apparently quiescent illness (e.g. metastases in cancer). Clinically significant change is an important criterion, because there may be long periods of illness when significant change is unlikely and monitoring therefore unnecessary. Substantial resources are wasted in clinical practice by monitoring stable conditions.

The second criterion differentiates a monitoring test from a test used simply for diagnosis. This is illustrated by the example of carbimazole therapy for hyperthyroidism. Carbimazole can cause a catastrophic fall in the white blood cell count in a small number of patients, usually within the first 6 months of treatment [3]. This is undeniably a clinically significant adverse effect of treatment, for which a straightforward diagnostic test (a full blood count) is available. However, a monitoring strategy involving scheduled full blood counts in patients taking carbimazole is not likely to be worthwhile, because the fall in blood count is rapid and unpredictable and likely to occur between scheduled monitoring tests. Hence, monitoring the full blood count regularly is unlikely to improve the safety of treatment. A different example, which makes the same point, is scheduled clinical follow-up after treatment for breast cancer. Although clinical examination can detect recurrence, most recurrences present symptomatically between clinic visits [4]. Clinical follow-up after breast surgery may meet a number of other needs and objectives, but it is a poor monitoring strategy for detecting recurrence.

The third criterion requires not only that the clinical change identified by the test is amenable to remedial action, but also that this action can be pre-specified and is thought to be cost-effective. This must apply to test results across the range—as with screening tests, most problems arise not from extreme values but from values that are in the grey area just outside the reference range or target range. In some cases, criterion 3 can only be fully assessed by a clinical trial. A good example is the use of CT scanning to detect isolated hepatic metastases in the follow-up of patients after surgical resection of colorectal cancer. We know that surgical resection of isolated hepatic metastases is associated with long-term survival in some patients. However, as with screening, the potential for lead-time and selection bias means that the cost-effectiveness of resecting liver metastases detected by monitoring can only be assessed by a randomized trial [5].

Specifying minimum criteria for monitoring raises the question of whether we can take a decision not to monitor if the criteria are not met. The example of colorectal cancer is one in which a decision needs to be made about whether or not to monitor. Similarly, a review of the evidence in relation to criterion 1 may suggest that it should be possible to predict and avoid a clinically important change over time rather than monitoring for its occurrence. For example, the need for drug monitoring may be substantially reduced or eliminated by alternative strategies to avoid treatment in individuals at high risk of adverse events (for example, identified by age or by genetic variants of cytochrome P450 enzymes) and/or if the drug dosage is individually titrated at the start of therapy (for example, by initially determining digoxin therapy by weight and creatinine clearance).

However, in most cases the important clinical question is when and how to monitor, rather than whether to monitor. Taking the example of carbimazole above, it is essential to detect a falling white cell count, but criterion 2 is likely to be better met by choosing a symptomatic test (e.g. self-monitoring for a minor illness such as a sore throat), which can trigger an immediate full blood count measurement, rather than monitoring by scheduled periodic blood counts.

2.3. Choosing a monitoring test

Once you have decided that monitoring a specific outcome in a defined population is justifiable in principle, the next step is to decide how this objective can be best achieved in practice. The most important step in this process is to choose the best monitoring target (i.e. the feature of the condition that needs to be monitored, which may not be the outcome itself) and the best test to measure this target. This question is considered in more detail in Chapter 4 on biomarkers and surrogate endpoints. The four criteria that need to be met (validity, high signal-to-noise ratio, responsiveness and practicality) are discussed briefly below and are listed in Table 2.3. The first criterion of validity highlights the importance of making the decision based on a sound understanding of the illness and treatment pathway.

2.3.1. Validity

A common monitoring objective is to avoid an adverse outcome. It might be thought that the adverse outcome should itself be the best (i.e. the most valid) monitoring target. However, it seldom is, because once it is detected it is usually too late to take effective remedial action. It is usually better to monitor

Table 2.3 Criteria for choosing a test

Criterion	Description
1. Validity	How well does the test measure or predict clinically significant events?
2. Responsiveness	How quickly does the test respond to changes in the condition or treatment?
3. High signal-to-noise ratio	Is a single test result easy to interpret or is it subject to substantial random variation that makes interpretation difficult?
4. Practicality	Is the test simple, non-invasive and affordable?

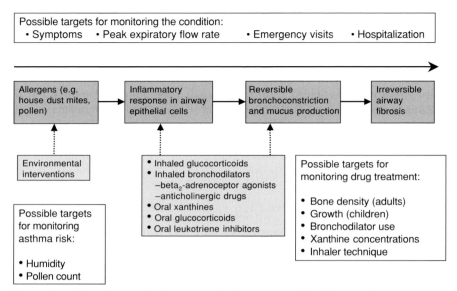

Figure 2.1 Choosing monitoring targets in the context of the illness and treatment pathway: the example of asthma.

a target (a biomarker) that indicates a prior risk of the adverse outcome and that can be detected at a stage at which remedial action can be taken. One way to clarify the choice of monitoring target is to draw a simple figure that sets out the disease pathway on the horizontal axis and the treatment pathways on the vertical axis. This is done in Figure 2.1, again taking asthma as an example. Possible monitoring targets are shown in red.

There is not always a simple linear progression in either the condition or the treatment, but it is usually possible to characterize possible monitoring targets as either 'proximal' (i.e. closely related to the adverse outcome to be avoided) or 'distal' (i.e. early in the pathophysiological or treatment pathway). A more proximal target will usually give a more reliable prediction of outcome, but as it occurs later in the disease or treatment pathway, effective remedial action may be more difficult. This progression is discussed in more detail in Chapter 3 on mechanisms (see especially Figure 3.3 and related figures in that chapter).

It will be obvious that when the illness and treatment pathways are mapped out, there may be a long causal chain between risk factors and final outcomes; hence, there are several points along the chain that measure or predict outcome and might potentially be monitored. The example of asthma has been discussed above. Another example is hypertension, in which we routinely monitor mean blood pressure (as a predictor of both condition and effectiveness of treatment), but could feasibly also monitor blood pressure variability, left ventricular hypertrophy, markers of renal function, or even cerebral blood flow.

In the proximal–distal continuum introduced above, blood pressure would be a relatively distal test, left ventricular hypertrophy an intermediate test, and cerebral blood flow a relatively proximal test. Distal tests are used earlier and usually offer greatest scope for effective intervention, but may only poorly predict outcome (for example, the early trials of treatment of mild hypertension reported an NNT (number needed to treat) to prevent one stroke of about 800). In contrast, intermediate and proximal tests tend to predict outcome more strongly, but may be impractical to measure and may document pathophysiological changes at a stage when they are more difficult to reverse (e.g. left ventricular hypertrophy). Tests that are of the greatest value are earliest in time and most strongly associated with the outcome. However, earliness and association with outcome are often inversely related, and hence a trade-off between the two is usually necessary.

2.3.2. Responsiveness

A good monitoring test must be sensitive to changes in the condition and to adjustments in treatment. This is true whether one monitors the condition or the treatment itself, although the required degree of responsiveness varies. For example, it is important that a cancer marker used to monitor recurrence (such as the blood concentration of carcinoembryonic antigen) rises sufficiently quickly to allow diagnosis at a stage when remedial action is possible. It is not important that the cancer marker falls rapidly with treatment. In contrast, in monitoring oral anticoagulation therapy, it is important to choose a monitoring target that is rapidly responsive to both upward and downward adjustments in treatment.

Assessment of responsiveness is not always straightforward. For example, the effect of antihypertensive medication is mediated by both *pharmacokinetic* and *pharmacodynamic* mechanisms. These effects tend to occur within different time frames, and therefore the effect of treatment is not easily captured by a measurement at a single time point [6]. Similarly, in monitoring oral therapy in diabetes, blood glucose concentration may be too time-responsive a target—it has a low signal-to-noise ratio in assessing treatment effect (see below) and it is probably better to adjust therapy using a less time-responsive measure, such as glycosylated haemoglobin (Hb_{A1c}), which reflects the degree of glycaemia over the lifespan of the circulating erythrocytes.

2.3.3. Signal-to-noise ratio

A good monitoring test must be able to differentiate changes in the condition or treatment from background measurement variability (short-term biological fluctuations and technical measurement error). The most frequently used monitoring test in medicine is probably measurement of blood pressure, and it is now widely understood that variability over time makes a single measurement of blood pressure a poor monitoring test—the signal-to-noise ratio is too low.

The two important sources of noise are biological variability and measurement error. Biological variability is likely to have three components:

1 Predictable short-term physiological variation (e.g. diurnal variation or time from drug administration).

2 Less predictable short-term variation due to external events (e.g. stress, diet, exercise).

3 Long-term variation due to changes (often deterioration) in the underlying condition or the development of co-morbidity.

In assessing a test, it is important to take account of all three components. Variability can often be reduced by strategies such as measuring at the same time of day, taking measurements at rest and taking more than one measurement. Measurement error can be minimized by standardizing the measurement process (in taking the measurement, transporting specimens and laboratory practices) and by instituting quality-assurance measures.

It is important to note that the signal-to-noise ratio must be assessed in the context of the way in which the test is going to be used. A single blood pressure reading may have a low signal-to-noise ratio but it is a good monitoring test when therapy adjustment is based on clustered measurements or a mean of a series of measurements. The problem is whether a high signal-to-noise ratio can be achieved, not whether noise is an inherent characteristic of the test itself. It is also possible that in choosing test options, the achievable signal-to-noise ratio may be the key issue in determining the validity of the test.

2.3.4. Practicality

The ideal monitoring test should be non-invasive, simple to conduct and easily interpretable. It must also be affordable in the health-care setting in which it is to be used. Tests that are suitable for self-monitoring are becoming increasingly important. Tests that are used at the point of care (see Chapter 14) need to meet the added criterion that they give rapid results and are reliable when used by non-experts under a range of different operating conditions.

2.4. Taking account of changes in the condition over time

One specific reason why it is critical to understand the illness pathway is that the optimal monitoring test interval, and the optimal action to take on the basis of the test result, will change over time as the condition changes [7]. This is shown in Figure 2.2, which illustrates the phases of a monitoring strategy designed to maintain a condition (e.g. blood pressure, drug concentration) within a target range over time. It adopts a control chart approach (see Chapter 7) and describes five phases. The black line indicates the test value and the coloured bars indicate the action that needs to be taken in response to the result of each monitoring test (defined in terms of the number of standard deviations of the result from a target value). The usual approach is to adjust

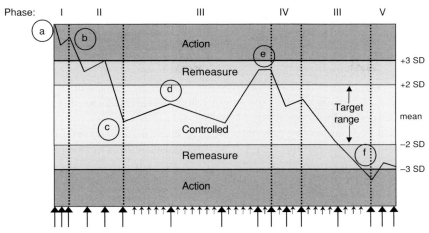

Figure 2.2 The five different phases of monitoring.

treatment if a single test result is 3 standard deviations (SDs), or if a repeat measurement is 2 SDs, from a target value.

The letters in the figure indicate key points in the time course of the condition:

1 the point at which the condition is first suspected;
2 when treatment is begun;
3 when initial titration of treatment is completed;
4–5 when treatment is being monitored.

At point (e) two consecutive test results have been more than 2 SDs from the target and therapy is adjusted to bring the monitoring value to within the ±2 SD target range. The final letter (f) illustrates the possibility that changes with time (through evolution of the condition, age-related changes in sensitivity to treatment, co-morbidity and/or co-treatment with other interventions) may also create circumstances in which a decision needs to be made whether or not to continue treatment. Although this particular figure depicts the problem of keeping the test result within a target range (e.g. in monitoring blood pressure), in other circumstances the treatment aim might be to increase the value of the test result (e.g. monitoring haemoglobin in anaemia) or to reduce it (e.g. in monitoring viral load).

This schematic time course defines five possible phases of monitoring, reflecting two separate time-related observations that

1 the processes of diagnosis, initiation of treatment and response to treatment of any clinical condition take place over time;
2 the natural history of almost all clinical conditions changes over time, in many cases (diabetes, for example) worsening progressively.

The large arrows along the bottom axis are scheduled tests; the small arrows illustrate the need for additional discretionary tests when adjusting therapy.

For the individual patient, the specific objectives of monitoring in each phase are as follows:

- Phase I: to decide whether to initiate treatment based on a (series of) measurements.
- Phase II: to determine whether the expected response to treatment (benefit) has been achieved and to identify any short-term harms.
- Phase III: to check that the condition and/or treatment remains 'under control' (i.e. within predefined limits).
- Phase IV: to adjust treatment in order to move back to phase III.
- Phase V: to determine whether to withdraw treatment in order to avoid harm.

The optimal monitoring strategy therefore varies with the stage of monitoring. One particular problem that needs to be made explicit is that the frequency, and sometimes the specific target, of monitoring may need to be 'stepped up' or 'stepped down' between stages. For example, when the test result falls outside the control limits in phase III and it is necessary to move to phase IV to regain therapeutic control, the optimal frequency of testing is likely to increase. In clinical terms, a patient with hypertension, who may be seen yearly while the blood pressure remains within the therapeutic target range, may need to be seen at weekly intervals while treatment is being adjusted. If the adjustment to treatment involves the introduction of an ACE inhibitor, it would be necessary to initiate monitoring of serum creatinine concentration (a new target).

In the case of blood pressure, the monitoring test result (usually the mean of a series of clustered measurements) is often sufficient to guide treatment. In many other circumstances, a positive monitoring test will trigger a series of further investigations before treatment is initiated. For example, a positive protein dipstick test in antenatal care indicates the need for a battery of further investigations, some of which are more precise measurements of the same target (e.g. repeat blood pressure, 24-hour urine protein) to confirm pre-eclampsia, while others are new targets used to characterize the severity of pre-eclampsia (e.g. platelet count, inflammatory markers, liver function tests). Whether these further investigations are usefully characterized as monitoring tests depends on whether they continue to be measured over time.

2.5. Moving from a monitoring test to a monitoring strategy

This chapter began by highlighting the importance of focusing on an overall monitoring strategy rather than an individual monitoring test. Having decided on objectives and chosen the test, there are necessary components in the final stage in specifying, implementing and evaluating the strategy, summarized in Table 2.4.

Table 2.4 Steps in developing, evaluating and
implementing a monitoring strategy

---

1 Decide on the test frequency

2 Predefine the clinical actions to be taken on test results

3 Evaluate and confirm the cost-effectiveness of the strategy

4 Implement a training and quality-assurance scheme

2.5.1. Deciding on the testing frequency

Once the monitoring test has been chosen, a measurement scheme must be drawn up, specifying the frequency of testing (as stated above, the 'test' may need to be a cluster of more than one measurement to maximize the signal-to-noise ratio). The optimal interval between tests will depend on four factors discussed above:

1 the phase of monitoring;
2 the probability that clinically important changes will develop during each phase;
3 the speed with which important clinical changes develop;
4 the responsiveness of the test.

For example, the risk of deterioration in renal function with up-titration of ACE inhibitors is greatest in the first weeks of treatment (during phase II of monitoring), during which time the onset may be rapid and monitoring should therefore be frequent (e.g. weekly). In phase III, further sudden deterioration in renal function is unlikely, the rate of change reflecting deterioration in the underlying condition rather than change in the effect of treatment. So monitoring could either cease, be reduced to a much longer interval (e.g. 6 monthly), or be triggered by external events, such as an intercurrent illness that might precipitate more rapid change. Similarly, the most effective mechanism for monitoring asthma in the group of patients most at risk of acute admission to hospital appears to be to ask them to start monitoring their peak expiratory flow rate only during high-risk periods rather than to monitor continuously [8]. The primary monitoring test (i.e. the target that needs to be monitored to signal the need to start testing the peak expiratory flow rate) could be changes in symptoms, increased frequency of bronchodilator usage, or even environmental factors such as weather or pollen count. By contrast, the risk of bleeding with warfarin is time independent (see Chapter 17); it remains high throughout treatment, with a constant risk of rapid onset of loss of haemostatic function, so it is necessary to continue to measure the INR frequently while treatment continues.

2.5.2. Pre-defining the clinical actions to be taken on test results

The point of monitoring is to decide if action needs to be taken to initiate, adjust, or withdraw treatment. If no action is planned, there is no point in monitoring. Although this might seem self-evident, difficulties arise when the results of monitoring are not clear-cut. The range of test values that should not precipitate adjustment in therapy has to be defined, and a difficult decision often has to be made on how to respond to values that are slightly above or below these values (for example, when to remeasure). Given inevitable measurement variability and error, we shall not want to adjust therapy with every minor fluctuation. As shown in Chapter 9, this has the potential to precipitate more random variation and worsen clinical management.

One option that is particularly useful when the monitoring objective is to maintain a biological variable within an optimal range (e.g. achieving a target INR, plasma drug concentration or blood pressure) is illustrated in Figure 2.2. This is to set 'control limits' that define when a monitoring test value is sufficiently far from target that it requires a change (i.e. an adjustment of dose or a change of treatment). In the absence of better information, these can be defined probabilistically in terms of SDs from the mean or multiples of the median [9]. Normal practice would be to initiate change in response to a single value 3 SDs from the mean or two consecutive values 2 SDs from the mean (again, see Chapters 7 and 9 for more details).

The extent to which the dose should be adjusted in response to measurements must also be defined. This requires a clear understanding of the relation between the treatment and the monitoring target. The degree of precision required depends on the therapeutic target range—when the safe range is wide (e.g. most types of inhaled therapy for asthma) guidance can be less precise than when the therapeutic range is narrow and substantial between-person variation in drug response is common (e.g. warfarin and insulin). This process can be facilitated if individual markers of drug response (e.g. the effect of CYP2C9 genetic polymorphisms on warfarin metabolism) can be identified [10], although the use of genetic tests to predict treatment response remains uncommon in practice. However, one modern technology that has been used to customize treatment adjustment plans is computer software, which has been used successfully to improve control of patients taking a number of drugs [11].

2.5.3. Evaluating and confirming the cost-effectiveness of the strategy

Modern health economies demand evidence of cost-effectiveness before adopting new technologies. Although most monitoring strategies will involve tests that are not new, having been used as diagnostic tests for many years, the monitoring strategy as a whole should be seen as a new technology that merits formal evaluation. In most cases, the cost of the evaluation is likely to be far exceeded by the cost of national implementation of an ineffective strategy. The three sequential questions that need to be asked are as follows:

1 Does monitoring improve the percentage of patients who achieve a value within a given target range or state, compared with treating all patients in the same way without monitoring?

2 Does improving the percentage of patients within the target range result in improved benefits and/or reduced harms?

3 Does the net benefit of monitoring vary between subgroups of patients?

Questions 1 and 2 concern the 'per cent in range'. This is a useful surrogate and precondition for patients to benefit from monitoring. Sometimes we may accept this as sufficient, provided there is a clear link between the 'per cent in range' and the outcome; for example, a scheme that improved the Hb_{A1c} concentration in a patient with diabetes might be accepted as sufficient evidence of effectiveness. However, in other cases it may be necessary to conduct a randomized controlled trial. In choosing trial outcomes, it is important to remember that benefits and harms arise from more than one source. First are those that are related to therapy and flow from improved control of therapy achieved by monitoring. Second are those that arise directly from the monitoring itself; for example, learning about self-management, benefits such as a sense of control, and harms such as inconvenience, anxiety and adverse effects of an invasive procedure [12]. Thirdly, we should remember that one of the harms in a state-funded heath economy may be the opportunity costs that arise from waste of resources from excessive monitoring. We therefore need to assess whether the monitoring strategy is not only effective but also cost-effective.

Question 3 takes us back to the discussion of monitoring objectives. In some cases monitoring may not be beneficial for all patients, but only for a subgroup of susceptible individuals. This is because individual susceptibility to the beneficial and harmful effects of an intervention varies from subject to subject, depending on factors such as genetic constitution, age, sex, physiological variability (e.g. body weight, pregnancy), other therapy (especially drugs) and co-morbidities [13]. Similarly, some patients are likely to thrive on self-monitoring, while others will find it impossible and their health will deteriorate (see Chapter 11). As already discussed, it may be possible to predict these issues in designing the monitoring strategy. However, this variable susceptibility to harm or benefit may only be assessable (or become apparent) post hoc in the evaluation process. The importance of looking for heterogeneity of effect in the evaluation, and of providing as much information as possible to allow individual customization of care, is as important for monitoring as for other therapeutic interventions.

2.5.4. Implementing a training and quality-assurance scheme

Finally, and to come full circle to the problem raised at the beginning of the chapter, it is important to be clear that no matter how well a monitoring strategy has been developed, and how well it performs in trial conditions, if it is implemented poorly in everyday clinical practice it will fail. The initial failure of the cervical screening programme in the UK partly reflected lack of care in undertaking the steps outlined above to develop the strategy, but above all it reflected poor implementation. These problems of development and implementation overlap. An ineffective strategy will remain ineffective

Table 2.5 Implementing the monitoring strategy: TTQA

Feature	Requirement
Training	Individuals who undertake monitoring (patients or professionals) need to be clear about their responsibilities; they must understand what is important in achieving a reliable test result and what action to take on the result
Technology	Do not assume that tests that sound the same are the same; measurement technologies need to be constantly compared and standardized; information technologies will also need to be put in place to implement call and recall
Quality assurance	Achievement of planned population coverage, test interval and adjustment action need themselves to be monitored and remedial action taken if necessary; the strategy needs to be sensitive to the patient's concerns

even if implemented well. An implementation and quality-assurance plan cannot be put in place unless the characteristics of an effective strategy have been defined (i.e. the target population, test interval and adjustment action).

So for each monitoring strategy developed, an implementation plan needs to be put in place (at national and local levels). This will usually have three elements: training, technology and quality assurance (TTQA) (Table 2.5).

Most of the above steps are discussed in depth in other contexts, particularly in relation to screening [2]. The key step at a local clinical level is usually to agree individual responsibility (i.e. to decide who should be responsible for call and recall, who should do the monitoring tests, and who should be in control of actions in response to abnormal results). The key steps at a management level are to set up the information technology and quality-control systems that allow the success of the monitoring strategy to be itself monitored.

It is beyond the scope of this chapter to discuss TTQA in detail. However, it should be stressed that a laboratory technology can differ significantly depending on the laboratory that performs it. Doctors are not always aware of analytical quality and biological variation when interpreting laboratory results [14]. Furthermore, they may think that if they ask for, for example, a carcinoembryonic antigen test to monitor colorectal cancer, or for ferritin to monitor renal anaemia in a patient taking epoetin, they will get the same type of result from each laboratory. However, tests are not by any means standardized; different technologies can measure different values or even differing forms of the given molecule. For example, measurements of blood ciclosporin concentrations differ according to whether they are measured by radioimmunoassay of high-performance liquid chromatography [15]. If a monitoring scheme has been developed using a particular technology it is best reproduced elsewhere using the same technology, so that the results are likely to be comparable.

Table 2.6 An overall framework for developing and evaluating a monitoring strategy

Step	Action
1	Ask whether your monitoring objective can meet the three minimum criteria • clinically significant change over time • a possible test to detect that change • an intervention that can ameliorate the change detected
2	Choose the best monitoring test • choose the best test for the monitoring objective and treatment pathway • anticipate the different phases of monitoring • decide who should test (i.e. the patient or a health professional)
3	Specify and assess the monitoring strategy • decide when to test (i.e. the scheduled interval, step-ups and step-downs) • specify what action will be taken on the test result • check whether the strategy works and is cost-effective in practice
4	Implement the monitoring strategy • set up a training programme • commission the necessary information technology (for example, for call/recall) • establish quality assurance

2.6. Conclusions

The overall framework for developing and evaluating monitoring tests is summarized in Table 2.6 in four steps.

Other chapters in this book expand many of the concepts introduced by this framework and show how they can be applied to different conditions. It will become clear that for many monitoring procedures already in common use the evidence to underpin step 2 has yet to be collected, the evaluation of effectiveness of monitoring recommended in step 3 has not been undertaken, and the quality-assurance procedures recommended in step 4 have not been put in place. The objective of the contributors to this book is to change this.

References

1 Anonymous. Cancer of the cervix: death by incompetence. *Lancet* 1985; **ii**: 363–4.
2 Mant D. Prevention. *Lancet* 1994; **344**: 1343–6.
3 Pearce SH. Spontaneous reporting of adverse reactions to carbimazole and propylthiouracil in the UK. *Clin Endocrinol* 2004; **61**: 589–94.
4 Grunfeld E, Mant D, Yudkin P, et al. Routine follow-up of breast cancer in primary care: a randomised trial. *BMJ* 1996; **313**: 665–9.
5 Renehan AG, Egger M, Saunders MP, O'Dwyer ST. Impact on survival of intensive follow up after curative resection for colorectal cancer: systematic review and meta-analysis of randomised trials. *BMJ* 2002; **324**: 813.

6 Aronson JK. Biomarkers and surrogate endpoints. *Br J Clin Pharmacol* 2005; **59**: 491–4.

7 Glasziou P, Irwig L, Mant D. Monitoring in chronic disease: a rational approach. *BMJ* 2005; **330**: 644–8.

8 Yoos HL, Kitzman H, McMullen A, Henderson C, Sidora K. Symptom monitoring in childhood asthma: a randomized clinical trial comparing peak expiratory flow rate with symptom monitoring. *Ann Allergy Asthma Immunol* 2002; **88**: 283–91.

9 Wald N. Use of MoMs. *Lancet* 1993; **341**: 440.

10 Sanderson S, Emery J, Higgins J. CYP2C9 gene variants, drug dose, and bleeding risk in warfarin-treated patients: systematic review and meta-analysis. *Genet Med* 2005; **7**: 97–104.

11 Walton RT, Harvey E, Dovey S, Freemantle N. Computerised advice on drug dosage to improve prescribing practice. *Cochrane Database Syst Rev* 2001; (1): CD002894.

12 Pierach CA. Did Ulysses have porphyria? *J Lab Clin Med* 2004; **144**: 7–10.

13 Aronson J, Ferner R. Joining the DoTS: new approach to classifying adverse drug reactions. *BMJ* 2003; **327**: 1222–5.

14 Skeie S, Thue G, Sandberg S. Use and interpretation of HbA1c testing in general practice. Implications for quality of care. *Scand J Clin Lab Invest* 2000; **60**: 349–56.

15 Reynolds DJ, Aronson JK. ABC of monitoring drug therapy. Cyclosporin. *BMJ* 1992; **305**: 1491–4.

CHAPTER 3

Developing monitoring tools: integrating the pathophysiology of disease and the mechanisms of action of therapeutic interventions

Jeffrey K. Aronson, Susan Michie

A 55-year-old woman who developed an acute pneumonia was admitted to hospital for treatment. The admitting doctor gave her oral co-amoxiclav. She failed to improve. The consultant (attending) physician added erythromycin to her treatment regimen and she soon recovered. The consultant had appreciated what the admitting doctor had failed to do—that although community-acquired pneumonia is most often due to *Streptococcus pneumonia* (which would respond to co-amoxiclav) it is not infrequently due to an atypical organism such as *Legionella pneumophila* (which would not) [1].

This case illustrates in the simplest possible way (and more complex examples are possible [2]) how failure to understand the pathophysiology of a disease can lead to inappropriate or inadequate therapy.

3.1. Understanding pathophysiology

Misunderstanding the pathophysiology of a disease can lead to the wrong choice of monitoring test. Take the example of hypothyroidism.

3.1.1. Monitoring subclinical hypothyroidism

In subclinical hypothyroidism, the serum concentrations of triiodothyronine (T3) and thyroxine (T4) may seem to be normal, but there is already some change in the serum concentration of thyrotrophin (TSH). This is because each individual has his or her own genetically determined set point for free T4/T3,

Evidence-based Medical Monitoring: from Principles to Practice. Edited by Paul Glasziou,
Les Irwig and Jeffrey K. Aronson. © 2008 Blackwell Publishing, ISBN: 978-1-4051-5399-7.

within the population reference range, at which they maintain euthyroidism and thus a normal TSH. In addition, there is a log-linear relation between TSH and free T4/T3. This means that, for example, a small decrease in free T4/T3 from the individual set point, even within the population reference range, may have positive feedback on pituitary TSH secretion, and small deviations in free hormone concentrations (linear response) produce a much larger change in TSH (logarithmic response) [3]. Therefore, when monitoring the progress of subclinical hypothyroidism without therapeutic intervention, the serum T3 or T4 and TSH concentration should be measured; TSH alone will be unhelpful.

3.1.2. Monitoring clinical hypothyroidism

When clinical hypothyroidism occurs, feedback from serum T3 falls below the lower limit of the reference range, and positive feedback to the hypothalamic–pituitary axis leads to an increase in serum TSH. Exogenous T4 during levothyroxine replacement is peripherally converted to T3 and there is a discordant response of peripheral and pituitary target tissues to levothyroxine. Small changes in serum thyroid hormone concentrations that occur within the usual reference range produce large changes in TSH [3]. Since serum free T3 is the biologically active hormone at the tissue level, one could argue that this should be the test of choice for monitoring the effects of levothyroxine replacement. However, T3 and particularly free T3 are difficult and more expensive to measure, and although serum TSH concentration does not correlate well with tissue markers of hypothyroidism, it is generally used in the long-term monitoring of levothyroxine treatment of primary hypothyroidism. Better clinical markers are being sought (see Chapter 19).

3.1.3. Monitoring the long-term adverse effects of hypothyroidism

In monitoring the long-term adverse effects of hypothyroidism, markers that are relevant to the adverse outcomes are more appropriate (e.g. serum lipids for the risk of ischaemic heart disease, pulse rate or systolic time intervals for cardiac effects of thyroxine).

3.1.4. Monitoring the treatment of overt hypothyroidism

In treating overt hypothyroidism, the choice of the monitoring test also depends on the phase of therapy. In the initial phase (the first 2–3 months), TSH is slow in responding to treatment as it takes about 6–12 weeks for the pituitary gland to re-equilibrate to the new hormone status. Later in treatment, however, TSH can be used as a marker with higher confidence, but one must be aware that TSH still responds with some delay when the dose of levothyroxine is adjusted. Pathophysiological features therefore define not only the selection of monitoring tests but also the monitoring intervals in treated hypothyroidism.

These examples show how specific factors can be important. In this chapter, we describe how an understanding of the pathophysiology of a disease can in

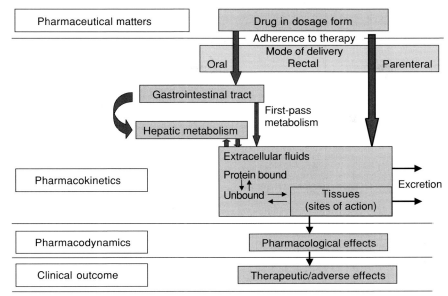

Figure 3.1 The four processes of drug therapy. The pharmaceutical process is not relevant to monitoring. The pharmacokinetic and pharmacodynamic processes are described in this chapter, along with a description of how the pharmacodynamic actions of a drug are translated into therapeutic or adverse outcomes.

general be integrated with an understanding of the mechanism of action of a drug that is used to treat it, in order to develop appropriate monitoring tests. We then extend these concepts to monitoring behavioural interventions.

3.2. The processes of drug therapy: relevance to monitoring the effects of interventions

After a drug has been administered, by whatever route, it has to reach its site of action; this is the *pharmacokinetic* process of drug therapy. At the site of action it has a pharmacological effect, which is eventually translated into a therapeutic or adverse outcome; this is the *pharmacodynamic* process of drug therapy. These processes are shown in Figure 3.1 [4], and the types of monitoring tests that are appropriate to these levels of effect are shown in Figure 3.2.

3.2.1. The pharmacokinetic process of drug therapy
The pharmacokinetic process comprises
- drug absorption and systemic availability,
- drug distribution,
- drug metabolism,
- drug excretion.

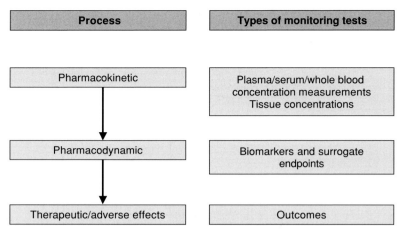

Figure 3.2 The types of monitoring tests that are appropriate to the different levels of pharmacological actions of a drug.

After oral administration a drug reaches the systemic circulation if it is absorbed from the gastrointestinal tract and escapes metabolism (so-called first-pass metabolism) in the gastrointestinal tract, the liver and the lungs. The fraction of the dose that reaches the systemic circulation after running this gauntlet is called the systemic availability or bioavailability. Direct entry of the drug into the systemic circulation can be achieved by giving the drug parenterally. Once in the systemic circulation the drug is distributed to tissues and may be bound by plasma proteins. It is eliminated by one or more of many mechanisms; the main ones being liver metabolism and renal excretion.

3.2.1.1. Plasma drug concentration measurement in monitoring

Measurement of plasma, serum or whole blood drug concentrations can be used to monitor drug therapy.

In monitoring therapy you would ideally try to measure the clinical response directly. If that is difficult to measure, or is not related directly in time to a dose of the drug, some measure of the pharmacological effect of the drug may be required (see the pharmacodynamic process below). If measurement of the pharmacological effect of the drug is difficult you may have to resort to measuring the plasma concentration of the drug. The more information you can gather about drug concentrations in various body tissues, particularly at the site of action, the more able you will be to relate those concentrations to the clinical therapeutic response. Only rarely can one measure the concentration of the drug at its site of action (measuring concentrations of diuretics, such as furosemide and bumetanide, in the urine being an exception [5]), but in a few cases the concentration of drug in the blood (i.e. in the serum, plasma or whole blood) can be used as a surrogate marker of tissue concentration.

Table 3.1 Drugs for which blood concentration
measurement is a suitable monitoring strategy

Aminoglycoside antibiotics (e.g. gentamicin, kanamycin)
Anticonvulsants (principally carbamazepine, phenytoin)
Cardiac glycosides (digitoxin and digoxin)
Immunosuppressants (e.g. ciclosporin, tacrolimus)
Lithium
Theophylline
Vancomycin

Note: For more details, see [5].

There is a combination of criteria that determine whether measuring the blood concentration of a particular drug may be useful in practice:

- Drugs for which the relation between dose and concentration is unpredictable.
- Drugs for which there is a good relation between concentration and effect.
- Drugs with a low toxic:therapeutic ratio (i.e. therapeutic dose close to toxic dose).
- Drugs that are not metabolized to active metabolites.
- Drugs for which there is difficulty in measuring or interpreting the clinical evidence of therapeutic or toxic effects.

The reasons for these criteria are discussed in detail elsewhere [4, 6]. Only a few drugs fulfil these criteria sufficiently to justify blood concentration measurement as a monitoring tool. The major examples are listed in Table 3.1.

3.2.2. The pharmacodynamic process of drug therapy

The pharmacodynamic process describes all those matters concerned with the pharmacological actions of a drug, whether they are determinants of therapeutic effects or of adverse effects [4]. There are many different types of pharmacological actions at the molecular level, including actions on receptors, indirect effects on endogenous agonists (e.g. neurotransmitters and hormones), inhibition of transport processes (e.g. pumps, transporters, channels) and actions on enzymes (inhibition, replacement or activation). However, whatever the primary action is, in all cases the action at the molecular level is sequentially translated into actions at the cellular, tissue and organ levels and finally into a therapeutic or adverse effect (see Figure 3.3).

For example, cardiac glycosides (such as digoxin; Figure 3.4) inhibit the plasma membrane-bound Na/K-ATPase (the sodium/potassium pump) (a molecular effect), which results in reduced cellular sodium efflux, secondarily causing an increase in intracellular calcium (cellular effects). The consequent increase in the rate of myocardial contractility (a tissue effect) leads to an increase in cardiac output (an effect at the organ level), which causes

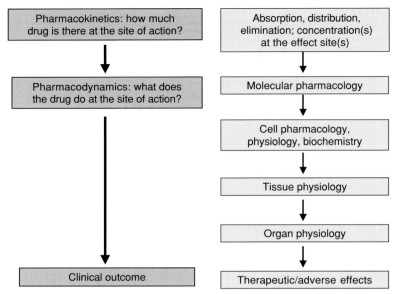

Figure 3.3 The nature of the events in the pharmacokinetic process and the chain of events linking the pharmacological action of a drug at the molecular level to the final therapeutic or adverse outcome (the pharmacodynamic process).

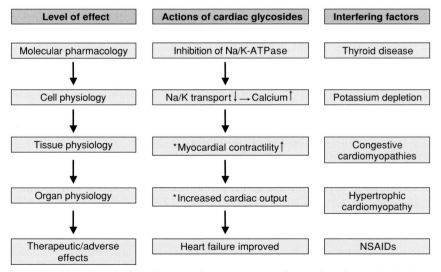

Figure 3.4 The chain in the pharmacodynamic process for cardiac glycosides in the treatment of congestive heart failure and the factors that can disrupt the chain at different levels.

improvement in the signs and symptoms of cardiac failure. This mode of action fits the pathophysiology of ischaemic cardiac failure, which is associated with reduced cardiac contractility and reduced cardiac output (Table 3.2). However, in some cases different forms of pathophysiology or concurrent interfering factors can disrupt this logical chain of events (Figure 3.4):

- In hyperthyroidism the nature of the Na/K-ATPase is changed and there is a poor response to cardiac glycosides (interference at the molecular level).
- Potassium depletion increases the affinity of cardiac glycosides for the Na/K-ATPase, and toxicity occurs more readily (interference at the cellular level).
- Congestive cardiomyopathies, for reasons that are not understood, increase the sensitivity of the myocardium to cardiac glycosides (interference at the tissue level).
- Hypertrophic cardiomyopathy provides a fixed obstruction to ventricular outflow; when cardiac contractility is increased by a cardiac glycoside cardiac output falls instead of rising (interference at the organ level).
- The use of non-steroidal anti-inflammatory drugs in patients with cardiac failure exacerbates fluid retention, vitiating the beneficial effect of cardiac glycosides (interference at the whole body level).

It should be possible to devise methods for studying the action of the drug at each of these levels, methods that could be candidates for use as monitoring tools, either in research or in day-to-day therapy. For example, techniques that have been used in patients with heart failure taking cardiac glycosides include the following:

- Molecular level: Na/K-ATPase activity or receptor function [7].
- Cellular level: intracellular sodium concentration [7].
- Tissue level: rate of myocardial contractility [8].
- Organ level: systolic time intervals [7].
- Whole body level: signs and symptoms of heart failure [9].

However, it is not always possible to devise tests that can be applied at each level. Take for example the coumarin anticoagulants, such as warfarin (Figure 3.5). Although therapy can potentially be monitored at each level, only the international normalized ratio, an effect at the level of tissue physiology, is routinely used (see also Chapter 17).

In the clinical examples given in the second part of this book, we discuss measurements that can be used for monitoring purposes, aimed at different levels in the pharmacological chain.

3.2.3. Dose–response curves (concentration–effect curves) for benefit and harms

The pharmacodynamic effect of a drug is summed up in its dose–response curve (or concentration–effect curve), which is the central dogma of pharmacology [10], as important, for example, as the central limit theorem is to statistics. Figures 3.6–3.8 illustrate different types of dose–response curves.

Table 3.2 The relevance of the pathophysiology of ischaemic congestive cardiac failure to monitoring interventions; the 4 stages are in a time-related progression, as shown by the arrows (cf Figure 5.1)

	Susceptibility factors	→ Early intermediate pathophysiology	→ Later intermediate pathophysiology	Outcome/result of test
→ Pathophysiological features	Age Smoking Cholesterol Blood pressure Homocysteine	Ischaemic heart disease	Reduced cardiac contractility	Cardiac failure
Biomarkers	As above	Angiography	Echocardiography	Atheroma Poor LV function
Interventions	Modify risk factors if possible	Angioplasty (Drug-eluting) stents Treat symptoms (e.g. nitrates)	ACE inhibitors Diuretics Vasodilators Beta-blockers	Reduce mortality Relieve signs and symptoms
Monitoring	Measure modifiable risk factors	Symptoms Nitrate consumption	LV size/function Adverse drug effects	Body weight, breathlessness, oedema Adverse drug effects
Interfering factors	Non-steroidal anti-inflammatory drugs cause fluid retention; calcium channel blockers cause ankle swelling; obesity affects body weight; co-morbidities can cause breathlessness			

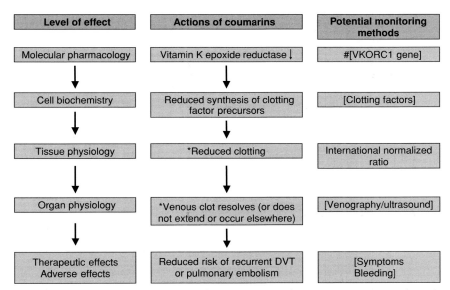

Level of effect	Actions of coumarins	Potential monitoring methods
Molecular pharmacology	Vitamin K epoxide reductase ↓	#[VKORC1 gene]
Cell biochemistry	Reduced synthesis of clotting factor precursors	[Clotting factors]
Tissue physiology	*Reduced clotting	International normalized ratio
Organ physiology	*Venous clot resolves (or does not extend or occur elsewhere)	[Venography/ultrasound]
Therapeutic effects Adverse effects	Reduced risk of recurrent DVT or pulmonary embolism	[Symptoms Bleeding]

Figure 3.5 The chain in the pharmacodynamic process for coumarin anticoagulants in the treatment of venous thromboembolism and the potential monitoring measurements that might be made at each pharmacodynamic level. (*Relevant to the pathophysiology of the condition (items in brackets are not actually used in monitoring); #predictive of dose (also CYP2C9 genotype—pharmacokinetic.)

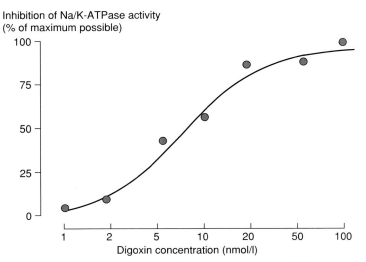

Figure 3.6 A logarithmic concentration–effect curve showing inhibition of the Na/K-ATPase in erythrocyte membranes by the cardiac glycoside digoxin.

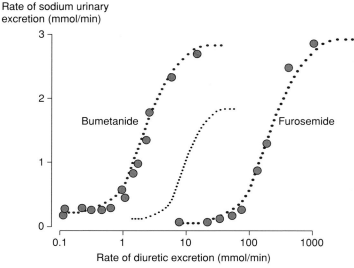

Figure 3.7 Logarithmic concentration–effect curves for the natriuretic effects of the loop diuretics bumetanide and furosemide; the dotted curve is a theoretical curve for a thiazide diuretic (Redrawn from data in [12, 13]).

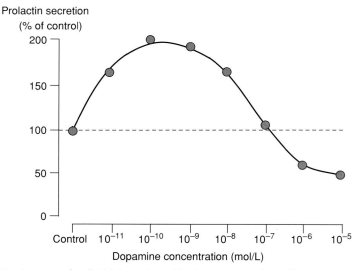

Figure 3.8 An example of a biphasic logarithmic concentration–effect curve (hormesis) (Redrawn from data in [14]).

Inhibition of the Na/K-ATPase in erythrocyte membranes by the cardiac glycoside digoxin can be measured by quantifying the influx of ^{86}Rb into erythrocytes in vitro [11]. The range of effects, from no inhibition to maximum possible inhibition, occurs over two orders of magnitude (i.e. in this case from 1 nmol/l to 100 nmol/l) (Figure 3.6). This is a typical concentration–effect curve, as predicted by theory [10].

However, some concentration–effect curves are steeper. For example, the natriuretic effects of the loop diuretics bumetanide and furosemide occur over about only one order of magnitude (Figure 3.7) [12, 13]. Note that although the shapes of the curves for the two loop diuretics are identical (i.e. they have the same efficacy), bumetanide is more potent than furosemide (its curve is to the left). The corresponding curve for a thiazide diuretic might look like the middle curve in Figure 3.7, with a similar slope but a lower maximum efficacy.

Some concentration–effect curves are biphasic, with opposite effects at low and high concentrations (Figure 3.8 [14]). This phenomenon is known as hormesis [15].

The concentration–effect curves that define different types of adverse drug reactions are discussed in Chapter 15 and shown in Figures 15.2–15.4.

3.3. Monitoring behavioural interventions

Not all therapeutic interventions are pharmacological. The role of behaviours in health and health care is being increasingly understood and recognized [16]. For example, in a US epidemiological study 48% of mortality was caused by preventable behaviours, such as smoking, diet, physical activity and unsafe sex [17]. In a direct placebo-controlled comparison of the impact of a pharmacological and a behavioural intervention on the incidence of diabetes among non-diabetic individuals at high risk, improved diet and increased physical activity produced a 58% reduction, which was significantly greater than the 31% reduction produced by metformin [18]. Interventions that are aimed at changing behaviours associated with health may target lifestyle behaviours in healthy subjects, behaviours of those who are ill (e.g. adherence to medication), and behaviours of those who provide health care; for a critical review of behaviour change interventions, see [19].

Monitoring is a behavioural intervention that can improve health, whether conducted preventively by those who are well, curatively by those who are ill, or by health professionals making decisions about when and how to intervene. Here we discuss a schema (Figure 3.9) for considering the mechanisms of action of behavioural interventions (Figures 3.10 and 3.11) and for monitoring an intervention (Figure 3.12). In this schema pharmacodynamics are replaced by psychodynamics, and the chosen intervention changes behaviour by altering the individual's cognitive processes and emotions, through interactions with environmental factors, both material and social. We recognize that other models are possible [20].

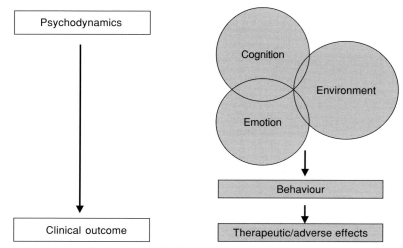

Figure 3.9 The psychodynamics of behavioural interventions.

Behavioural therapy can be considered as an analogy of pharmacological therapy. The behavioural intervention is analogous to the active drug in a formulation. The manner in which a pharmacological intervention is delivered depends on factors other than the active drug (such as the nature of the formulation, the inactive excipients that it contains, the route of administration).

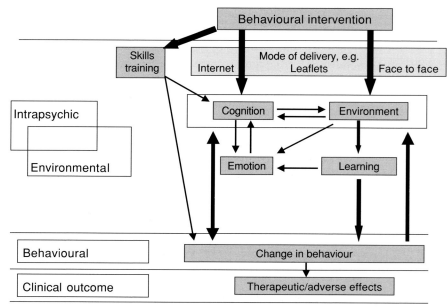

Figure 3.10 The cognitive, emotional, behavioural and environmental processes involved in responses to behavioural interventions.

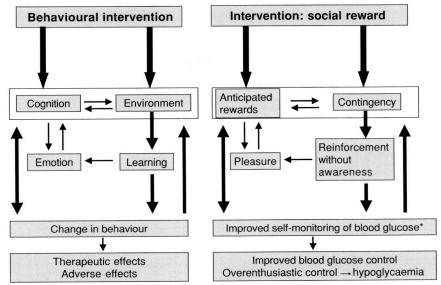

Figure 3.11 Example of behavioural intervention 1: social reward to improve blood glucose control in diabetes mellitus, showing the mechanisms of the intervention. (*The label 'Improved self-monitoring of blood glucose' encompasses several outcomes, including timely injections of insulin, measurement of the blood glucose concentration at appropriate times, the maintenance of accurate records of the results and adjustment of the insulin dosage appropriately; the intervention might affect each of these outcomes differently and multiple interventions might be necessary.)

Analogously, the setting and mode of delivery of a behavioural intervention differ from the intervention itself and are likely to influence its effect. Interventions can be delivered in many different ways, such as via the Internet, by leaflets, via broadcast and print media (e.g. advertising), or face to face. They can be delivered to single individuals, groups, organizations, communities or even whole populations (analogous to mass immunization programmes). The mode of delivery will depend on factors such as the nature of the techniques, the aim of the intervention, the target group, the setting and feasibility (e.g. the available time, funding and skills).

Behavioural interventions work by a variety of mechanisms, explained by a multitude of theories [21]. For example, interventions based on social cognitive theory may target self-efficacy (confidence in changing behaviour), using techniques to increase it, such as persuasive communication, graded mastery (the process of learning gradually) and modelling (observing the behaviour of others) [22]. Other cognitive functions that can be targeted by interventions are expectations of outcome, risk perceptions and perceptions about what other people think. Changing cognitive processes can also in turn change both emotional responses (for example, increasing self-efficacy

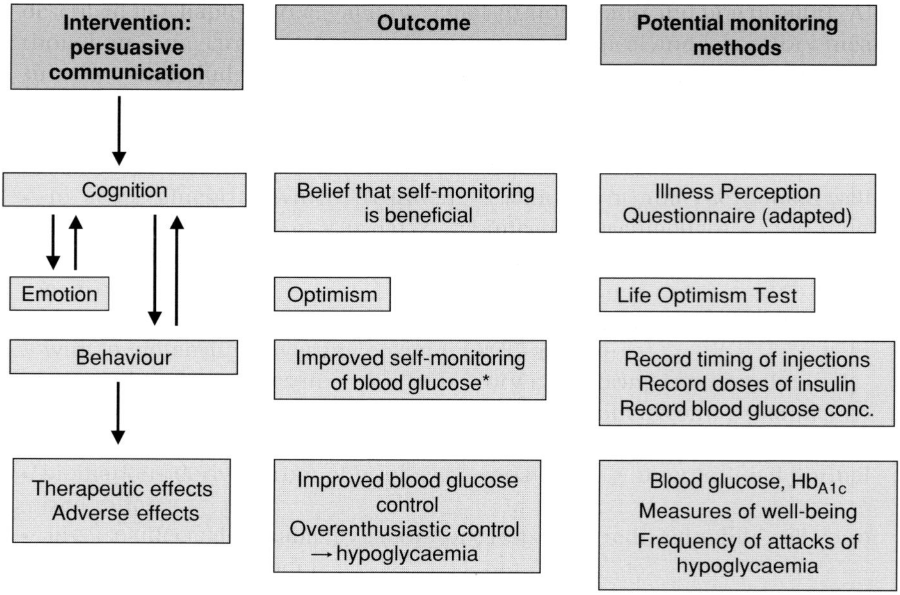

Intervention: persuasive communication	Outcome	Potential monitoring methods

Cognition → Belief that self-monitoring is beneficial → Illness Perception Questionnaire (adapted)

Emotion / Optimism / Life Optimism Test

Behaviour → Improved self-monitoring of blood glucose* → Record timing of injections / Record doses of insulin / Record blood glucose conc.

Therapeutic effects / Adverse effects → Improved blood glucose control / Overenthusiastic control → hypoglycaemia → Blood glucose, Hb_{A1c} / Measures of well-being / Frequency of attacks of hypoglycaemia

Figure 3.12 Example of behavioural intervention 2: persuasive communication to improve blood glucose control in diabetes mellitus, showing the mechanisms of the intervention and the monitoring tools that can be used. (See the explanation of 'Improved self-monitoring of blood glucose' in the caption to Figure 3.11.)

tends to reduce feelings of hopelessness) and behaviours that change the environment.

Environmental factors can change behaviour through operant conditioning, by serving as both contingent reinforcers of behaviour and cues to signal the likelihood of these reinforcers [23, 24]. For example, social rewards, such as praise, increase the frequency of the rewarded behaviours (Figure 3.11). Environmental factors can also produce emotional effects by classical conditioning, in which previously neutral events or circumstances are associated with emotionally charged ones [25, 26].

Using this model, we can explore how behavioural interventions produce beneficial effects, and devise monitoring tests accordingly. Monitoring can be used to assess both whether a change has occurred and how it has occurred (i.e. whether it has been mediated by cognitive or environmental changes). Two examples are given in Figures 3.11 and 3.12 in relation to diabetes mellitus (see also Chapter 16).

The first example deals with the ways in which social reward (for example, telling the patient that they are doing well) might improve blood glucose control (Figure 3.11). The reward increases the likelihood of the behaviour, providing more opportunities for reward, giving a positive feedback loop of reinforcement. The hoped-for results are that the patient will self-administer timely injections of insulin, measure the blood glucose concentration at appropriate times, record the results accurately, and adjust the insulin dosage appropriately. This behaviour should result in improved blood glucose control (a beneficial effect), but an overenthusiastic patient might produce such tight control that attacks of hypoglycaemia become more common (an adverse effect). Various monitoring methods are possible (not illustrated). For example, cognition and emotion can be monitored by validated self-report questionnaires and behaviour can be monitored by keeping records in diaries, palm-held computers or mobile phones [27]. Rewards can be directed at both the patient and the health professional; in a small study, when doctors were financially rewarded there were improvements in objective measurements of quality of care in their patients with diabetes mellitus [28].

The second example deals with the effect of persuasive communication on self-monitoring behaviour in diabetes mellitus [29]. The main aim of the intervention is to persuade the patient that self-monitoring is efficacious and will improve blood glucose control, so that the patient becomes optimistic about the potential results of self-monitoring and is encouraged to use it. The result is improved blood glucose control, as in the previous example. Methods of monitoring this behaviour are available at the different levels shown in Figure 3.12. These include various questionnaires and measures of blood glucose control. For more details, see Chapter 16.

3.4. Conclusions

A full understanding of the pathophysiology and behavioural pathways of disease linked to the mechanism of action of the relevant intervention is necessary in order to develop and use proper monitoring tools. Incomplete knowledge of either vitiates this. In the next chapter, we shall consider biomarkers and surrogate endpoints used to monitor the effects of interventions.

Acknowledgements

Susan Michie is supported by the MRC Health Services Research Collaboration.

References

1 Lim WS, Macfarlane JT, Boswell TC, et al. Study of community acquired pneumonia aetiology (SCAPA) in adults admitted to hospital: implications for management guidelines. *Thorax* 2001; **56**: 296–301.
2 Aronson JK. Rational prescribing, appropriate prescribing. *Br J Clin Pharmacol* 2004; **57**: 229–30.
3 Demers LM, Spencer CA. The National Academy of Clinical Biochemistry laboratory medicine practice guidelines: laboratory support for the diagnosis and monitoring of

thyroid disease. Available from http://www.nacb.org/lmpg/thyroid_lmpg_pub.stm (last accessed 26 December 2006).

4 Grahame-Smith DG, Aronson JK. *The Oxford Textbook of Clinical Pharmacology and Drug Therapy*, 3rd edn. Oxford: Oxford University Press, 2002.

5 Brater DC, Chennavasin P, Day B, Burdette A, Anderson S. Bumetanide and furosemide. *Clin Pharmacol Ther* 1983; **34**: 207–13.

6 Aronson JK, Hardman M, Reynolds DJM. *ABC of Monitoring Drug Therapy*. London: BMJ Publishing Group, 1993.

7 Ford AR, Aronson JK, Grahame-Smith DG, Carver JG. Changes in cardiac glycoside receptor sites, [86]rubidium uptake and intracellular sodium concentrations in the erythrocytes of patients receiving digoxin during the early phases of treatment of cardiac failure in regular rhythm and of atrial fibrillation. *Br J Clin Pharmacol* 1979; **8**: 125–34.

8 Braunwald E. Effects of digitalis on the normal and the failing heart. *J Am Coll Cardiol* 1985; **5** (5 Suppl A): 51A–59A.

9 Pugh SE, White NJ, Aronson JK, Grahame-Smith DG, Bloomfield JG. The clinical, haemodynamic, and pharmacological effects of withdrawal and reintroduction of digoxin in patients with heart failure in sinus rhythm after long-term treatment. *Br Heart J* 1989; **61**: 529–39.

10 Aronson JK. Concentration–effect and dose–response relations in clinical pharmacology. *Br J Clin Pharmacol* 2007; **63**: 255–7.

11 Aronson JK, Grahame-Smith DG, Hallis KF, Hibble A, Wigley F. Monitoring digoxin therapy: I. Plasma concentrations and an in vitro assay of tissue response. *Br J Clin Pharmacol* 1977; **4**: 213–21.

12 Chennavasin P, Seiwell R, Brater DC. Pharmacokinetic–dynamic analysis of the indomethacin-furosemide interaction in man. *J Pharmacol Exp Ther* 1980; **215**: 77–81.

13 Brater DC, Chennavasin P, Day B, Burdette A, Anderson S. Bumetanide and furosemide. *Clin Pharmacol Ther* 1983; **34**: 207–13.

14 Burris TP. The stimulatory and inhibitory effects of dopamine on prolactin secretion involve different G-proteins. *Endocrinology* 1992; **130**: 926–32.

15 Calabrese EJ, Baldwin LA. Hormesis: U-shaped dose responses and their centrality in toxicology. *Trends Pharmacol Sci* 2001; **22**: 285–91.

16 Marteau TM, Dieppe P, Foy R, Kinmonth A-L, Schneiderman N. Behavioural medicine: changing our behaviour. *BMJ* 2006; **332**: 437–8.

17 Mokdad AH, Marks JS, Stroup DF, Gerberding JL. Actual causes of death in the United States, 2000. *JAMA* 2004; **291**: 1238–45. Erratum 2005; **293**: 293–4.

18 Knowler WC, Barrett-Connor E, Fowler SE, et al. Diabetes Prevention Program Research Group. Reduction in the incidence of type 2 diabetes with lifestyle intervention or metformin. *N Engl J Med* 2002; **346**: 393–403.

19 Michie S, Abraham C. Identifying techniques that promote health behaviour change. Evidence based or evidence inspired? *Psychol Health* 2004; **19**: 29–49.

20 Lee C. Arguing with the cognitivists. *J Behav Ther Exp Psychiatry* 1996; **27**: 357–61.

21 Michie S, Johnston M, Abraham C, Lawton R, Parker D, Walker A. Making psychological theory useful for implementing evidence based practice: a consensus approach. *Qual Saf Health Care* 2005; **14**: 26–33.

22 Bandura A. *Self-Efficacy: The Exercise of Control*. New York: W.H. Freeman, 1997.

23 Skinner BF. *Science and Human Behavior*. New York: Free Press, 1953.

24 Nemeroff CJ, Karoly P. Operant methods. In: Kanfer FH, Goldstein AP (eds), *Helping People Change: A Textbook of Methods*. London: Allyn and Bacon, 1991.

25 Wolpe J. *The Practice of Behavior Therapy*, 2nd edn. New York: Pergamon, 1973.

26 Bouton ME. Context, time, and memory retrieval in the interference paradigms of Pavlovian learning. *Psychol Bull* 1993; **114**: 80–99.

27 Farmer A, Gibson O, Hayton P, et al. A real-time, mobile phone-based telemedicine system to support young adults with type 1 diabetes. *Inform Prim Care* 2005; **13**: 171–7.

28 Beaulieu ND, Horrigan DR. Putting smart money to work for quality improvement. *Health Serv Res* 2005; **40** (5 Pt 1): 1318–34.

29 Farmer A, Wade A, French DP, Goyder E, Kinmonth AL, Neil A. The DiGEM trial protocol—a randomised controlled trial to determine the effect on glycaemic control of different strategies of blood glucose self-monitoring in people with type 2 diabetes. *BMC Fam Pract* 2005; **6**: 25.

CHAPTER 4

Biomarkers and surrogate endpoints in monitoring therapeutic interventions

Jeffrey K. Aronson

In Chapter 3 we saw that it is important, when devising monitoring strategies, to establish, as far as possible, the pathophysiology of a disease and the mechanisms of action of the interventions used to treat it, and to integrate the two.

The ideal monitoring test is one that measures the final outcome of the intervention. For example, the final outcome in the management of pneumonia is resolution of the signs and symptoms of the disease (such as fever, breathlessness, chest pain, auscultatory signs), and those can be monitored during treatment. Other measures related to effects of the infection can also be measured, such as the chest x-ray, inflammatory markers in the blood, and the presence of the organism in the sputum or antibodies to it in the blood, but since they are not the actual endpoints they are regarded as surrogate endpoints. Although in this case the surrogate endpoints are very close in the pathophysiological chain to the true clinical endpoints, there are important differences. For example, the time course of changes in a chest x-ray is not the same as the time course of changes in the clinical features of pneumonia: the former can take longer to show evidence of pneumonia and may take longer to resolve [1]. In some infections (e.g. typhoid) an individual can continue to carry the organism long after recovery from the infection [2]; after recovery from infection with *Clostridium difficile* the toxin can be detected in the stools [3], and after recovery from viral diseases serum antibodies can persist for years. These differences reduce the value of such markers in monitoring the disease and its response to treatment.

Intermittent disorders. Intermittent disorders can be very difficult to monitor. For example, it is possible for a patient with epilepsy to keep a diary of the number of seizures. However, the absence of seizures over a period of time

Evidence-based Medical Monitoring: from Principles to Practice. Edited by Paul Glasziou,
Les Irwig and Jeffrey K. Aronson. © 2008 Blackwell Publishing, ISBN: 978-1-4051-5399-7.

during therapy cannot necessarily be attributed to the treatment but might simply be a reflection of periodicity. Measuring the plasma concentration of an antiepileptic drug will tell you whether there is enough drug in the body to have a putative effect but not that it is the drug that is having the apparent beneficial effect. Some other marker might be better, although in this case none has been developed. However, measuring the plasma drug concentration will at least tell you whether there is any drug in the body, whether the amount that is there is likely to be beneficial, and whether there is a risk of overdose and toxicity [4].

Preventive therapies.   In some cases it is not feasible to measure the final outcome. For example, in the management of hypertension the final outcome is prevention of the long-term complications, such as a heart attack or a stroke. But when an intervention is aimed at preventing the endpoint, the endpoint is not itself suitable for monitoring. The best that one can do is to find an event that can be monitored in advance of the endpoint and that predicts the efficacy of the preventive intervention, in other words a surrogate endpoint. In hypertension the blood pressure is a surrogate endpoint, changes in which predict the success or failure of antihypertensive therapy in preventing heart attacks and strokes.

4.1. History and definitions

The word surrogate comes from the Latin surrogare (sub + rogare; supine surrogatus), literally meaning asked in place of. It was first defined as 'A deputie in another place' (1604), and the current definition is 'a person or thing that acts for or takes the place of another'.

The use of the term 'surrogate' relating to a biomedical marker or endpoint dates from the early 1980s. The earliest example of 'surrogate endpoint' that I have found is from 1983, but there it is in the context of competitive strategy [5]: 'this means that at any point of time... it is necessary and desirable that a surrogate endpoint be assigned together with a measurement criterion which enables the planners to view what they have been doing up to that point in time and to be able to state whether or not their long-term strategic plan met their criteria of success'. The first use in a biomedical sense is from 1985, in a textbook on clinical trials, in which the term 'surrogate response variable' was used and the example given of change in tumour size as a surrogate for mortality [6]; the text that contains this description was not in the first edition of the same textbook, published in 1981. The first use of the term 'surrogate marker' dates from 1988 [7] and of 'surrogate endpoint' from 1989 [8].

The term 'biomarker' dates from a little earlier, in the 1970s, although it is not until 1980 that it appears in a human context. The first instance that I have found is in the title of a paper published in 1973: 'A search for porphyrin biomarkers in Nonesuch Shale and extraterrestrial samples' [9]. The earliest biological usage that I have found is from 1977 [10]: 'Characterization of selected

Table 4.1 Examples of circulating biomarkers in clinical oncology

Level	Biomarker	Examples
Susceptibility factors	Genetic susceptibility	BRCA1 and BRCA2, MSH, MLH1
	Environmental susceptibility	Steroid hormones, insulin-like growth factors and their binding proteins, gene polymorphisms (lactate dehydrogenase gene)
Molecular pathology	DNA repair	MGMT and hMLH1 promoter hypermethylation
Cell pathology	Immune responses	Auto-antibodies against MUC1 protein, p53 mutated protein, overexpressed erbB2/neu protein
	Tumour burden	Carcinoembryonic antigen, prostate-specific antigen, mucin markers (CA15.3, CA19.9, CA125), alpha-fetoprotein, human chorionic gonadotropin, cell-free DNA
	Oncogene or oncosuppressor gene deregulation	p53, soluble HER2neu, soluble epidermal growth factor receptor, APC, RAR, p73, FHIT, RASSF1A, LKB1, VHL, BRCA1 promoter hypermethylation
	Cell-cycle regulation	Cyclin D1 mRNA, p14, p15, p16 promoter hypermethylation
	Apoptosis	Survivin, M30 antigen
	Extracellular matrix modification	TIMP2, MMP, uPA, DAPK1, E-cadherin, TIMP3 promoter hypermethylation
	Detoxification	GSTP1 promoter hypermethylation
Tissue pathology	Angiogenesis	Vascular endothelial growth factor, fibroblast growth factor
Organ pathology	Organ damage	Tissue-specific enzymes, acute-phase proteins, markers of inflammation, haemoglobin

Note: Adapted from [13].

viral isolates indicated that hemagglutination elution was the most consistent biomarker for CO[lorado] P[sittacine] I[solate] and subsequent N[ewcastle] D[isease] V[irus] pet-bird isolates'. The earliest usage in relation to humans is from 1980, in relation to the use of serum UDP-galactosyl transferase activity as a potential biomarker for breast carcinoma [11].

To see where the terms biomarker and surrogate endpoint stand in relation to each other, we need to define them from the bottom up.

A surrogate endpoint has been defined as 'a biomarker intended to substitute for a clinical endpoint', the latter being 'a characteristic or variable that reflects how a patient feels, functions, or survives' [12]. And a biomarker has been defined as 'a characteristic that is objectively measured and evaluated as an indication of normal biologic processes, pathogenic processes, or pharmacologic responses to a therapeutic intervention' [8]. So all surrogate endpoints are biomarkers, but not all biomarkers are surrogate endpoints, since biomarkers can substitute for endpoints that are not clinical. A surrogate marker can be defined as a surrogate that substitutes not for an endpoint but for some other measure. For example, the plasma concentration of a drug is a surrogate marker for the concentration of the drug at its site of action.

4.2. Uses and advantages of surrogate endpoints

Surrogate endpoints can be used for different purposes, in screening, diagnosing, staging and monitoring diseases, or in monitoring responses to interventions. They can also be used in various aspects of drug discovery and development:

- as targets for drug actions in drug discovery (e.g. COX-2 activity as a target for anti-inflammatory drugs);
- as endpoints for pharmacodynamic studies of drug action (for example, serum cholesterol as a marker for the action of a drug that is intended to be used to prevent cardiovascular disease) and in pharmacokinetic/pharmacodynamic studies;
- in studying concentration–effect (dose–response) relations (see Chapters 1 and 3);
- in clinical trials;
- for studying adverse effects (see Chapter 15).

In clinical oncology, for example, it has been suggested that there are four uses of biomarkers [13]:

- to assess the risk of cancer;
- to study tumour–host interactions;
- to reflect tumour burden;
- to reflect function.

The tumour markers that have been identified in these categories can also be classified according to the pharmacodynamic schema outlined in Chapter 3, as shown in Table 4.1, and this is a more logical way to approach the question.

The principal advantages of surrogate endpoints are that they are easier to measure than clinical endpoints and can be measured over a shorter time span. Biomarkers are often cheaper and easier to measure than 'true' endpoints. For example, it is easier to measure a patient's blood pressure than to use echocardiography to measure left ventricular function, and it is much easier to do echocardiography than to measure morbidity and mortality from hypertension in the long term. Biomarkers can also be measured more quickly and earlier. Blood pressure can be measured today, whereas it takes several years to collect mortality data. In clinical trials, the use of biomarkers leads to smaller sample sizes. For example, to determine the effect of a new drug on blood pressure a relatively small sample size of say 100–200 patients would be needed and the trial would be relatively quick (1–2 years). To study the prevention of deaths from strokes a much larger study group would be needed and the trial would take many years. There may also be ethical problems associated with measuring true endpoints. For example, in paracetamol overdose it is unethical to wait for evidence of liver damage before deciding whether or not to treat a patient; instead a pharmacological biomarker, the plasma paracetamol concentration, is used to predict whether treatment is required [14].

4.3. Taxonomies of surrogate endpoints

There are different ways of classifying surrogate endpoints.

4.3.1. By the pathophysiology of the disorder or illness

A general approach to considering surrogate endpoints in terms of the pathophysiology of a disorder or illness is illustrated in Figure 4.1. A susceptibility

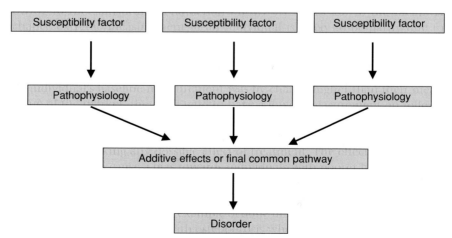

Figure 4.1 A schematic representation of the pathways whereby susceptibility factors contribute to disease.

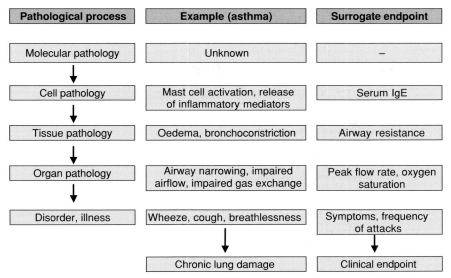

Figure 4.2 Surrogate endpoints in the pathophysiology of asthma.

factor can trigger a pathophysiological process, and for each disorder there may be more than one such susceptibility factor and more than one corresponding pathophysiological process. Eventually, through additive effects or a final common pathway, the disorder or illness results. Each primary pathophysiological process can be considered to occur through an effect at the molecular level, which results, through a chain of events at the cellular, tissue and organ levels, in the signs and symptoms of the disease. There may also be secondary pathology and complications, and each of those can be analysed analogously. Figure 4.2 illustrates an example (asthma) that is restricted to primary pathology, showing the chain of events and the surrogate endpoints that could be used to monitor its progress or changes in response to interventions.

4.3.2. By the mechanism of action of the intervention
Classification of surrogate endpoints according to the level at which they occur in the pharmacological chain (see Chapter 3) is illustrated in Figure 4.3. The nearer the therapeutic or adverse effect a surrogate endpoint is, the better a measure of the true endpoint it is likely to be.

4.3.3. By the nature of the measurement
A taxonomy of this sort is shown in Table 4.2. A biomarker can be extrinsic to the individual, for example cigarette smoking as a surrogate endpoint for lung cancer, or intrinsic. Intrinsic endpoints can be physical (signs and symptoms), psychological or laboratory measurements. Examples are shown in the table. The categories in Table 4.2 could be further subdivided according to whether

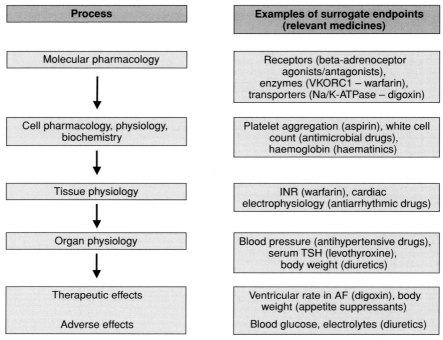

Figure 4.3 Examples of surrogate endpoints at different pharmacodynamic levels (from molecular to whole body) in the management of diseases.

the markers are being used for diagnosis, staging or monitoring of disease or for determining its response to an intervention. They could also be divided according to the level at which they occur (molecular, cellular, etc.) and according to whether they relate to susceptibility factors, primary or secondary pathology, or complications of the disease.

4.4. Criteria for useful biomarkers

There are many links in the chain of events that leads from the pathogenesis of a disease to its clinical manifestations (see Figures 4.2–4.4); biomarkers can be used at any point in the chain, at the molecular, cellular, tissue or organ levels. Likewise, a therapy might be developed to attack any one of these links, in order to try to manipulate the disease, symptomatically or therapeutically. Any measurement short of the actual outcome could be regarded as a biomarker.

However, there are different scenarios that link the biomarker or surrogate endpoint to the disease and its outcome, as illustrated in Figure 4.5. These examples are not exhaustive.

Scenario (a).   The ideal surrogate is one through which the disease comes about or through which an intervention alters the disease (see also Chapter 5).

Table 4.2 Classifying biomarkers by the type of measurement

Types of biomarker	Examples of surrogate endpoints	The relevant clinical endpoints
A. Extrinsic markers	Cigarette consumption	Lung cancer
	Daily defined dose	Drug consumption
B. Intrinsic markers		
1. Physical evaluation	Breathlessness	Heart failure
a. Symptoms	Lid lag	Hyperthyroidism
b. Signs		
2. Psychological evaluation	Likert scales	Pain
	Questionnaires	Self harm
3. Laboratory evaluation		
a. Physiological	Blood pressure	Heart attacks and strokes
b. Pharmacological		
i. Exogenous	Inhibition of CYP enzymes	Routes of drug metabolism
ii. Endogenous	Docetaxel clearance	Febrile neutropenia
c. Biochemical	Blood glucose concentration	Complications of diabetes
d. Haematological	INR with warfarin	Pulmonary embolism
e. Immunological	Autoantibodies	Autoimmune diseases
f. Microbiological	*Clostridium difficile* toxin	Pseudomembranous colitis
g. Histological	Jejunal biopsy	Gluten-sensitive enteropathy
h. Radiographic	White dots on MRI scan	Lesions of multiple sclerosis
i. Genetic	CYP2C19 isozymes/VKORC1 genotype	Warfarin dosage

For example, the serum cholesterol concentration should be an excellent diagnostic marker for cardiovascular disease; however, there is no clear cut-off point, and only about 10% of those who are going to have a stroke or heart attack have a serum cholesterol concentration above the reference range (see Chapter 18) [15]. But even if cholesterol is not a good diagnostic marker, it can still be used as a biomarker of the therapeutic response to cholesterol-lowering drugs.

Scenario (b).   Even if a surrogate is in the pathway leading from the pathophysiology of the disease to its final outcomes, the intervention may not alter it. For example, most antihypertensive drugs lower the blood pressure by mechanisms that are probably not directed specifically at the prime cause of hypertension, whatever that is. Any surrogate marker earlier in the pathway than the raised blood pressure itself is therefore unlikely to be a good surrogate.

Scenario (c).   In some cases, the surrogate comes after the outcome rather than before it, which is just as good. For example carcinoembryonic antigen, which

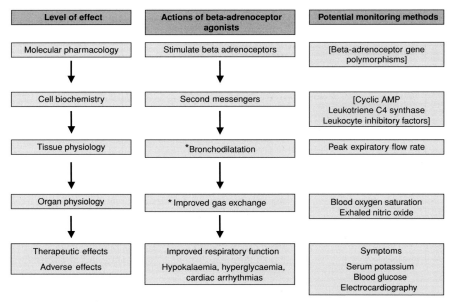

Level of effect	Actions of beta-adrenoceptor agonists	Potential monitoring methods
Molecular pharmacology	Stimulate beta adrenoceptors	[Beta-adrenoceptor gene polymorphisms]
Cell biochemistry	Second messengers	[Cyclic AMP Leukotriene C4 synthase Leukocyte inhibitory factors]
Tissue physiology	*Bronchodilatation	Peak expiratory flow rate
Organ physiology	* Improved gas exchange	Blood oxygen saturation Exhaled nitric oxide
Therapeutic effects Adverse effects	Improved respiratory function Hypokalaemia, hyperglycaemia, cardiac arrhythmias	Symptoms Serum potassium Blood glucose Electrocardiography

Figure 4.4 The chain in the pharmacodynamic process for beta-adrenoceptor agonists in the treatment of acute severe asthma and the potential monitoring measurements that might be made at each pharmacodynamic level. (*Relevant to the pathophysiology of the condition; items in parentheses are not actually used in monitoring.)

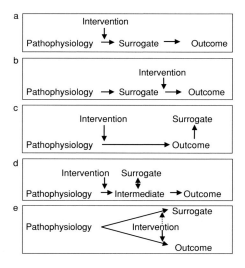

Figure 4.5 Five different scenarios relating pathophysiology, surrogate endpoints and primary outcomes (see text for discussion).

is produced by cancer cells, is not useful in diagnosing ovarian carcinoma, since it is non-specific, but can be used to monitor its response to treatment [16].

Scenario (d). In some cases, a surrogate is closely related to an intermediary that mediates the effect of the pathophysiology but is not itself suitable as a biomarker. In this case the surrogate is a kind of meta-marker—it is a marker of a marker. For example, in Gram-negative septicaemia the release of cytokines can cause a major primary outcome, such as hypotension. Cytokines are not suitable as biomarkers, but fever, another effect of cytokines, can be used as a biomarker of the response to antimicrobial drug therapy.

Scenario (e). An important pitfall to avoid is to assume that an epiphenomenon or secondary outcome is a good surrogate marker. If the pathophysiology produces an effect by a different mechanism than that by which it produces the disease outcome, that effect (the epiphenomenon or secondary outcome) will not be a useful surrogate unless it is affected in the same way by the intervention as the primary outcome is. There are many examples of epiphenomena.

In order to understand the value of a biomarker in monitoring therapy, it is necessary to known which type of model fits the disease best.

4.4.1. Bradford Hill's guidelines

In looking for criteria for deciding which biomarkers are good candidates for surrogate endpoints, we can turn to the guidelines that Austin Bradford Hill propounded for helping to analyse associations in determining causation (Table 4.3) [17, 18]. He propounded these guidelines (sometimes mistakenly called criteria) in the context of environmental causes of disease, but they can be used in other spheres [19]. Whenever a biomarker conforms to these guidelines, it is more likely to be useful. Note that simply because a biomarker fulfils the guidelines it will not necessarily be useful; it merely makes it more likely to be useful.

4.5. Identifying biomarkers

The first step in identifying suitable biomarkers is to understand the pathophysiology of the disease and to find factors that determine it. For example (Figure 4.2), understanding the pathophysiology of asthma allows one to identify factors that might be useful as biomarkers. In a study of the use of biomarkers in heart failure, biomarkers that were linked to mechanisms involved in the aetiology seemed to be best suited to serve as early markers to predict and diagnose disease, select therapy or assess progression [20].

The next step is to identify potential biomarkers based on the mechanism of action of the intervention related to the pathophysiology of the disease. This is illustrated for the case of asthma in Figure 4.4.

Table 4.3 Austin Bradford Hill's guidelines that increase the likelihood that an association is causative, as applied to biomarkers

Guideline	Characteristics of useful biomarkers
Strength	A strong association between marker and outcome, or between the effects of a treatment on each
Consistency	The association persists in different individuals, in different places, in different circumstances, and at different times
Specificity	The marker is associated with a specific disease
Temporality	The time courses of changes in the marker and outcome occur in parallel
Biological gradient (dose responsiveness)	Increasing exposure to an intervention produces increasing effects on the marker and the disease
Plausibility	Credible mechanisms connect the marker, the pathogenesis of the disease and the mode of action of the intervention
Coherence	The association is consistent with the natural history of the disease and the marker
Experimental evidence	An intervention gives results consistent with the association
Analogy	There is a similar result to which we can adduce a relationship

Finally, one must determine the extent to which the putative marker actually correlates with the process. For example, it has been suggested that in searching for useful biomarkers of ageing the following requirements must be fulfilled [21]:

- the biomarker should have a significant cross-sectional correlation with age;
- there should be a significant longitudinal change in the same direction as the cross-sectional correlation;
- there should be significant stability of individual differences over time;
- the rate of change in a biomarker of ageing should be predictive of lifespan.

Barriers to the development of biomarkers have been discussed in relation to cancers [22]:

- the methods of collecting data are different in different places and may be less easy in places where health care is not centralized or where there are no standardized methods of collecting and storing data;
- many patient records are incomplete or the databases are not searchable;
- the sample size may be too small;
- intellectual property rights and informed-consent agreements can restrict the future use of stored samples;
- funding may be hard to obtain, because investors may be concerned that a biomarker will not work or because the expected financial returns are poor.

4.6. Pitfalls and problems in using biomarkers

A major problem in the use of biomarkers is the failure to understand the relation between the pathophysiology of the problem and the mechanism of action of the intervention (see Section 4.4 above). For example, smoking causes lung cancer, and a trial of the benefit of education in preventing lung cancer might use smoking as a surrogate endpoint rather than the occurrence of the cancer itself. On the other hand, if chemotherapy is used as a measure for treating lung cancer, smoking could not be used as a surrogate endpoint. This is obvious, but alerts us to the possibility of similar but less obvious examples, in which the mechanisms are not understood.

For example, ventricular arrhythmias cause sudden death, and antiarrhythmic drugs prevent ventricular arrhythmias. It was therefore expected that antiarrhythmic drugs would prevent sudden death. In fact, in the Cardiac Arrhythmia Suppression Trial [23], Class I antiarrhythmic drugs *increased* sudden death significantly in patients with asymptomatic ventricular arrhythmias after a myocardial infarction, and the trial was stopped prematurely. The mechanisms were not understood and the hypothesis was wrong.

Another good example is enalapril and vasodilators, such as hydralazine and isosorbide, whose haemodynamic effects and effects on mortality associated with heart failure are dissociated. Vasodilators improved exercise capacity and improved left ventricular function to a greater extent than enalapril; however, enalapril reduced mortality significantly more than vasodilators [24]. So in this case haemodynamic effects are not a good surrogate.

Confounding factors, particularly the use of drugs, can nullify the value of surrogate endpoints. For example, serum T3 is used as a marker of the tissue damage that thyroid hormone causes in patients with hyperthyroidism (see Chapter 19). However, its usefulness is blunted in patients taking amiodarone, which interferes with the peripheral conversion of T4 to T3 without necessarily altering thyroid function. In a patient with gastrointestinal bleeding the heart rate may not increase if the patient is also taking a beta-blocker, leading the clinician to underestimate the severity of the condition. Likewise, corticosteroids can mask the signs of an infection or inflammation.

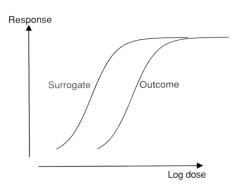

Figure 4.6 The concentration–effect curves for the effect of an intervention on a surrogate endpoint and the primary outcome may not be the same.

As a general principle, if the concentration–effect curves for the effects of an intervention on the primary outcome and the surrogate are different (Figure 4.6) a change in the surrogate may not truly reflect the degree of change in the outcome. This is true for any biomarker that does not lie on the same line as the pathophysiology and the outcome.

Proper application of useful biomarkers may be hindered by lack of reproducibility of the methods used to measure it. For example, there are differences between ciclosporin concentrations measured in serum and blood and between blood ciclosporin concentrations measured using radioimmunoassay and high-performance liquid chromatography [25]. Despite the fact that the association between thiopurine methyltransferase (TMPT) activity and the risk of adverse effects from mercaptopurine was described several years ago [26], methods for measuring the enzyme are not standardized [27] and optimal treatment is often not achieved [28]. Another problem with TMPT is that in someone who has had a recent transfusion the activity of the enzyme in the recipient's erythrocytes may be contaminated by that in the donor's [29].

It is unusual for a single biomarker to provide all the information one needs in monitoring interventions. For example, patients with asthma feel breathless if they have a low peak expiratory flow rate (PEFR). However, in one study different drugs produced different relationships between PEFR and breathlessness [30]. Patients taking beclomethasone did not feel as breathless as those taking theophylline for a given PEFR. So what should the surrogate marker be; the 'hard' endpoint of peak flow or the 'soft' marker of how the patients felt? Probably both should be used. How to choose the best tests to use is covered in Chapter 5.

Statistical problems can arise with biomarkers and surrogate endpoints. A surrogate endpoint has been defined statistically as 'a response variable for which a test of the null hypothesis of no relationship to the treatment groups under comparison is also a valid test of the corresponding null hypothesis based on the true endpoint' [31]. Often the surrogate endpoint is used as an entry criterion in clinical trials, and it is important to be aware that this can lead to statistical problems [8]. It introduces heterogeneous variance and the problem of regression to the mean. If someone is entered into a trial on the basis of an abnormal surrogate endpoint and then receives no treatment, the surrogate endpoint will still improve, simply because of the statistical variation in the measurement of variables. This reduces the power of a study. There is also a high likelihood of missing data when surrogate endpoints are used. Using a small sample size when using a surrogate endpoint may also mean that a study is not big enough to detect adverse effects of drugs.

4.7. Conclusions

There are clear potential benefits in using biomarkers. Information can be obtained earlier, more quickly and more cheaply. However, the chain of events in a disease process linking pathogenesis to outcome is fragile and the better we understand the nature of the path a disease takes and the mechanism of action of an intervention that affects it the better biomarkers we will be able to develop in diagnosing, staging and monitoring disease and its response to therapy.

References

1 Kuru T, Lynch JP, III. Nonresolving or slowly resolving pneumonia. *Clin Chest Med* 1999; **20**(3): 623–51.

2 Bourdain A. *Typhoid Mary: An Urban Historical.* New York: Bloomsbury, 2001.

3 Johnson S, Homann SR, Bettin KM, et al. Treatment of asymptomatic *Clostridium difficile* carriers (fecal excretors) with vancomycin or metronidazole. A randomized, placebo-controlled trial. *Ann Intern Med* 1992; **117**(4): 297–302.

4 Aronson JK, Hardman M, Reynolds DJ. ABC of monitoring drug therapy. Phenytoin. *BMJ* 1992; **305**: 1215–8.

5 Shubik M. The strategic audit: a game theoretic approach to corporate competitive strategy. *Manage Decis Econ* 1983; **4**: 160–1.

6 Friedman LM, Furberg CD, De Mets DL. *Fundamentals of Clinical Trials*, 2nd edn. Littleton, MA: PSG Publications Company, 1985, p. 17.

7 Brotman B, Prince AM. Gamma-glutamyltransferase as a potential surrogate marker for detection of the non-A, non-B carrier state. *Vox Sang* 1988; **54**: 144–7.

8 Wittes J, Lakatos E, Probstfield J. Surrogate endpoints in clinical trials: cardiovascular diseases. *Stat Med* 1989; **8**: 415–25.

9 Rho JH, Bauman AJ, Boettger HG, Yen TF. A search for porphyrin biomarkers in Nonesuch Shale and extraterrestrial samples. *Space Life Sci* 1973; **4**: 69–77.

10 Erickson GA, Maré CJ, Gustafson GA, Miller LD, Carbrey EA. Interactions between viscerotropic velogenic Newcastle disease virus and pet birds of six species. II. Viral evolution through bird passage. *Avian Dis* 1977; **21**: 655–69.

11 Paone JF, Waalkes TP, Baker RR, Shaper JH. Serum UDP-galactosyl transferase as a potential biomarker for breast carcinoma. *J Surg Oncol* 1980; **15**: 59–66.

12 NIH Definitions Working Group. Biomarkers and surrogate endpoints in clinical research: definitions and conceptual model. In: Downing GJ (ed), *Biomarkers and Surrogate Endpoints*. Amsterdam: Elsevier, 2000, pp. 1–9.

13 Gion M, Daidone MG. Circulating biomarkers from tumour bulk to tumour machinery: promises and pitfalls. *Eur J Cancer* 2004; **40**(17): 2613–22.

14 Wallace CI, Dargan PI, Jones AL. Paracetamol overdose: an evidence based flowchart to guide management. *Emerg Med J* 2002; **19**(3): 202–5. Erratum 2002; **19**(3):376.

15 Wald NJ, Hacksaw AK, Frost CD. When can a risk factor be used as a worthwhile screening test? *BMJ* 1999; **319**: 1562–5.

16 Gargano G, Correale M, Abbate I, et al. The role of tumour markers in ovarian cancer. *Clin Exp Obstet Gynecol* 1990; **17**(1): 23–9.

17 Hill AB. The environment and disease: association or causation? *Proc R Soc Med* 1965; **58**: 295–300.

18 Legator MS, Morris DL. What did Sir Bradford Hill really say? *Arch Environ Health* 2003; **58**: 718–20.

19 Shakir SA, Layton D. Causal association in pharmacovigilance and pharmacoepidemiology: thoughts on the application of the Austin Bradford Hill criteria. *Drug Saf* 2002; **25**: 467–71.

20 Jortani SA, Prabhu SD, Valdes R, Jr. Strategies for developing biomarkers of heart failure. *Clin Chem* 2004; **50**(2): 265–78.

21 Ingram DK, Nakamura E, Smucny D, Roth GS, Lane MA. Strategy for identifying biomarkers of aging in long-lived species. *Exp Gerontol* 2001; **36**(7): 1025–34.

22 Nelson NJ. Experts wrestle with problems developing biomarkers, search for new tests. *J Natl Cancer Inst* 2006; **98**(9): 578–9.

23 The Cardiac Arrhythmia Suppression Trial Investigators. Preliminary report: effect of encainide and flecainide on mortality in a randomised trial of arrhythmia suppression after myocardial infarction. *N Engl J Med* 1989; **321**: 406–12.

24 Cohn J. Lessons from V-HeFT: questions for V-HeFT11 and the future therapy of heart failure. *Herz* 1991; **16**: 267–71.

25 Reynolds DJ, Aronson JK. ABC of monitoring drug therapy. Cyclosporin. *BMJ* 1992; **305**: 1491–4.

26 Lennard L, Rees CA, Lilleyman JS, Maddocks JL. Childhood leukaemia: a relationship between intracellular 6-mercaptopurine metabolites and neutropenia. *Br J Clin Pharmacol* 2004; **58**: S867–S871.

27 Armstrong VW, Shipkova M, von Ahsen N, Oellerich M. Analytic aspects of monitoring therapy with thiopurine medications. *Ther Drug Monit* 2004; **26**: 220–6.

28 Coulthard SA, Matheson EC, Hall AG, Hogarth LA. The clinical impact of thiopurine methyltransferase polymorphisms on thiopurine treatment. *Nucleosides Nucleotides Nucleic Acids* 2004; **23**: 1385–91.

29 Ford L, Prout C, Gaffney D, Berg J. Whose TPMT activity is it anyway? *Ann Clin Biochem* 2004; **41**(Pt 6): 498–500.

30 Higgs CMB, Laszlo G. Influence of treatment with beclomethasone, cromoglycate and theophylline on perception of bronchoconstriction in patients with bronchial asthma. *Clin Sci* 1996; **90**: 227–34.

31 Prentice RL. Surrogate endpoints in clinical trials: definition and operational criteria. *Stat Med* 1989; **8**: 431–40.

CHAPTER 5

Choosing the best monitoring tests

Les Irwig, Paul P. Glasziou

Often several tests may be available to monitor a clinical condition. How do we decide which of the tests to use? To aid this decision, several criteria are helpful:

1 *Clinical validity.* The test should be either a measure of the clinically relevant outcome or a good predictor of the clinically relevant outcome.
2 *Responsiveness.* The test should change promptly in response to changes in therapy.
3 *Large signal-to-noise ratio.* The test should differentiate clinically important changes over time from background measurement variability (short-term biological fluctuations and technical measurement error).
4 *Practicality.* The test should be non-invasive, cheap and simple to do. Results should be immediately available and suitable for patient self-monitoring.

It is unlikely that any test will entirely fulfil all these criteria. Which test to choose depends on deciding the objectives of monitoring, then identifying which criteria are most important for the objectives, and finally assessing the extent to which the alternative tests fulfil the criteria. Not uncommonly, fulfilling the objectives may require several monitoring tests, for example one for monitoring the short-term response to therapy and another for long-term effects, or one for monitoring benefits and another for monitoring harms.

Later in this chapter, we shall explain each of these criteria. To understand them, it is helpful to first consider what tests might be measured along the pathway that leads from the administration of the treatment to the outcome that the treatment aims to produce (Figure 5.1).

Figure 5.1 shows the natural history of disease from risk factors to the outcome via intermediate pathology, both early and late. Juxtaposed is a pathway (lower box) starting from giving a drug (or another type of intervention) aimed at altering that natural history or ameliorating the disease at different stages.

Evidence-based Medical Monitoring: from Principles to Practice. Edited by Paul Glasziou, Les Irwig and Jeffrey K. Aronson. © 2008 Blackwell Publishing, ISBN: 978-1-4051-5399-7.

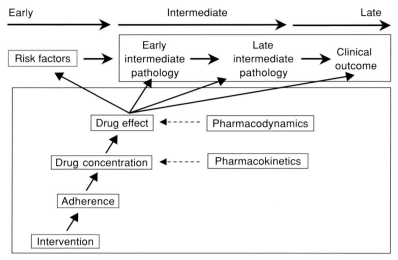

Figure 5.1 A flow diagram of disease and the effects of treatment. Left top box: risk factors/natural history; right top box: progression; bottom box: intervention.

In Figure 5.2 the development of hypertension is shown as an example. Over time, hypertension can lead to subclinical end-organ effects, such as left ventricular hypertrophy and hypertensive retinopathy. Eventually clinical events, such as stroke or myocardial infarction, can occur. There may be other possible pathways to the clinical event, for example from serum cholesterol, obesity or smoking; however, for simplicity we shall restrict the example to the single factor of raised blood pressure. We could use tests to monitor the natural history from risk factor to the clinical outcome and the effects of treatment at each step along the pathway. To foreshadow the criteria that we shall present later in this chapter, we point out here that monitoring tests later in the pathway, for example evidence of end-organ damage, have the advantage of validity or relevance: they are closer to the clinical outcome that the intervention aims to prevent and they may be the most useful ways to monitor the long-term effects of treatment. Monitoring tests earlier in the pathway, for example blood pressure, have the advantage of responsiveness: they change quickly in response to treatment and may be most useful for the initial phase of monitoring. For example, inadequate blood pressure reduction in response to an antihypertensive drug in an adequate dosage is sufficient to decide that an alternative drug should be tried.

Examples of the use of different monitoring tests for assessing initial response to treatment and long-term monitoring are as follows:

- *Depression treated with lithium.* The initial response is measured by serum lithium concentration, but monitoring thereafter should also assess features of depression and the adverse effects of lithium (for example, on renal function).

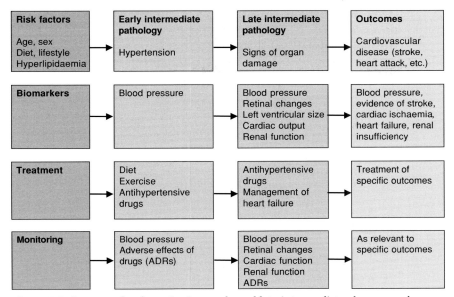

Figure 5.2 An example of monitoring: early and late intermediate changes and outcomes in hypertension.

- *Diabetes.* The initial response can be monitored by fasting blood sugar concentration (days), the early intermediate response by Hb_{A1c} concentration (months) and later response by clinical changes such as diabetic retinopathy (years).

Although we are discussing monitoring the anticipated beneficial effects of an intervention, similar flow diagrams can be drawn to help decide on tests for monitoring the adverse effects of a disease or its treatment (see Chapter 15).

Whether monitoring is being done for treatment effectiveness or for adverse effects, the criteria used to choose the best test fall into four main categories:
- Clinical validity,
- Responsiveness;
- Signal-to-noise ratio,
- Practicality.

5.1. Clinical validity

The first question is whether the test actually measures what we are interested in therapeutically. It may do so directly (by monitoring the disease itself) or indirectly (by monitoring something on the pathway between treatment and outcomes). Hence the important questions to ask are the following:

5.1.1. Is the test a measure of the clinically relevant outcome or a proxy for or good predictor of the clinically relevant outcomes?

Because monitoring consists in assessing changes over time, clinical validity is achieved if changes in the test reflect or predict changes in the clinically relevant outcome [1].

5.1.2. Is the test free of important bias (systematic variability)?

If the clinical state does not alter over time, there should be no systematic difference in test measurements over that time. A striking example is subjective measurement, such as patient self-reporting, which may be consciously or unconsciously over-reported or under-reported. For example, patients may under-report improvements in arthritic symptoms if monitoring is being used to decide whether to continue first-line therapy or switch to alternative drugs whose use is restricted because of costs to the health service. On the other hand, they may over-report improvements if they are already taking the restricted drugs and think that they may be withdrawn unless there is a response (see also Chapter 3). If sources of systematic variability or bias are known, they should be avoided or reduced. This applies at a clinical stage, and for laboratory measurements also at the pre-analytical and analytical stages.

Clinical standardization includes the correct use of calibrated instruments and the timing and circumstances of measurement. For example, diurnal variation can be dealt with by measuring at the same time each day. Variability due to the timing of treatment can be dealt with by taking measurements at a set time after the last dose, or timing the dose for a set time before measurement. Pre-analytical standardization includes ensuring that specimens are taken, stored, and handled in a way that preserves the stability of the specimen. Analytic standardization includes calibrating laboratory instruments, using the same methods and instrument on several monitoring occasions, training staff and quality control.

There are almost always several sources of variation; it is important to identify the most important remediable ones and give them priority. For example, in monitoring glaucoma, the variation in intraocular pressure during office hours is probably less than the variation induced by drugs given three times a day, so standardizing measurements at a set time after the last dose is more important than ensuring that measurements are made at the same time on each occasion.

5.2. Responsiveness

Responsiveness can be thought of as having several components.

5.2.1. The test should be on the pathway between the intervention and the outcome

For example, consider treating hypertension to prevent stroke or coronary heart disease (Figure 5.2). If we are considering only antihypertensive treatment, blood pressure is on the pathway. On the other hand, serum cholesterol also predicts the outcome but is unsuitable for monitoring the response to antihypertensive treatment as it is not on the appropriate pathway.

5.2.2. Reversibility

The test needs to be reversible, or at least its progression should be halted or slowed by the intervention. Test results should change monotonically as the treatment dose is changed. For this reason, continuous measures are usually preferred, for example blood pressure or myocardial wall thickness in the case of hypertension. Dichotomous events, such as myocardial infarction, are irreversible and therefore too late to give useful feedback about how to change management.

Sometimes one can measure function related to clinically relevant outcome events; for example, renal function may be monitored to predict the onset of renal insufficiency (see Chapter 20). In this case, the monitoring measure is a good predictor of outcome, as it is in fact the same variable.

5.2.3. Rapid response to changes in treatment

The test should change rapidly in response to changes in treatment. A rapid response is clearly most important when there are large variations in the dose or intensity of treatment required by different patients, for whom monitoring allows appropriate dose titration. The more rapid the response, the more helpful the test. If the response time is an order of magnitude less than the duration of the illness, it enables decisions about treatment, such as titrating the dose of a drug, to be made sufficiently early in the illness. Sometimes the response time can be very short; for example, intraocular pressure responds to topical medications within hours.

5.3. Large signal-to-noise ratio

In a good monitoring test, the Signal (the meaningful biological change we are aiming to detect) needs to be large relative to the Noise (the short-term variability in the measurement). Measurement variability refers to the random variation, usually for unknown reasons, around the true value, which can be estimated by the mean of a large set of measurements. Measurement variability includes short-term biological variability and technical measurement variability. Biological variability refers to real short-term changes in the measured variable around its mean or true value. Technical measurement variability refers to random differences in test results attributable to the measurement technique. Technical variability in laboratory tests may be due to the way the

Response

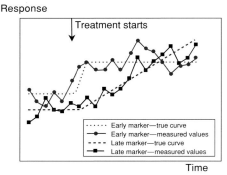

Time

Figure 5.3 Signal-to-noise ratios in early and late markers of treatment response.

sample is taken (pre-analytical) or the way it is analysed in the laboratory (analytical). For example, technical measurement variability causes cholesterol measurements that are repeated at different times on the same sample to differ from one another. Biological variability in cholesterol measurement is the additional variation found when samples are taken from the same patient a few days apart, i.e. sufficiently far apart to encompass short-term fluctuations in measurement but not so far apart that there is a true change in the underlying value. About 80% of the measurement variability in cholesterol measurements is biological and 20% occurs for technical reasons.

To help understand these questions when assessing test validity, Figure 5.3 shows how two hypothetical test results change over a time during which treatment is introduced and kept steady. The early marker is a drug concentration or responsive physiological variable, such as blood pressure reduction in response to antihypertensive drugs or bone turnover markers in osteoporosis. Its true value increases shortly after treatment is started. The late marker shows gradual improvement in a pathophysiological measure, for example reduction in myocardial wall thickness in hypertension or change in bone mineral density in osteoporosis. Both early and late markers are subject to measurement variability, as shown by the data points around the lines for each marker. The points are generated randomly from a normal distribution of the same variance for the early and late marker. Soon after treatment is started, the signal component of the late marker is very small relative to its noise, and it is difficult to assess whether an observed change—or lack of change—is real or attributable to measurement variability. On the other hand, the signal of the early marker is large and easily discernible from its measurement variability. With a longer duration of treatment, the signal-to-noise ratio of the late marker becomes larger and the effect more obvious, as the size of the signal in the late marker depends on an effect that accumulates over time.

Clearly, the estimates of the likely range of magnitudes of signal and noise are critical in the choice of monitoring tests. We now discuss how to quantify it, reduce its magnitude, and further understand its role in the choice of monitoring tests.

5.3.1. Estimation of signal and noise

Although one would hope to get estimates of treatment response and measurement variability from the published literature, studies are often not designed and analysed in a way that is helpful for monitoring. For example, randomized trials commonly report the mean change in outcome in the treatment arms without providing information on the distribution of observed responses around the mean. It is then difficult to determine whether there truly is variability between patients in their response to treatment or whether all the observed variability is simply due to noise (measurement variability). The ideal study would take patients before they start treatment, establish a baseline value and its variation with several measurements, then start a fixed amount of treatment in the treatment arm and measure the early response and long-term changes by making repeated measurements over months or even years. Further development of this concept is given in the chapter on initial response monitoring (Chapter 6) and examples in the later clinical chapters, such as the chapter on cholesterol monitoring (Chapter 18).

5.3.2. Estimation of noise

In the absence of studies in which signal and noise are simultaneously assessed, decisions about monitoring can be assisted by short-term studies of measurement variability. To construct the control limits around a target for the type of control chart used in the clinical chapter on glaucoma monitoring (Chapter 23), measurement variability can be assessed by repeating measurements in an individual over a time that is sufficiently long that the errors are not correlated but sufficiently short that there is no change in the true underlying value. For example, when measuring blood pressure, several measurements on one occasion do not adequately capture short-term variability. Short-term variability is best assessed by measurements a few days apart, after which the variability does not increase further over the next weeks [2, 3]. Measurement variability can also be estimated by examining the difference between two measurements in each of a series of patients [4].

There are certain requirements of studies of measurement variability to assist monitoring decisions about patients taking treatments. They should

- be in-patients taking stable treatment, because the measurement variability may be different to that in unaffected people or patients not taking treatment [5, 6];
- include biological variability, not just technical variability, by doing repeat measurements within a short period (usually days or weeks), rather than on just one occasion;
- show the distribution of within-person variability, not just provide estimates of the standard deviation, to assess asymmetry and normality;

• provide Bland–Altman plots to assess whether the measurement variability (the difference between measurements in each individual) depends on the value of the test (the mean of the two measurements in each individual); variability increases with the value of the measurement for many biological measures.

5.3.3. How to reduce noise

If the analyses above suggest that the 'noise' of a potential test is too great for that test to be able to discern the signal, i.e. the noise swamps the signal, several methods can be used to try to reduce the noise. Methods include the following.

5.3.3.1. Identify and reduce the sources of biological and technical variability

This needs to be done for two reasons. Firstly, sources of variability can cause bias in a measurement. Secondly, if randomly distributed, so that they do not cause bias, they will add to the measurement variability or noise of the test. Noise can be reduced by standardizing the testing, as discussed in Section 5.1.2.

5.3.3.2. Use multiple measurements or multiple measures

Further reduction in noise can be achieved by the following:
• Using the mean of multiple measurements.
• Clustering the measurements.
• Repeating the same test if one measure is suggestive rather than conclusive, for example beyond 1 or 2 SDs; the time interval for remeasurement should be chosen so that tests have independent errors, for example blood pressure measurement is more useful a few days later rather than on the same visit.
• Doing another test, for example a triage and follow-up sequence.

When clustering tests, if one is going to make four measurements and it is unlikely that important effects of treatment occur in less than say 3 months, there will be greater value in making two measurements at both the start and the end of the 3-month period rather than four spread over the 3 months. For monitoring that depends on a change from baseline, multiple measurements at baseline, before treatment starts, are particularly important. In both examples, the multiple measurements must be sufficiently far apart to capture all sources—biological as well as technical—of short-term measurement variability. In other words, the multiple measurements should be so far apart that their errors are not correlated.

5.3.4. How the size of the signal and noise affects the choice of monitoring test

To understand how signal and noise affect the choice of monitoring test, consider a hypothetical scenario of several continuous normally distributed monitoring test results (Table 5.1). The scenarios in the table build up progressively more complex variability structures.

Table 5.1 Correlation of tests with a perfectly measured outcome in scenarios in which the test is measured with random measurement variability

Scenario	Drug concentration (early)	Pharmacodynamic marker	Risk predictor of outcome (late)
1: No measurement error in any test	0.60	0.70	**0.80**
2: Some measurement error in all tests	0.53	0.62	**0.72**
3: Progressively more measurement error in tests later in the sequence	**0.53**	0.44	0.44
4: As in scenario 3, but the pharmacodynamic marker is the mean of multiple measurements	0.53	**0.57**	0.44

Note: In this hypothetical example, all tests are continuous and normally distributed; the highest correlation in each scenario is shown in bold; for estimation of correlation coefficients attenuated by measurement error, see the Appendix.

Scenario 1.   If tests are made without any measurement variability, one would expect measurements later in the sequence (such as a risk predictor of outcome) to be more highly correlated with outcome, and early markers (such as the drug concentration) to be less highly correlated. For example, in scenario 1, the correlation between the risk predictor and outcome is 0.8, whereas the correlation between the drug concentration and outcome is 0.6.

Scenario 2.   However, when there is measurement variability, the expected correlation with a perfectly measured outcome will be smaller [7, 8]. For example, in scenario 2, in which there is some measurement variability in all of the tests, the correlations are all smaller than in scenario 1. If the variability was reduced (for example by using some of the techniques outlined in Section 5.3.3, on how to reduce noise) the correlations would move closer to those in scenario 1.

Scenario 3.   Measurement variability may be greater for some tests, which will result in greater attenuation of the correlation of tests with outcome. If the measurement error is much greater for tests later in the sequence, an earlier test could be more highly correlated with outcome, as when the drug concentration has a higher correlation with outcome than either the pharmacodynamic marker or risk predictor.

Scenario 4.   The above scenarios are based on a single measurement of each test at a particular time. If a test is intrinsically predictive but has a lot of measurement variability, the variability can be overcome by averaging multiple measurements at that time. As the number of tests approaches infinity, the correlation approaches that in scenario 1, in which there is no measurement

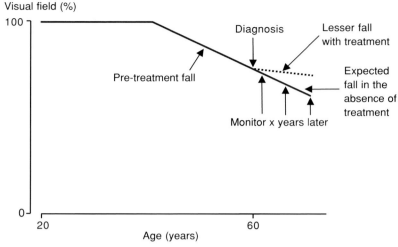

Figure 5.4 Monitoring tests based on change in function from that expected from the natural history of the disease, using glaucoma as an example.

error. In scenario 5, the average of multiple measurements of the pharmaco-dynamic marker is more highly correlated with outcome than a single measurement of any of the other tests.

5.3.5. Monitoring interventions in the presence of a changing baseline

Often tests are based on an abnormality that would normally worsen with time, in which improvement is sought; for example loss of renal function or lung function with age. One such example, visual field defects in glaucoma, is illustrated in Figure 5.4.

In this example, glaucoma is diagnosed because of a 25% defect in visual fields in a patient aged 60 years. The visual field test is good for diagnosis for three reasons. Firstly, there is very little between-person variability in visual fields in healthy people. Secondly, the diagnosis is based on the current value, i.e. the test represents the accumulation of loss over many years (a large signal). Thirdly, the measurement variability of a test at age 60 is small compared with the signal.

Now consider the same visual field test when used for monitoring. At a given age, patients with the greatest visual field loss are likely to progress the fastest in the future. This phenomenon has been called the horse-racing effect: the horse furthest in front got there by being faster and is therefore likely to be faster in the future [9]. If we assume that the 25% loss occurred over 20 years and that this history is predictive of future expected loss, we would expect an annual loss of 1.25% per year. In monitoring, one is trying to discern whether progression, as shown by the dotted line in Figure 5.4, deviates from the expected decline (solid line). The benefit of treatment is the difference between the observed (dotted) line and the expected or predicted (solid) line. Clearly, this requires previous testing to be highly predictive of future decline and observations of decline during treatment to have high signal-to-noise ratios, despite the relatively short time interval over which the decline is measured. Monitoring for deviation from expected functional decline, for example assessing whether a treatment is slowing the decline of renal function or lung function, is therefore fraught with difficulty.

5.4. Practicality

Finally, once all the above have been considered, and there are still several possible tests that could be used to monitor the effect of treatment for a disease, the choice will depend on which has most practical advantages. Practical issues include that the test
- is not invasive,
- is cheap,
- is simple to perform, and
- can be done by the patient.

The last of these is important, since self-monitoring in general seems to have advantages [10]; if two measures are otherwise equal, choose one that patients can do themselves.

5.5. Conclusions

We have suggested several criteria that drive the choice of monitoring tests: clinical validity, responsiveness, large signal-to-noise ratio and practicality. It is unlikely that any test will entirely fulfil all these criteria. Which test to choose will depend on the objectives of monitoring. If the objective is to assess initial response, responsiveness may be the main criterion. For example, that an adequate dose of an antihypertensive drug does not lower the blood pressure sufficiently can be rapidly assessed and the drug replaced by another. On the other hand, assessment of the success of long-term treatment may place more emphasis on clinical validity—the assessment of measures that are more predictive of clinical outcome. There will often be trade-offs between the extent to which different potential monitoring tests fulfil the criteria. Assessing the extent to which the criteria are fulfilled and the importance of each criterion for the objective of monitoring should result in better selection of what and when to monitor.

Acknowledgements

This work was partly funded by program grants (211205 and 402764) from the National Health and Medical Research Council of Australia. We are grateful to Katy Bell, Martin Turner, Andrea Horvarth, Patrick Bossuyt, Petra Macaskill and Fiona Stanaway for helpful comments, and to Martin Turner for help with preparation of the figures.

Appendix

Correlation coefficients have been estimated using the formula

$$R_o = R_t \sqrt{G}$$

where R_o is the observed correlation, R_t is the true underlying correlation in the absence of measurement error, as shown in scenario 1, G is the generalizability or reliability coefficient, obtained, for example, as the correlation of two measurements in each of a series of patients.

For scenario 2, the generalizability coefficient is 0.8 for each of the tests.

For scenario 3, the generalizability coefficient is 0.8 for drug concentration, 0.4 for the pharmacodynamic marker and 0.3 for the risk predictor of outcome.

For scenario 4, the generalizability coefficients are as for scenario 3, but the pharmacodynamic marker is the mean of three measurements.

References

1 Begg C, Leung D. On the use of surrogate end points in randomized trials. *J R Stat Soc* 2000; **163**(1): 15–28.
2 Rosner B, Polk F. The implications of blood pressure variability for clinical and screening purposes. *J Chronic Dis* 1979; **32**: 451–6.
3 Kardia SL, Turner ST, Schwartz GL, Moore JH. Linear dynamic features of ambulatory blood pressure in a population-based study. *Blood Press Monit* 2004; **9**(5): 259–67.
4 Bland JM, Altman DG. Statistical methods for assessing agreement between two methods of clinical measurement. *Lancet* 1986; **i**: 307–10.
5 Lassen JF, Brandslund I, Antonsen S. International normalised ratio for prothrombin times in patients taking oral anticoagulants: critical difference and probability of significant change in consecutive measurements. *Clin Chem* 1995; **41**: 444–7.
6 Lassen JF, Kjeldsen J, Antonsen S, Petersen PH, Brandslund I. Interpretation of serial measurements of INR for prothrombin times in monitoring oral anticoagulant therapy. *Clin Chem* 1995; **41**: 1171–6.
7 Gardner MJ, Heady JA. Some effects of within-person variability in epidemiological studies. *J Chronic Dis* 1973; **26**: 781–95.
8 Kupper LL. Effects of the use of unreliable surrogate variables on the validity of epidemiological research studies. *Am J Epidemiol* 1984; **120**: 643–8.
9 Fletcher C, Peto R, Tinker C, Speizer F. Appendix B10. Epidemiological studies of rates of change of FEV (or other factors) in a general, non-clinical population. In: *The Natural History of Chronic Bronchitis and Emphysema*. Oxford: Oxford University Press, 1976, pp. 199–208.
10 Heneghan C, Alonso-Coello P, Garcia-Alamino JM, Perera R, Meats E, Glasziou P. Self-monitoring of oral anticoagulation: a systematic review and meta-analysis. *Lancet* 2006; **367**: 404–11.

CHAPTER 6

Monitoring the initial response to treatment

Katy Bell, Jonathan Craig, Les Irwig

In this chapter, we provide a conceptual framework within which an initial response can be evaluated. It is structured in three parts:

1 Introduction: why and how do we monitor an initial response?

2 Should we monitor the initial response to therapy: what is the response distribution at a population level?

3 How can we monitor the response at the individual level?

Other questions that are relevant to monitoring the initial response are covered elsewhere (for example, timing of measurement during the initial response is covered in Chapter 9).

6.1. Introduction

6.1.1. Why do we monitor an initial response to therapy?

When a therapy is used we must decide whether the potential benefits outweigh the harms of the treatment in that individual patient. If variability of response will affect the decision to continue therapy, initial monitoring is desirable. That is, initial monitoring is appropriate when (i) there is clinically relevant variability in treatment effects (both desired and adverse) and (ii) there is a suitable marker for estimating the initial response.

Monitoring of the initial response to therapy is not needed if variability of the response will not affect the decision to continue therapy. This may be the case when there is thought to be no variation in the response or variation does not matter. Alternatively, there may be no suitable marker with which to monitor the initial response (see below and Chapter 5 for discussion of desirable test attributes).

6.1.2. How do we monitor initial response to a therapy?

When initial monitoring is required, we shall need to choose the clinical and/or laboratory measures to use based on the properties of a 'desirable test', as

Evidence-based Medical Monitoring: from Principles to Practice. Edited by Paul Glasziou, Les Irwig and Jeffrey K. Aronson. © 2008 Blackwell Publishing, ISBN: 978-1-4051-5399-7.

described in Chapter 5 (i.e. validity, signal-to-noise ratio and practicality). Although in some circumstances a combination of clinical and laboratory measures is used to judge the initial response, often most importance is placed on one measure.

Here are some examples of cases in which clinical monitoring is primarily used:

- an acute illness in which treatment is short term and the patient self-monitors the effect (e.g. a urinary tract infection or impetigo);
- the outcome of interest is also what is monitored (e.g. depression, asthma, pain);
- clinical adverse effects of therapy (e.g. wheeze with beta-blockers, cough with angiotensin converting enzyme (ACE) inhibitors).

Here are some examples in which laboratory monitoring is primarily used:

- target drug concentrations (e.g. digoxin, lithium, phenytoin, gentamicin);
- physiological variables (e.g. blood pressure, cholesterol, creatinine);
- biomarkers derived from physiological variables (e.g. international normalized ratio);
- adverse effects detectable by laboratory tests (e.g. reduced white cell count with cyclophosphamide).

6.1.3. Initial monitoring of commonly prescribed therapies

The most frequently prescribed medications in three developed countries are presented in Table 6.1. For about half of these drugs a laboratory outcome is primarily used when judging effectiveness (e.g. lipid-modifying agents, medications for diabetes mellitus, levothyroxine). For most of the others a clinical outcome is used (e.g. analgesics, bronchodilators, psychotropic drugs). In a few cases no initial measurement of the intended therapeutic effect is made, e.g. aspirin: the lack of a suitable marker of response means that therapy is given at the same dose to everyone. Other examples of cases in which there is no monitoring of the initial effect include folate supplementation in pregnancy and childhood immunizations; in both of these cases no measurement of response is made because any variation in serum folate or antibody levels is thought unimportant. Even for the few drugs that do not require initial monitoring of the intended therapeutic effect, it may be necessary to monitor for adverse effects.

6.2. Is monitoring for initial response needed?

Monitoring to check response is often done, but not always needed.

6.2.1. Factors that contribute to an apparent variation in response

The apparent variability in a biomarker of response seen in trials is likely to be only partly due to true variability between individuals in the therapeutic response [4–6]. Table 6.2 summarizes the main sources of such variability.

Table 6.1 The 20 most frequently prescribed pharmaceutical formulations in Australia, England and the USA* (with outcome measures used to judge the therapeutic response).

Australia†	England‡	USA§
Atorvastatin (cholesterol)	Paracetamol‖ 500 mg (pain)	Acetaminophen‖ (pain)
Simvastatin (cholesterol)	Salbutamol 100 µg (shortness of breath)	Amoxicillin (symptoms and signs of infection)
Paracetamol (pain)	Furosemide 40 mg (shortness of breath; other)	Hydrochlorothiazide (blood pressure)
Omeprazole (gastrointestinal symptoms)	Co-proxamol 32.5/325 mg (pain)	Albuterol¶ (shortness of breath)
Irbesartan (blood pressure)	Atorvastatin 10 mg (cholesterol)	Aspirin (none)
Atenolol (blood pressure/pulse rate)	Levothyroxine 50 µg (TSH)	Hydrocodone (pain)
Salbutamol¶ (shortness of breath)	Metformin 500 mg (blood glucose and HbA_{1c})	Fluticasone (frequency of exacerbations)
Irbesartan + hydrochlorothiazide (blood pressure)	Simvastatin 20 mg (cholesterol)	Levothyroxine (TSH)
Esomeprazole (gastrointestinal symptoms)	Amoxicillin 250 mg (symptoms and signs of infection)	Atorvastatin (cholesterol)
Celecoxib (pain)	Levothyroxine 60 µg (TSH)	Ibuprofen (pain)
Ramipril (blood pressure)	Lansoprazole 15 mg (gastrointestinal symptoms)	Lisinopril (blood pressure)
Salmeterol + fluticasone (shortness of breath and frequency of exacerbations)	Aspirin 75 mg (none)	Pseudoephedrine (symptoms of allergy)
Perindopril (blood pressure)	Lactulose (bowel movements)	Furosemide (shortness of breath)
Metformin (blood glucose and HbA_{1c})	Atenolol 25 mg (blood pressure/pulse rate)	Guaifenesin (cough)
Codeine + paracetamol (pain)	Lansoprazole 30 mg (gastrointestinal symptoms)	Metoprolol (blood pressure/pulse rate)
Sertraline (depression)	Fluoxetine 20 mg (depression)	Amlodipine (blood pressure)
Pantoprazole (gastrointestinal symptoms)	Simvastatin 40 mg (cholesterol)	Azithromycin (symptoms/signs of infection)
Amoxicillin (symptoms and signs of infection)	Levothyroxine 25 µg (TSH)	Estrogens (menopausal symptoms)
Amlodipine	Diclofenac 50 mg (pain)	Celecoxib (pain)
Temazepam (insomnia, anxiety)	Amoxicillin 500 mg (symptoms/signs of infection)	Triamcinolone (symptoms/signs of inflammation)

Note: *Differences between countries are partly explained by differences in funding. These data are for all clinic prescriptions (USA), all publicly subsidized prescriptions (Australia) or publicly funded subscriptions (England). Note also that the English data reflect individual dose formulations, so that one drug can appear multiple times.

†The number of prescriptions for drugs subsidized by government (through PBS) for the year ending June 2005, as measured by the Department of Health and Ageing [1].

‡The number of prescriptions for any therapeutic preparation in England for the year 2004, as measured by the Department of Health [2].

§The number of prescriptions in ambulatory care for the year 2002, as measured by the National Ambulatory Medical Care Survey [3].

‖Paracetamol (rINN) = acetaminophen (USAN).

¶Salbutamol (rINN) = albuterol (USAN).

Table 6.2 Sources of variation in a biomarker of response seen in a clinical trial*

Label	Source	Description
T	Between treatments	Variation due to the average effect of therapy
B	Between patients	Variation due to differences between patients unrelated to therapy
W	Within patients	Variation due to differences between measurements in an individual patient
R	Between patients in treatment effect	Variation due to differences in the effects of treatment between patients

Note: *Adapted from [4].

These are as follows: the average treatment effect (T), differences between patients overall B), differences in active treatment effect between individuals (R), and intra-individual variation (W). As an illustration, there is substantial variability in outcome in the placebo arms of trials, when there is no active effect of therapy in any of the participants. In this scenario there is no variation from T and R; all the variation is from sources B and W. In order to gain an accurate estimate of the true variability in therapeutic response (R) from observations of a biomarker of response in a trial, attempts must be made to control for these other sources of variation.

The timing of measurement is also important. If measurements are made too early, between-person differences in pharmacokinetic processes will increase the variation observed. Lack of standardization of timing of measurement is another potential source of variation. To avoid these problems, measurements need to be made at a standardized time after treatment, and this needs to be long enough after treatment to ensure that everyone has reached the new steady state. This and other issues relevant to timing of measurement are discussed in Chapter 9. For now, we shall assume that there is no variation due to suboptimal timing of measurement.

6.2.2. Methods of estimating variation in individual response

We shall describe two approaches for estimating the variation in a biomarker of response that is due to differing response to treatment (R) rather than other sources (T, B and W). These are (i) to analyse data from a series of n-of-1 trials and (ii) to compare the relative variability of treatment arms in a randomized placebo-controlled trial.

6.2.2.1. Series of n-of-1 trials

Analysing data from a series of n-of-1 trials is a direct method of examining the variability in the therapeutic response to a particular drug [4]. By this method, measurements are collected on a series of patients, each of whom undergoes trials of the active intervention and the control intervention (usually three periods of each). The sequence, which is determined randomly, is kept secret from both the clinician/investigator and the patient until the last trial is completed. Using a mixed-effects model, data from the series of patients can be analysed so that the four different sources of variation are separated. Thus, the variation in outcome due to source R from Table 6.2 can be estimated. The area in which this was first used was that of population pharmacokinetics [7] and it is now also of interest in the field of pharmacogenetics [8–10]. Estimation of variability in treatment effect is of particular interest here, as it represents the maximum effect that genetic differences can be expected to have.

Another area of application has been in studies of bioequivalence; we use one such study (comparing the systemic availability of two formulations of phenytoin) to illustrate the method [11]. In this study 26 subjects were allocated to two replicates of each treatment and outcomes were measured at four time points. Mixed-effects models were then fitted (using SAS PROC MIXED) with the following terms: sequence, formulation, period, subject (nested within sequence and fitted as random effects) and formulation*subject interaction. The model without the interaction term allows estimation of an overall mean effect of the two formulations (T in Table 6.2, represented by the formulation). Inclusion of the interaction term allows the effect to vary between individuals (R, represented by formulation*subject). Fitting subject as a random effect allows for differences between individuals (B). Time period effects (period) and carry-over effects (sequence) are also allowed for in the model. Within-individual variability (W) is represented by the error term. There were no differences in effect, either overall or between individuals, suggesting bioequivalence.

6.2.2.2. Comparison of variance in randomized controlled trials

Another alternative is to consider whether the variance of the outcome measure in the treatment arm of a randomized controlled trial differs from that expected if R from Table 6.1 was absent or negligible (i.e. if the variation could be explained by B and W). The variance of the placebo arm of the randomized controlled trial can provide an estimate of what this expected variance would be. The 'comparison of variance' method compares the variances seen in the active and placebo arms to see if there is a difference greater than that expected by chance. This is only possible if there is a multi-category or continuous outcome measure.

Increased variance in the active arm relative to the placebo arm suggests variation in the true treatment effect. Reduced variance in the active arm is also possible; here the variation in treatment effect negates some of the naturally occurring variation in the outcome. If the variances in the active and placebo groups are similar, there is no evidence of variation in the true treatment effect. All of the variation in outcome seen in the active arm can be explained by other sources of variability (B and W from Table 6.2), and the

Frequency

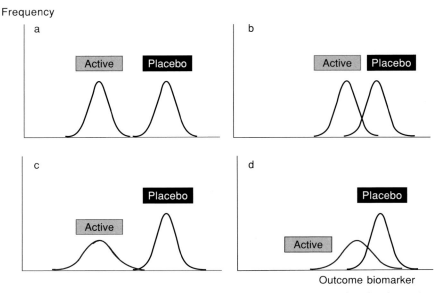

Figure 6.1 Hypothetical distribution curves of an outcome measure for placebo and active arms in large randomized controlled trials. (a) Separate curves, same variance (monitoring not needed); (b) overlapping curves, same variance (monitoring not needed); (c) separated curves, increased variance (monitoring may not be needed); (d) overlapping curves, increased variance (monitoring needed).

average therapeutic effect (T from Table 6.2) will be applicable to all individuals. Hence, initial response monitoring will not be helpful; in fact, it will be misleading, as we may misinterpret random variations as variations in the true response.

Comparing the distributions of outcomes seen in the placebo and active groups may identify instances in which the effect of therapy is of such magnitude that there is almost a complete separation of the curves. This provides evidence that active treatment had an effect on all individuals. Again, initial response monitoring may not be needed.

Figure 6.1 illustrates four types of frequency distribution that may be seen in trials when there is evidence that the treatment is effective overall (i.e. T from Table 6.2 is significant for all four). The first two scenarios (Figures 6.1a and 6.1b) represent trials in which there is no evidence that the therapeutic response differs between individuals. As the variances in the placebo and active arms are the same, all of the variability in the outcome can be explained by other sources. The separation of curves seen in Figure 6.1a provides further evidence of a universal effect of therapy. In neither of these scenarios is it necessary to monitor the initial response.

The separation of curves in Figure 6.1c again provides evidence of a universal effect. However, in this case there is increased variance in the active treatment arm, indicating a variation in response to treatment between individuals. The need to monitor the initial response in this case will depend on the harms/costs associated with treatment. If these are minimal, it may be decided that there is no need to monitor response, as therapy can be continued for everyone. If there are significant harms/costs then we may want to continue therapy only for those patients with a response above a certain level. In this case we shall need to monitor the initial response.

In the fourth scenario (Figure 6.1d) there is again evidence of variation in the therapeutic response between individuals, with increased variance in the active arm. In this case there is also overlap of the frequency curves, so it is uncertain whether therapy had an effect in all individuals or whether for some there was actually no effect. Monitoring for an initial response is needed in this case.

There is a caveat about using the above method. If there is a difference in variance between the treatment groups, alternative explanations should be investigated before concluding that there is evidence of variation in the treatment effect. Often variables naturally display increased variance with an increase in mean; alternatively, there may be increased variance at lower values of the variable. A Bland–Altman plot (plotting the difference in measures against the average of the measures) will help identify if this is the case [12]. If the variance depends on the value, this will need to be dealt with before comparing the active and placebo groups. Transformation of the data to a scale that exhibits a constant variance is one possibility. Another approach when standard deviation is proportional to the value is to use the coefficient of variation as the comparative measure.

6.3. Individual initial response monitoring

If there is variation in the therapeutic response at the population level, the next question is how we should estimate the therapeutic response in the individual. Two timings of measurement may help in this: measurement of predictors before trialling therapy and measurement of a biomarker of the response after therapy has started. For a continuous variable, the response can be estimated by measuring the biomarker after therapy, by measuring the change (either absolute or proportionate) in the biomarker or by modelling the follow-up measurement adjusted for the baseline measurement using analysis of co-variance. If feasible, ANCOVA modelling may be the preferred method of estimating the initial response: this method provides unbiased estimates of treatment effects in randomized controlled trials. However, for simplicity of explanation here, we shall use changes in the biomarker after therapy or follow-up of the biomarker alone (i.e. the target measurement) to illustrate how to judge an individual's response.

6.3.1. Predictors of outcome

Usually, the distribution of a response to therapy is considered to be unimodal; that is, there is a universal therapeutic effect that varies in magnitude between individuals. This relies on the assumption that responses are unimodally distributed when the outcome variable is unimodally distributed. Although it is possible that variability from other sources (see the previous section) masks a subtle non-unimodal response, this is unlikely to be substantial if the assumption of a unimodal distribution is reasonable.

On the other hand, if the observed outcome distribution is clearly not unimodal, the true response distribution is unlikely to be unimodal. Statistical evidence of a non-unimodal distribution will usually require study of a sizeable population, unless there is clear separation of response curves. A non-unimodal distribution is likely when there are categorical factors that modify the response to treatment. Sometimes these may not be known; for example, hypersusceptibility drug reactions only occur in a subset of those given a therapy, but we are usually unable to predict those who are likely to be affected (e.g. angio-oedema with ACE inhibitors).

In other cases, there may be effect modifiers that account for the non-unimodal distribution. These may be characteristics of the disease. Examples include oestrogen receptor status in patients with breast cancer for the effect of tamoxifen, the time since onset of chest pain for the effect of thrombolysis in acute myocardial infarction (both of these have bimodal response distributions). Or they may be characteristics of the individual separate from the disease, in which case they are often genetically determined. Genetic factors that modify the effect of treatment are most likely when there is no redundancy in the genetic determinants of key pharmacokinetic and pharmacodynamic processes (such as metabolizing enzymes, transporters and target receptors). For example, variant genes for a metabolizing enzyme may result in no active effect of therapy (e.g. codeine—7% of white individuals are unable to form the active metabolite morphine) or an enhanced therapeutic effect (e.g. isoniazid—slow metabolizers have increased drug concentrations; azathioprine—homozygotes for thiopurine methyltransferase (TPMT) variant have greatly increased concentrations of active metabolites). The distribution may be trimodal if there are different effects in homozygous variants, heterozygotes and homozygous wild type (e.g. pseudocholinesterase deficiency causing prolonged muscle relaxation after suxamethonium). Or there may be an even more complex distribution of response, such as occurs with nortriptyline metabolism, mediated by CYP2D6, the number of whose functional genes varies from 0 to 13; the lower the number of functional genes, the higher the individual's plasma drug concentration (and by implication the greater the response to the drug) [13].

If measurement of the effect modifier in the individual is practical, it may be possible to identify non-responders for whom treatment should not be trialled (e.g. oestrogen receptor-negative breast cancer and tamoxifen). Alternatively, over-responders may be identified in whom the starting dose of drug should be

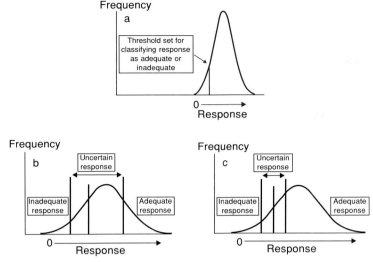

Figure 6.2 (a) The true response of individuals to a treatment with a sufficiency threshold; (b) the observed response of individuals to a treatment with random measurement error (one measurement before and one after); (c) the observed response of individuals to a treatment with random measurement error (multiple measurements taken).

much reduced (e.g. TPMT and azathioprine). Or there may be differing initial doses that should be trialled for different individuals (e.g. CYP2D6 activity and nortriptyline).

Even if effect modifiers are known for a particular therapy, the magnitude of the effect in responders still needs to be estimated by trialling the intervention. In the more common case, when no effect modifiers are known, the magnitude of response must also be estimated after therapy is begun.

6.3.2. Measuring outcome after therapy

6.3.2.1. True change/follow-up value

If it were possible to measure the true change in a biomarker (or only the follow-up value) after treatment in different individuals, the distribution of responses might be represented by Figure 6.2a, in which increasing values indicate an increasing response. Trial data may be used to decide on a contin-uation threshold—the average response needed for the benefits of treatment to outweigh the harms. Responses to the left of the threshold are categorized as 'inadequate' and those to the right as 'adequate'. If an individual does not show an adequate response, the clinician may decide to increase the dose of drug, to add another therapy, or to change to another therapy. The clinician may also decide that the benefit to harm balance for a particular individual differs substantially from the average and may want to individualize the continuation threshold. For example, if the patient is likely to derive substantial benefit from the treatment, a smaller response may be accepted and the threshold moved to the left; alternatively, if the patient is more susceptible to an adverse effect of treatment, it may be decided that a larger response is needed and the continuation threshold would be shifted to the right.

6.3.2.2. Effects of measurement error (component W from Table 6.2)

The observed measurements are determined by both the true underlying value and an additional factor, the measurement error. Measurement error may be systematic—bias that occurs on average for all measured subjects; for example, diurnal fluctuation in an outcome biomarker will cause a systematic error if measurements are made at different times of the day. Standardizing how measurement is done, with regular checks for bias, will help to eliminate most sources of systematic measurement error. These steps will not help to reduce measurement error that is non-systematic, in other words the random error that occurs for each individual because of technical error as well as short-term fluctuations in the individual.

The effect of random error in the measurement is to increase the variance of the response distribution. Figure 6.2b reflects the effect of introducing random error to the measurement of response seen in Figure 6.2a. Because of measurement error and the resultant uncertainty about an individual's true response, decisions on whether to change therapy can only be made for patients who are at the extremes of the distribution. This is because for the patients with a measured response that is in the middle of the range, we cannot be certain about which side of the threshold they truly occupy.

Random measurement error may lead to a biased assessment of response, owing to the statistical phenomenon known as regression to the mean. A chance extreme measurement in an individual is likely to be partly due to measurement error and will be followed by one that is closer to the mean value (which represents the true response). At a population level, extreme measurements tend to be nearer the population mean on remeasurement. If an individual's baseline measurement was by chance higher than their mean value of the marker, they will tend to have a lower measurement on follow-up, which will exaggerate the treatment effect. If the baseline measurement was lower than the individual's mean, the measurement at follow-up will tend to increase, masking any possible effect of treatment. The effect of regression to the mean is to cause a bias towards individuals with poorer baseline scores [14].

An illustration of the relevance of regression to the mean to initial response monitoring is provided by the example of bone mineral density measurements in postmenopausal women with osteoporosis who start to take a bisphosphonate [15, 16]. Most women who appeared to lose bone mineral density in the first year of treatment gained it on the next measurement. The benefit of bisphosphonate therapy (in terms of a reduction in risk of fracture) was found to apply to women who lost bone mineral density as well as to those who gained it.

6.3.2.3. Use of multiple measurements

One method of minimizing random measurement error in a continuous variable is to make multiple measurements of the outcome marker both before and after treatment and to use the difference in means to estimate the true change. Using the mean of multiple measurements enhances the accuracy of the estimate for that time period, but there is less additional gain with each extra measurement. For this reason, the most accurate estimate of change will be possible if there is a balance in the number of measurements done before and after starting treatment. For example, there is minimal gain in the accuracy of the change estimate if multiple measurements are done after treatment but only one measurement is done before. (These concerns are not as important if the outcome measure is the follow-up value alone irrespective of the baseline value.)

The effect of multiple measurements on random measurement error is illustrated in Figure 6.2c. Note that the variance has fallen compared with Figure 6.2b. Decisions on the sufficiency of response are now possible for a higher proportion of the population.

A more sophisticated alternative to requiring all individuals to undergo multiple measurements is to require this only of those who fall within the uncertainty band initially (although if the change in the biomarker is being used to estimate the response, multiple baseline measurements would still be required). People who are beyond these uncertainty limits would not require further testing, as one can decide about the adequacy of treatment with the information already available. For those who require re-testing, since the measurement error in their response falls with more measurements, the uncertainty band around the threshold narrows. Thus, one will be able to make decisions about the adequacy of treatment for all patients except those whose true response is too close to the threshold for the uncertainty to be resolved.

6.3.3. Bayesian methods of estimating individual responses

In the above discussion, we have examined ways in which measurements can be used to estimate the response to therapy. These include both predictor variables before starting treatment and measurements of change in an outcome biomarker. However, even with the opportunity to make these measurements, there will still be some uncertainty about the response status of some individuals. In addition, in many instances it may not be possible to make all the measurements that we would ideally like to. In these circumstances, a method that translates the uncertainty about these estimates into the probability of a response is useful.

Such a method has been described for estimating the true response to the intervention of dietary advice for cholesterol reduction [17]. The estimates were based on a Bayesian model that used information from two sources: the measurement of change in that individual and the change reported for the population (in trial data). All individuals had their baseline value estimated from the mean of three measurements. Measurements made after treatment were based on either one measurement or the mean of three. The information from the two sources (individual and population) was then converted into the probability of a reduction of 5 or 10% in cholesterol in that individual. By presenting the probability of a response, the authors were able to make the uncertainty of a true change explicit. Consumers and clinicians are then much better placed to judge for themselves whether the individual has had a sufficient response to the intervention.

6.3.4. Individual n-of-1 trials

An alternative method to the use of multiple measurements before and after an intervention is to have multiple trials of the intervention versus placebo, the n-of-1 trial. This technique has been used to judge the therapeutic effect in an individual (rather than the use of series of n-of-1 trials in the population, discussed above). Applications include osteoarthritis (non-steroidal anti-inflammatory drugs versus paracetamol) [18], ADHD (methylphenidate versus placebo) [19], chronic airflow limitation [20] and fibromyalgia (amitriptyline versus placebo) [21]. There are some disadvantages to n-of-1 trials. Because the method requires repeated crossover of treatments to determine superiority, it is only suited to diseases that are chronic and relatively stable and to treatments that do not have significant carry-over effects. There are also practical barriers to implementation of the method, for example many clinicians finding the time and resources required prohibitive; the establishment of n-of-1 trial centres that serve clinicians in the surrounding area addresses this problem [22–24].

6.3.5. Statistical process control

Statistical process control (SPC) is another technique that makes use of multiple measurements. A detailed theoretical framework and potential applications for this method are provided in Chapter 7. To illustrate how SPC can be used to judge the initial response using this method, we give the example of an individual with a high serum LDL cholesterol concentration for whom centre line and control limits are drawn for the cholesterol measurements both before and after the start of therapy with a statin (Figure 6.3) [25]. The mean of the measurements taken after treatment has started is compared with that taken before to provide an estimate of the change in cholesterol concentration. Adequacy of therapy can be judged by the proportion of measurements that have met the target of under 100 mg/dl (the specification limit, equivalent to 2.6 mmol/l).

SPC has not yet been widely adopted in clinical practice. The development of software packages that allow easy construction of control charts and the use of (sub-)population data to substitute for some of the individual data are

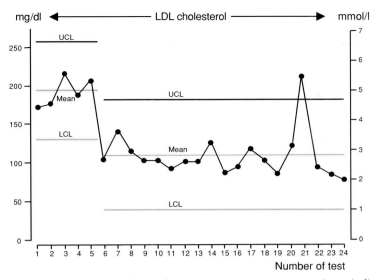

Figure 6.3 Control chart of cholesterol concentration measurements in an individual subject, demonstrating considerable variability between individual measurements. There is a mean reduction of 84 mg/dl (2.2 mmol/l) after simvastatin therapy is started (point 6) but failure to consistently reach the target concentration of 100 mg/dl (2.6 mmol/l). (Adapted from [25].) UCL, upper control limit; LCL, lower control limit.

possible solutions to problems of practicality. Perhaps more important to the implementation of SPC and the other methods described is the need for champions in clinical practice. Clinicians who trial these methods will appreciate an improved capacity to make informed therapeutic decisions. If they are able to convince others of the merit of these techniques, more widespread adoption is likely.

6.4. Conclusions

There are many unanswered questions about the early monitoring of an individual's response to therapy. Currently, there are too few published data on response distributions to enable an informed decision about whether initial monitoring is indicated for a particular intervention. There are also no structures in place to generate data needed to inform decision-making for the individual patient. Furthermore, the benefits of these monitoring strategies are at this stage largely theoretical—to date there have been no comparisons of conventional and novel/sophisticated methods of monitoring. Despite these uncertainties, the methods for monitoring the initial response described in this chapter represent exciting new areas of research. If conventional methods can be improved, even marginally, it is likely that there will be substantial benefits for both patients and clinicians.

Acknowledgements

This work was funded by program grant 402764 from the National Health and Medical Research Council of Australia.

References

1 *Expenditure and Prescriptions Twelve Months to 30 June 2005*. Australia: Department of Health and Aging, 2005.
2 *Prescription Cost Analysis: England 2004*. United Kingdom: Department of Health, 2004.
3 *Advance Data No. 346 National Ambulatory Medical Care Survey: 2002 Summary*. Atlanta: National Centre for Health Statistics, Centre of Disease Control and Prevention, 2002.
4 Senn S. Individual therapy: new dawn or false dawn? *Drug Inform J* 2001; **35**: 1479–94.
5 Senn S. Controversies concerning randomization and additivity in clinical trials. *Stat Med* 2004; **23**: 3729–53.
6 Senn S. Individual response to treatment: is it a valid assumption? *BMJ* 2004; **329**: 966–8.
7 Sheiner L, Rosenberg B, Melmon K. Modelling of individual pharmacokinetics for computer-aided drug dosage. *Comput Biomed Res* 1972; **5**: 411–59.
8 Kalow W, Ozdemir V, Tang B, Tothfalusi L, Endrenyi L. The science of pharmacological variability. *Clin Pharmacol Ther* 1999; **66**: 445–7.
9 Ozdemir V, Kalowa W, Tang BK, et al. Evaluation of the genetic component of variability in CYP3A4 activity: a repeated drug administration method. *Pharmacogenetics* 2000; **10**: 373–88.
10 Kalow W, Tang B, Endrenyi L. Hypothesis: comparisons of inter- and intra-individual variation can substitute for twin studies in drug research. *Pharmacogenetics* 1998; **58**: 281–4.
11 Shumaker R, Metzler C. The phenytoin trial is a case study of "individual" bioequivalence. *Drug Inform J* 1998; **32**: 1063–72.
12 Bland JM, Altman DG. Measurement error. *BMJ* 1996; **313**: 744.
13 Weinshilboum R. Inheritance and drug response. *N Engl J Med* 2003; **348**: 529–37.
14 Vickers A, Altman DG. Statistics notes: analysing controlled trials with baseline and follow up measurements. *BMJ* 2001; **323**: 1123–4.
15 Cummings SR, Palermo L, Browner W, et al. Monitoring osteoporosis therapy with bone densitometry: misleading changes and regression to the mean. *JAMA* 2000; **283**: 1318–21.
16 Cummings SR, Karpf DB, Harris F, et al. Improvement in spine bone density and reduction in risk of vertebral fractures during treatment with antiresorptive drugs. *Am J Med* 2002; **112**: 281–9.
17 Irwig L, Glasziou PP, Wilson A, Macaskill P. Estimating an individual's true cholesterol level and response to intervention. *JAMA* 1991; **266**: 1678–85.
18 March L, Irwig L, Schwarz J, Simpson J, Chock C, Brooks P. N of 1 trials comparing a non-steroidal anti-inflammatory drug with paracetamol in osteoarthritis. *BMJ* 1994; **309**: 1041–5.
19 Duggan CM, Mitchell G, Nikles CJ, Glasziou PP, Del Mar CB, Clavarino A. Managing ADHD in general practice. N of 1 trials can help! *Aust Fam Phys* 2000; **29**: 1205–9.

20 Patel A, Jaeschke R, Guyatt GH, Keller JL, Newhouse MT. Clinical usefulness of n-of-1 randomized controlled trials in patients with nonreversible chronic airflow limitation. *Am Rev Respir Dis* 1991; **144**: 962–4.

21 Jaeschke R, Adachi J, Guyatt G, Keller J, Wong B. Clinical usefulness of amitriptyline in fibromyalgia: the results of 23 n-of-1 randomized controlled trials. *J Rheumatol* 1991; 18: 447–51.

22 Guyatt G, Keller J, Jaeschke R, Rosenbloom D, Adachi J, Newhouse MT. The n-of-1 randomised controlled trial: clinical usefulness. Our three-year experience. *Ann Intern Med* 1990; **112**: 293–9.

23 Nikles C, Glasziou P, Del Mar CB, Duggan CM, Mitchell G. N of 1 trials. Practical tools for medication management. *Aust Fam Phys* 2000; **29**: 1108–12.

24 Nikles C, Clavarino A, Del Mar CB. Using n-of-1 trials as a clinical tool to improve prescribing. *Br J Gen Pract* 2005; **55**: 175–80.

25 Staker L. The use of run and control charts in the improvement of clinical practice. In: Carey RG (ed), *Improving Healthcare with Control Charts*. Milwaukee: American Society for Quality, 2003, p. 194.

CHAPTER 7

Control charts and control limits in long-term monitoring

Petra Macaskill

Most health-care monitoring guidelines specify a particular target that should be achieved, but this ignores the uncertainty and imprecision involved in making clinical measurements. Even if the true underlying value of a marker, such as cholesterol or blood pressure, in an individual patient is stable, we would expect to observe variability in the measurement over time. Hence, it is more appropriate to specify a range for which a measure may be considered to be stable or on target. This helps to differentiate which changes in measurement are likely to be due to random variability (noise) and which are likely to be real changes (signal) that may require action [1].

I shall discuss two approaches used to identify whether differences between successive (serial) measurements in an individual go beyond the limits of intrinsic variability. The first approach, in common use in laboratories, estimates a 'reference change value' (or 'critical difference') between two successive measurements, which if exceeded, indicates that the observed difference exceeds what would be expected through random variability [2, 3]. The second approach, used routinely in industrial settings to monitor the behaviour and performance of a process, is known as statistical process control (SPC). Although most applications of SPC are to be found in industry, SPC is now being adopted to monitor the performance of health services and also to monitor the health of individual patients [4]. This approach will be the major focus of this chapter, as it provides a powerful tool for investigating patterns of variability of multiple measurements taken over time.

7.1. Reference change value (critical difference)

In a laboratory, the variability between successive measurements (analytes) is attributed to a combination of pre-analytical variability (how and when

Evidence-based Medical Monitoring: from Principles to Practice. Edited by Paul Glasziou, Les Irwig and Jeffrey K. Aronson. © 2008 Blackwell Publishing, ISBN: 978-1-4051-5399-7.

the sample was collected, stored, etc.), analytical variability (the precision of the laboratory assay procedures) and individual (within-patient) biological variability, which represents the usual random variability (noise) in an analyte that one would expect to observe around the true underlying average value in an individual [2]. The overall (total) standard deviation is given by $S_T = \sqrt{S_P^2 + S_A^2 + S_I^2}$ where S_P^2, S_A^2 and S_I^2, respectively, represent three sources of variability: pre-analytical, analytical and individual. If, as would be expected, the pre-analytical variation has been minimized, its contribution is minimal and the formula simplifies to $S_T = \sqrt{S_A^2 + S_I^2}$.

Assuming approximate normality, the reference change value (RCV) is given by $\sqrt{2} \times z \times S_T$, where z is a 'standard normal deviate'. If the observed difference between two consecutive measurements is greater than the RCV, it is assumed that the observed difference has a low probability of occurring by chance based on analytical and the usual random within-person variability. The value of z determines the 'false alarm' rate and usually takes the value 1.96 or 2.58, corresponding to false alarm rates of 5 and 1% respectively. The coefficient of variation ($CV = S/mean$) is often used in place of the standard deviation (S) for each distribution in the above calculations to obtain a RCV for the percentage change instead of numerical change. The CV is preferable to S when there is dependence between the level of variability and underlying mean value.

7.1.1. Example: monitoring serum creatinine

Biological and analytical variation was estimated in a group of 12 healthy individuals [5]. Analytical variance was calculated using the difference between repeat results for the same specimen. A single analyst performed all assays and used the same batches of reagent. Within-subject and between-subject variabilities were computed using blood samples taken on 10 occasions 2 weeks apart for all participants, and samples were all taken at the same time of day. The mean creatinine concentration was 86 μmol/l and the estimated coefficient of variation for analytical and intra-individual variability was 3.1 and 4.9% respectively. The estimated RCV, assuming a 5% significance level, is $\sqrt{2} \times 1.96 \times \sqrt{CV_A^2 + CV_I^2} = 16\%$.

The RCV approach clearly relies on reasonably accurate estimates for the standard deviation (or CV) of A and I. Although reliable data are likely to be available in a laboratory [2] for analytical variability, within-person variability is often based on published estimates [6], which may not be applicable to a given individual [2, 3]. For instance, published estimates are often based on measurements in healthy people, whereas the individual being monitored has a condition that may have a different degree of variability. Even if the estimate is derived from a group of patients who have the same condition, this represents an 'average' variability, which does not take account of the fact that such variability may well differ across individuals. Inaccuracy in estimates of

S (or *CV*) will compromise the expected false alarm rates, which must then be regarded as approximate.

Although calculation of the RCV uses information from only two serial measurements, the approach is applied to successive pairs of measurements when multiple measurements are taken. In such circumstances, it is often better to use a method designed to identify changing patterns in serial measurements. One such approach is described below.

7.2. Statistical process control (SPC)

Control chart methods devised by Shewhart [7] are in widespread use in manufacturing. I shall focus here on how control charts can be used for long-term monitoring of individuals. I shall use standard SPC terminology, framed in the context of medical applications. More detailed discussion of the basic methods and more advanced approaches can be found in a range of texts [8–10] and other sources [11].

To apply SPC methods we require that the process, usually the medical condition or outcome we want to monitor, can be measured either directly or via a biomarker. As noted above, some variability between measurements over time is to be expected, even if the true underlying condition is stable. This variability over time can be divided into two major components, referred to as 'common cause' and 'special cause' (also referred to as 'assignable cause') variability.

7.2.1. Special-cause variability (signal)

Special-cause variability (signal) can also arise from a range of sources, including, most importantly, a true change in an individual's condition. Other special causes that can intentionally or unintentionally lead to a true change in the process include changes in medication, changes in dosage, behavioural interventions and environmental factors.

7.2.2. Common-cause variability (noise)

Common-cause variability (noise) is the random variability that can arise from a wide range of sources, including the following: usual within-person biological variation; minor daily variations in diet, alcohol intake and/or exercise; time of day; analytical error and measurement error. It can be thought of as background noise against which we want to detect a signal, such as a disruption or change in the process due to a special cause.

7.3. Control charts

A control chart is a graphical display of serial measurements of a biomarker, showing the changes that occur with time, which helps to distinguish special-cause from common-cause variability. By ensuring that measurements are taken so as to minimize common-cause variability, we can improve the ability to distinguish between true change in the patient's condition and background noise. Reductions in common-cause variability can be achieved by, for instance, reducing measurement error and standardizing how measurements are taken (time of day, use of the same instrument, use of a standardized method, etc.).

The major topics to be covered here include the following: graphical display of individual measurements collected over time; the calculation and interpretation of control limits; criteria for detecting special-cause variability; and target limits versus control limits. I shall describe and discuss Shewhart control chart methods and exponentially weighted moving average (EWMA) control chart methods for monitoring individual measurements. I shall illustrate key methods and concepts using hypothetical data and the example of diastolic blood pressure measurements.

7.4. Graphical displays for individual measurements

Graphical display of serial measurements is usually the first step in monitoring. This is generally done using a *run chart*, which represents the measurement on the vertical axis and serial order (time) on the horizontal axis. The run chart serves to illustrate the underlying variability in the process, extreme measurements, underlying trends and other patterns over time. For a process that is referred to as 'in control', the underlying mean value and variability of the measurements around the mean value will be stable over time, as shown in Figure 7.1a. In this context, 'in control' does not imply that the measurements lie within some ideal or target range for an individual patient, but it does indicate that the measurements lie within the intrinsic limits of random variability (noise) resulting from the common-cause variability for that individual. Figure 7.1b illustrates a shift in the mean of the process that is likely to be attributed to a special cause. Figure 7.1c shows a more subtle, gradual shift in the process mean over time.

Even though run charts provide helpful visualization of the behaviour of the measurements over time, there is potential for over-interpretation of the variation in the process. Criteria for concluding that there is some true change (special cause) affecting the process are necessary to limit the number of false alarms. Inappropriate 'tinkering' with the process is counterproductive, because it will lead to an increase in the variability. For instance, frequent adjustment of drug dosage in response to high or low plasma drug concentrations that are consistent with random variability around a stable mean level will lead to variation in the underlying mean concentration itself, in addition to the usual random fluctuations, thereby increasing overall variability. Hence, criteria must be established for deciding when there is sufficient evidence of a change or disruption in the process (special cause), and when it is appropriate to intervene.

a. Stable process

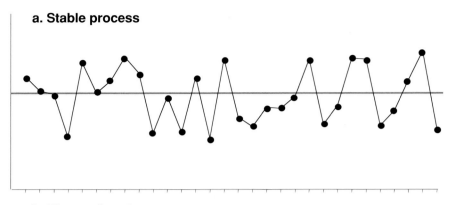

b. Change in value

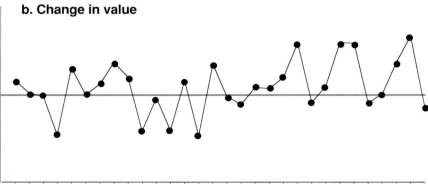

c. Underlying trend

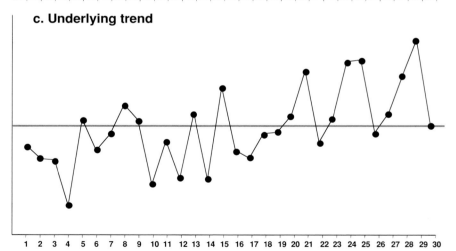

1 2 3 4 5 6 7 8 9 10 11 12 13 14 15 16 17 18 19 20 21 22 23 24 25 26 27 28 29 30

Figure 7.1 Run charts used to show patterns of variability in a process over time.

Control limits are often superimposed on a run chart. The resulting *control chart* then shows the range within which we expect the vast majority of measurements to lie, based on the expected common-cause variability of the measurements over time. Control limits, and criteria for using them, provide a means of identifying potential signs of change or instability in the underlying condition of the patient, which may be indicative of a special cause, such as sudden (or gradual) deterioration in their condition or problems related to the use of medications.

7.4.1. Constructing a control chart for individual measurements

7.4.1.1. X charts

If the measurements represented in the run chart are stable (in control), they will fluctuate around an underlying mean value (μ), and the variability (standard deviation σ) will be constant over time. When each point on the chart represents a single measurement at a point in time, the chart is referred to as an *individual's control chart* or *X chart*. Assuming that the process, i.e. the patient's condition, is stable, the process mean is estimated by the mean of the observed measurements ($\bar{x}$). However, computation of the standard deviation is less straightforward.

The sample standard deviation (s) provides a biased estimate of the process standard deviation (σ); particularly when the sample size is small. The process standard deviation for an individual's control chart is usually estimated using a moving range (MR), where MR is defined as the absolute difference between every pair of consecutive measurements. Hence, for n measurements there will be $n - 1$ MR values. Dividing the mean MR by the constant $d_2 = 1.128$ gives an unbiased estimate of σ. This estimate has the advantage that it is less likely to be affected by instability in the process than the sample standard deviation would be. Further explanation and discussion of the estimation of σ can be found in a range of publications [8, 9, 12].

7.4.1.2. Control limits

Assuming that estimates of μ and σ are based on a stable process that is 'in control', control limits can be established to identify when the process is likely to be changing or becoming unstable. Hence, each time a new measurement is available, we must assess whether that measurement is consistent with the expected 'noise'.

Shewhart initially suggested control limits at $\pm 3\sigma$ from the process mean, to signify the likely presence of special-cause variability. The centre line (mean) and '3 sigma' limits are marked routinely on control charts. Measurements that are outside control limits warrant investigation and possible action. The first step is to identify if a special cause is responsible for the extreme observation; for example, whether the patient has initiated some change in their life, such as another medication, a dietary change or a change in living conditions. This will help to identify the cause and establish what action, if any, should be

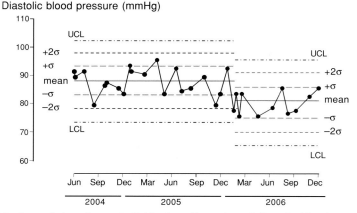

Figure 7.2   Control chart for an individual's self-monitored diastolic blood pressure.

taken, such as a modification to treatment or a change in drug dosage. Known special causes, such as changes in treatment, are often annotated on the chart.

Although control limits are sometimes centred on a target value rather than the sample mean, the control limits should nevertheless be based on an estimate of the underlying common-cause variation in the process. When it is not reasonable to estimate σ from the observed data, because there are insufficient observations or the process is unstable, historical or baseline data obtained when the process is in a stable state should be used. Basing the control limits on the data from an individual patient, when possible, has the advantage that the estimated variability is person specific. However, when multiple measurements are difficult or expensive to obtain, we shall usually have to rely on external data.

If an action such as a change in treatment or drug dosage is taken in response to process instability or because the process does not lie within a target range, the mean and standard deviation of the process must be re-established using post-intervention data. The resulting change in mean and/or standard deviation will lead to new control limits that are applicable to the modified process, and the monitoring process continues.

7.4.2. Example: monitoring diastolic blood pressure
The data in Figure 7.2 show a series of diastolic blood pressure measurements taken between May 2004 and January 2007 as part of self-monitoring. Methods of data collection were standardized to reduce noise by taking measurements at approximately the same time of day on the same day of the week. Measurement error was reduced on each occasion by taking the mean of two repeat measurements.

Until early 2006, what can be regarded as baseline measurements fluctuated around a mean of 88 mmHg. Upper and lower control limits (denoted by UCL and LCL respectively) were computed based on the measurements taken during this period. From the figure it is clear that none of the observations fall outside the control limits and the process appears to be reasonably stable. However, the mean of 88 mmHg is above what would be regarded as an acceptable average (target) value of 85 mmHg and several points are close to the upper target range of 75–95 mmHg. Hence, blood pressure lowering medication was begun in early 2006. Based on the subsequent measurements, we estimate that the mean of the process has reduced to 81 mmHg and the observations fall well within the revised control limits, and towards the lower end of the target limits. The post-intervention measurements appear to be stable, but some adjustment of drug dosage may be considered if the new mean value is deemed to be too low relative to the target of 85 mmHg.

7.5. Improved criteria for identifying special-cause variability

Assuming that the measurements are independent and approximately normally distributed, the 3 sigma (3σ) limits set the probability of a false alarm at 0.003 (a specificity of 0.997). However, in a clinical setting this rule is too insensitive, and thus too likely to miss important but more subtle changes in the true underlying condition of a patient. Several alternative rules have been developed for assessing whether the process is changing or becoming unstable; rules that are more sensitive to subtle shifts in the process but still retain an acceptably low probability of a false alarm. The most notable of these is the Western Electric Company (WECO) rules [11], which combine several criteria for identifying special-cause variability. WECO incorporates the 3σ rule, but also triggers an 'alarm' if

- two of the last three measurements are all more than 2σ above (or below) μ;
- four of the last five measurements are all more than σ above (or below) μ;
- or eight consecutive measurements are all above (or below) μ.

This set of rules increases the sensitivity to detect possible shifts in the process mean, but the probability of a false alarm is increased to 0.011. The additional 1σ and 2σ limits can be included on the control chart to aid implementation of the WECO rules (see Figure 7.2).

Even the WECO rules may be too insensitive for individual clinical monitoring, given the potential harm of missing a significant drift from 'control'. Hence, further work is needed in health care to develop rules with a more appropriate trade-off between false positives and false negatives. The level of stringency of the criteria adopted will depend on the relative seriousness of the implications of a false positive compared with a false negative. For instance,

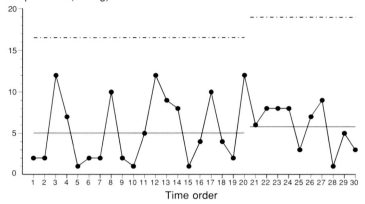

Difference between successive
measurements of diastolic
blood pressure (mmHg)

Time order

Figure 7.3 MR chart for an individual's self-monitored diastolic blood pressure.

less stringent rules are likely to be applied in circumstances such as monitoring transplant recipients, when the 'cost' of not detecting a change in the
patient's condition may be very high, as the damage of missing the 'special
cause' may be irreversible. In such cases, we require high sensitivity at the
expense of specificity, whereas for monitoring blood pressure or cholesterol
the implications of temporarily missing a 'special cause' will be relatively less
important, and we may favour specificity over sensitivity.

   Although not currently widespread, X charts and control limits have been
used in a number of areas in health care, including anticoagulation, asthma
and diabetes [4, 13]. Two additional charts are described below. The first is the
MR chart, which is used routinely in conjunction with the X chart to assess
the stability of the variability in the process, and the second is the EWMA
chart, which is useful in detecting more subtle shifts in the process mean.
More sophisticated and specialized charts have been developed for industrial
settings [10, 14], but they are rarely used in health care.

7.5.1. Moving range (MR) charts

Instability in the process can also be monitored by plotting the MRs over time.
The 'centre line' is the mean of the MR values. For individual measurements,
the upper control limit is 3.268 times the mean MR [8]. The lower bound is
zero, since the MR values are all absolute differences and hence must all be
greater than or equal to zero. It is worth noting that for individuals charts,
because the MR is based on two successive observations only, the chart does
not contain information that is not already contained in the X chart. Nevertheless, the chart serves to highlight instability in the variability over time.
Figure 7.3 shows the MR plot for the example data displayed in Figure 7.2.

Based on this plot, it appears that the variability in the process is stable in the pre-intervention period, but the variability may be decreasing over time in the post-intervention period.

7.5.2. Exponentially weighted moving average (EWMA) charts

The EWMA calculates a moving average at each time point that gives the highest weight to the measurement taken at that time, and successively less weight to the measurements that precede it. At a given point in time $(t, t = 1, \ldots, n)$, the EWMA is given by $EWMA_t = \lambda X_t + (1 - \lambda)EWMA_{t-1}$. $EWMA_0$ generally represents the historical mean of the process when stable (or target mean), X_t is the measurement at time t, and λ is a constant that determines the relative weight given to earlier measurements ($0 < \lambda \leq 1$). If $\lambda = 1$, the chart reduces to an X chart; the closer λ is to 0 the greater the contribution is from earlier measurements. In practice, λ usually takes a value between 0.2 and 0.4. The variance of the EWMA is given by $(\lambda/(1 - \lambda))s^2$, where s^2 is the estimated process variance. Three sigma or less stringent control limits for the EWMA are set in the usual way around a centre line at $EWMA_0$ [10, 11].

A combination of EWMA charts and X and MR charts is more sensitive to changes in the process than X and MR charts alone [15]. The sensitivity of these methods for detecting a change in the process is further enhanced by the adoption of a variable sampling interval, whereby the interval before the next measurement is very short if the process is close to a control limit (or some other rule for a special cause). The interval can be lengthened if the process is stable. A combination of these charts and varying intervals can reduce the time taken to detect change or instability in the process [15].

7.6. Target (specification) limits

As noted above, the primary purpose of a control chart is to differentiate between common-cause and special-cause variability. However, a process that is stable and fluctuating randomly within the control limits is not necessarily operating within limits that are clinically acceptable or desirable. For instance, the mean may be too high or low, and/or the variability may be too high.

Target limits, referred to in the SPC literature as specification limits, represent the range within which the process should ideally operate. These limits can be derived from population data, individual data such as 'best lung function' for an individual patient or clinical consensus. Such limits clearly need to account for the unavoidable intrinsic variability of the process (common-cause variability) but also to integrate this with information from epidemiological studies and clinical trials about the risk and impact of different target values. For example, in setting target limits we need to combine what is desirable, based on calculated risk reduction, with our knowledge of usual individual (within-person) variability.

The upper and lower target (specification) limits are used to define the acceptable range for the process. They are not control limits in the SPC context described above, because they are not derived from the actual variability of the process. A process that is not consistent with the target and/or target range may prompt action to shift the mean and/or reduce the variability of the process. Even if the mean is on target, a high underlying variability may produce an unacceptable number of observations outside the target limits. In that case, we would need to identify possible ways of reducing this variability, such as, for instance, reducing the variability in a patient's alcohol intake, diet, exercise or other environmental factors.

7.6.1. Process capability

Indices have been developed to compare the variability of the process with the target limits. The capability index (Cp index) is obtained by dividing the target range (upper limit – lower limit) by 6σ, which is the difference between the upper and lower 3σ control limits for the data that reflect the range within which we would expect almost all measurements to lie for that process. If the process mean is on target and Cp is greater than 1 (ideally above 1.3), the process will operate within target limits and we shall be likely to detect a change in the process before it moves outside the target limits [8, 9, 11]. However, even if the mean is on target, a Cp index less than 1 indicates that the underlying variability in the process (common-cause variability) must be reduced to ensure that most measurements will lie within the target limits.

The degree to which the process is centred on the target limits can be assessed using the *off target ratio*, $S_T = (\mu - T)/\sigma$, which measures how far the process mean is off target in standard deviation units. The C_{pk} index is also used to assess whether the process is centred within target limits. It is given by the absolute value of the difference between the process mean and the target limit closest to it, divided by 3σ.

7.7. Underlying assumptions

In constructing and using a control chart and control limits as described above, we assume that the observations are independent and normally distributed about the mean of the process. Skewness in the data will tend to lead to inflation of the number of false alarms on one side of the distribution. This will be more problematic for charts that are based on individual measurements, on which we have focused in this chapter, because individual measurements are plotted rather than means of (small) samples, as is usually the case in industrial settings. When there is clear evidence of non-normality, transformation may be possible to normalize the data. Control limits derived from the transformed data are more likely to result in the appropriate percentiles for the distribution. Autocorrelation in the data will compromise the assumption of independence and result in control limits that are too narrow. Such autocorrelation is likely to occur if measurements are taken too close together in time.

When calculating control limits it is often recommended that at least 20–25 serial measurements, usually comprising means of samples of size 4–5, should be used. Although this may be feasible in many industrial settings, it is probably unrealistic when monitoring an individual patient with a chronic condition. In practice, we often have to rely on a small number of measurements; particularly after some change in the process has occurred. Even if the number of observations is small, the data may nevertheless represent the best available information on the variability of the process. Wheeler [8, 9] has discussed this scenario and the available strategies for recalculating control limits as additional measurements are made.

7.8. Conclusions

Control charts are beginning to be introduced into medicine and clinical care. The most common application has been with control methods for monitoring warfarin by measuring the prothrombin time (INR; international normalized ratio), but they have been explored in other areas. However, much monitoring is currently done without an awareness of the within-person variation due to both analytic error and simple day-to-day variation. Greater use of control chart methods is likely to improve clinicians' awareness of within-person variation and will lead to more stable control. However, this will also require work to obtain the data needed to construct such charts and further work on the most appropriate charting methods and rules for clinical care.

References

1 Glasziou P, Irwig L, Mant D. Monitoring in chronic disease: a rational approach. *BMJ* 2005; **330**: 664–8.
2 Fraser CG. *Biological Variation: From Principles to Practice*. Washington, DC: AACC Press, 2001.
3 Fraser CG, Stevenson HP, Kennedy IMG. Biological variation data are necessary prerequisites for objective autoverification of clinical laboratory data. *Accredit Qual Assur* 2002; **7**: 455–60.
4 Carey RG. *Improving Health Care with Control Charts: Basic and Advanced SPC Methods and Case Studies*. Milwaukee: ASQ Quality Press, 2003.
5 Keevil BG, Kilpatrick ES, Nichols SP, Maylor PW. Biological variation of cystatin C: implications for the assessment of glomerular filtration rate. *Clin Chem* 1998; **44**: 1535–9.
6 Ricos C, Alvarez V, Cava F, et al. Biological Variation Database. Available from http://www.westgard.com/guest17.htm.
7 Shewhart WA. *Economic Control of Quality of Manufactured Product*. New York: Van Nostrand, 1931.
8 Wheeler DJ, Chambers DS. *Understanding Statistical Process Control*, 2nd edn. Knoxville, TN: SPC Press, 1992.
9 Wheeler DJ. *Advanced Topics in Statistical Process Control*. Knoxville, TN: SPC Press, 1995.

10 Box G, Luceno A. *Statistical Control by Monitoring and Feedback Adjustment*. New York: Wiley, 1997.

11 NIST/SEMATECH e-Handbook of Statistical Methods. Available from http://www.itl.nist.gov/div898/handbook (last accessed January 2007).

12 Roes KCB, Does RJM, Schurink Y. Shewart-type control charts for individual observations. *J Qual Technol* 1993; **25**: 188–98.

13 Boggs PB, Wheeler D, Washburne WF, Hayati F. Peak expiratory flow rate control chart in asthma care: chart construction and use in asthma care. *Ann Allergy Asthma Immunol* 1998; **81**: 552–62.

14 Stoumbos ZG, Reynolds MR, Ryan TP, Woodall WH. The state of statistical process control as we proceed into the 21st century. *J Am Stat Assoc* 2000; **95**: 992–8.

15 Reynolds MR, Stoumbos ZG. Monitoring the process mean and variance using individual observations and variable sampling intervals. *J Qual Technol* 2001; **33**: 181–205.

CHAPTER 8

Developing a monitoring schedule: frequency of measurement

Andrew J. Farmer

'It is important to monitor your blood sugar on a regular basis. Ask your doctor how often you should check your blood sugar and at what time of day. Many people start by checking their blood sugar two times a day: before breakfast and before supper. After a few weeks, some people are able to measure their blood sugar only two or three times a week.'
—American Academy of Family Practice Guidelines on Blood Glucose Self-Monitoring

Advice about the frequency with which monitoring tests should be carried out is often phrased in tentative language and given on a pragmatic basis with little research-based evidence. Attempts should be made to determine the optimum testing interval for a monitoring test for three main reasons. Firstly, carrying out tests too often or not often enough might lead to harms, either through adverse effects of the testing process (e.g. bruising from blood tests or reduced quality of life) or from failure to identify important changes. Secondly, carrying out and acting on test results when there is a degree of measurement or biological variability (see Chapter 7) may exacerbate poor control. Thirdly, carrying out tests more often than needed can lead to major increases in costs. For example, for each additional self-monitored blood glucose test per week recommended in the UK an additional £6.5 million in costs would be incurred for every 0.5 million of the population with diabetes.

In this chapter I shall cover some of the principles that are explored elsewhere in this book in relation to the frequency of monitoring tests. Previous publications have explored some of the factors that determine how often tests should be repeated when they are used to monitor disease progression or therapy. [1]. Here I shall expand on that work and examine its implications for future research and clinical practice.

Evidence-based Medical Monitoring: from Principles to Practice. Edited by Paul Glasziou, Les Irwig and Jeffrey K. Aronson. © 2008 Blackwell Publishing, ISBN: 978-1-4051-5399-7.

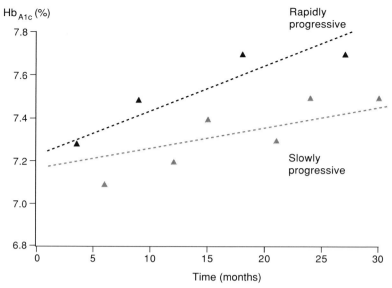

Figure 8.1 Serial Hb_{A1c} concentrations and the progression of diabetes.

8.1. Characteristics of surrogate markers and outcomes

Chapter 5 lays out the principles for choosing a test to monitor a condition or treatment. One of the most effective ways of doing this is to choose a disease outcome or a surrogate marker of that outcome to check for the response to the intervention, for disease progression, or for suspected changes in the condition, or to assess changes in management. The ways in which outcomes or surrogate markers of outcomes respond to the disease and its treatment will be among the most important factors that affect the schedule for testing.

8.1.1. How long does it take for a treatment to achieve a surrogate outcome?

The pharmacokinetic characteristics of a drug are an important determinant of the schedule for testing. The time it takes to reach a pharmacokinetic steady state depends on the half-life of the drug. Medications with long half-lives may take several days to achieve a steady state in the body, and this is reflected in their durations of action (Table 8.1) [2].

There are two key elements to be considered in making an overall assessment of the suitability of a disease marker for monitoring the progress of a treatment or a disease: (i) the rate of progression of the disease and (ii) the degree of random fluctuation in the measurement. These two elements provide an estimate of the signal-to-noise ratio (see Chapter 7), which helps in determining whether it might be possible to detect the likely change. Figure 8.1 provides an illustration, in which any individual measurement is unlikely to

Table 8.1 Half-lives of commonly used drugs*

<1 h	1–4 h	4–12 h	12–24 h	1–2 days	>2 days	Dose dependent
Adenosine	Azathioprine	Clozapine	Insulin (subcutaneous;	Carbamazepine	Amiodarone	Alcohol
Insulin (intravenous)	Beta-lactam	Epoetin	intermediate acting)	Chlorpropamide	Bisphosphonates	Fluoxetine
	antibiotics	Theophylline	Lithium	Ciclosporin	Digitoxin	Metoclopramide
	Carbimazole	Tolbutamide		Digoxin	Thyroxine	Phenytoin
	Heparin	Valproate		Insulin (subcutaneous;		Salicylates
	Levodopa			long acting)		
	Pravastatin			Triiodothyronine		
	Zidovudine			Warfarin		

Note: *Adapted from [2].

indicate the rate of glycaemic deterioration. Increasing the precision of any single measurement by repeated testing, or following progression over a period of time without a therapeutic change, may be required to establish whether medication changes are required.

8.2. The effect of the disease or treatment stage on monitoring frequency

8.2.1. Starting therapy

Testing should be more frequent during the start of treatment or initial disease monitoring (see Chapter 6). Reasons for this include checking the early response to therapy, identifying idiosyncratic responses and developing routines. Disease outcomes can occur rapidly or can take many years. High degrees of glycaemia are likely to lead to tissue damage and adverse effects such as retinopathy over a period of 5 years or more [3]. However, in some conditions, for example pregnancy, hypertension, or proteinuria, can rapidly progress to serious complications.

8.2.1.1. Checking the early response to therapy

Early and more frequent measurement will help monitor the response to therapy. For example, although published schedules for monitoring thyroid function tests suggest yearly or less frequent intervals, 6 weekly testing after the start of therapy and dosage changes is recommended to ensure that an adequate therapeutic effect is reached without delay.

8.2.1.2. Detecting idiosyncratic effects

Early testing may allow the detection of idiosyncratic results or adverse effects. For example, liver function tests are usually recommended after starting lipid-modifying therapy with statins, to ensure that no abnormalities of liver function have developed.

8.2.1.3. Developing self-help routines

Early testing may be helpful in developing self-help routines. For example, some clinicians recommend that all people with type 2 diabetes mellitus should undergo a period of blood glucose self-monitoring, although evidence that this improves outcomes is absent. They argue that frequent testing ensures that skills in self-monitoring are useful later in life, when regular testing may be required at short notice, and that the information provided helps ensure that attention is focused on the blood glucose concentration, which will require close future attention, whatever future methods of monitoring are used.

8.2.2. Stopping monitoring

For many conditions, monitoring, once started, is required for life. However, there is also a wide range of conditions in which, after the end of therapy, or after disease remission, monitoring can stop. For example, if anticoagulation with warfarin is stopped, for example 6 months after a pulmonary embolism, there is no further need for monitoring.

8.2.3. Determining the monitoring interval based on disease progression

Monitoring a disease needs to take account of the underlying time course of disease progression. While the eventual need for further therapy needs to be anticipated, the possibility of acute deterioration must also be taken into account. For example, the time course of an adverse outcome may be immediate, for example the risk of bleeding with excessive anticoagulation, or very slow, for example the development of microvascular disease with high concentrations of glucose. How long does the monitored measure take to change?

An individual with stable type 2 diabetes has underlying pathology of failure of pancreatic beta cells and a gradually failing endogenous supply of insulin. However, the decline in function is very slow. Follow-up of cohorts of people with type 2 diabetes has shown that there is a mean deterioration in HbA_{1c} of about 0.5% each year. The consequences of a slow drift over a period of 1 year from a target of HbA_{1c} to a measurement that is outside specified limits is not likely to be of great concern, provided further therapeutic action is undertaken.

Similarly, when using serum creatinine concentration to monitor progressive renal insufficiency, the rate of fall of creatinine predicts the time when renal replacement therapy is likely to be required. Any departure from the anticipated rate of fall requires further investigation.

The frequency of monitoring will also need to take account of the rate at which the test measurement changes after intervention. For example, blood glucose concentrations change within minutes as a result of endogenous insulin secretion or exogenous insulin administration. However, the concentration of HbA_{1c} (glycosylated haemoglobin) changes slowly over a period of up to 3 months, and reflects changes in glycaemia over that period (see Figure 5.3). Since the average lifespan of an erythrocyte is 3 months, measuring more often than monthly will not detect changes in HbA_{1c} that result from overall changes in blood glucose concentrations, and most guidelines suggest that 3 months should be the usual measurement interval; the most frequent interval recommended is about 8 weeks [4]. Other examples of different periods over which markers change are shown in Table 8.2. For example, the maximal changes in cholesterol synthesis will only begin to be observed once steady-state concentrations have been achieved, a process that can take several days [5].

The course of a disease is not always predictable. We need to know the chances that a clinically significant change will occur in any future time interval to determine a reasonable frequency of follow-up. Optimum intervals for follow-up for many cancers are uncertain after treatment, although there may be some descriptive data on which to make estimates of a range of likely

Table 8.2 Factors that affect monitoring intervals

Underlying condition	Test	How quickly the test changes with changes in the condition or treatment	Changes in the benefit to harm balance over time detected by monitoring	How the test is carried out	Changes that result from the test	Patient actions required	Frequency of testing
Adult onset (type 2) diabetes mellitus	Hb$_{A1c}$	The target measurement changes only slowly (over 6–8 weeks) with changes in treatment	Important changes in the underlying medical condition (e.g. retinopathy) occur only slowly	Laboratory	Intensify pharmacological treatment and general advice about lifestyle	Change treatment and lifestyle	Every 6–8 weeks minimum
Adult onset diabetes (type 2) diabetes	Fasting blood glucose	Changes occur from minute to minute; homoeostasis is achieved in the fasting state when not using insulin	Changes in the underlying condition occur only slowly	Laboratory testing is more accurate but less practical than self-testing for blood glucose	Intensify pharmacological treatment; the extent to which the information is useful in monitoring physical activity and diet in reducing glycaemia is not known	Change in amount of insulin therapy and lifestyle	Twice a week
Choriocarcinoma	Human chorionic gonadotrophin (HCG)	The measurement changes directly as a result of changes in the underlying problem	Detection of need for chemotherapy required	Laboratory	Chemotherapy if recurrence	Adherence to monitoring schedule	
Asthma	Peak flow	Rapid changes	Rapid changes	Patient	Use step changes in drug management (British Thoracic Society guidelines)	Adherence to treatment regimen	Very frequent, to establish minute to minute variability; looking for trends over 1–2 days

responses to therapy. Many schedules for follow-up of conditions such as bowel and prostate cancer have been based on providing reassurance (e.g. annual checks) rather than on an estimate of the likelihood of intervening to treat recurrence or to monitor disease progression.

When the disease course is stable, the rationale for regular monitoring is not always clear. For example, when people with bipolar illness are stable while taking lithium, there is little reason to monitor regularly. Regular monitoring is often defended on the grounds that it facilitates follow-up. However, it is not clear that setting up a schedule of regular tests in addition to appointments for psychological review is of additional benefit. In addition, complications are most likely to develop at times between scheduled visits, such as during a period of intercurrent illness or with co-administration of other medications, which is when monitoring *would* be justified.

People with type 2 diabetes who do not seek to achieve near-normal degrees of glycaemia do not need to measure the blood glucose concentration regularly. However, if an individual with diabetes is ill, timescales for monitoring are very tight. Blood glucose concentration can rise at a rate of 1 mmol/l in an hour, and hyperglycaemia and/or ketoacidosis can become problematic within hours. Prompt attention to monitoring and injecting corrective doses of insulin are essential. One should therefore use episodes of acute illness as a prompt to monitoring in some conditions.

8.2.4. High-risk groups and monitoring

Some individuals have a high risk of progression to adverse outcomes. For example, those with diabetes mellitus are at risk of sight-threatening retinopathy. The rate of progression from a normal retina to minor damage (background retinopathy) is low; most guidelines therefore recommend annual checks [6]. However, once background retinopathy is present, the incidence of sight-threatening complications increases and efforts to intensify glycaemic control (one of the main determinants of retinopathy) are intensified; in that case more frequent retinal inspection is recommended.

Regular monitoring is also justified when uncommon events are potentially serious. For example, the risk of neutropenia while taking methotrexate is low, but failure to identify this potentially life-threatening complication would be serious, and frequent testing is necessary.

A change of circumstances may dictate the need for monitoring, more frequent testing or even a change in the monitoring tests used. For example, pregnancy dictates the need to monitor regularly for evidence of raised blood pressure and proteinuria. However, once potential signs of pre-eclampsia are observed, observation becomes more frequent and is often accompanied by referral from primary care to a secondary care facility. A similar example, also relating to pregnancy, is the way in which an easily carried out, but less precise, method of monitoring foetal growth, such as symphysis-fundal height measurement, is followed by serial scans if concerns are raised about the growth pattern.

The final example listed above is an example of monitoring with a simple test but then switching to a more time- and resource-consuming test if problems arise. In essence, more frequent testing is justified when the sensitivity of the test needs to be high, but at the expense of an increased number of false-positive results.

8.2.5. Alterations in lifestyle or age that cause changes in frequency of monitoring

Frequency of monitoring needs to take into account the possibility of un-predictable events. For example, lifestyle changes, such as increased alcohol intake, are common among individuals taking warfarin. Two approaches may be necessary in these circumstances. The first is to ask the individual to notify the clinician of a change in circumstances (starting a new drug, increasing alcohol intake). The second, particularly when this approach has already failed, is to ensure that monitoring tests are carried out at more frequent intervals than would otherwise be indicated (see Table 8.3 for a list of circumstances in which monitoring intervals may need to be adjusted [2]).

8.3. Scheduling tests when results are outside control or specification limits

More frequent tests will be needed if test results show that the specified param-eter has moved away from the desired range, but has not crossed a threshold for intervention. Figure 8.1 shows two cases in which this might happen. For a test with a high degree of analytical variability (e.g. blood pressure measure-ment; Figure 8.2, upper panel), repeated tests would be appropriate to improve the accuracy of the test before progressing to a decision. There is no particular advantage of waiting for any possible biological variation to change, since the focus is on improving the accuracy of the measurement. An alternative case (Figure 8.2, lower panel) is the INR, a measure of blood coagulation, which has low analytical variability; in this case, a single measurement is sufficient on any occasion and the interval chosen for remeasurement should reflect the timescale for detecting any further trend in the change in the measure.

Another potential reason for scheduling more frequent tests is to investi-gate the possible causes of variation from the control or specification limits. Common causes (e.g. minor changes in lifestyle, timing of the test or minor variations in a self-testing regimen) are difficult to pick up, but variation can be reduced by careful attention to consistency in the circumstances surrounding the measurement. Special causes may be identifiable; for example, starting a new therapy or undertaking a major change in lifestyle (such as a new diet). In these circumstances, adjustment of therapy may be justified before remeasurement.

A third case in which increasing frequency of testing might be helpful with borderline results is when poor adherence to therapy and monitoring is a concern. Some clinicians set up a more intensive schedule for monitoring than

Table 8.3 Changes in the pharmacokinetics and pharmacodynamics of drugs that affect the frequency with which monitoring is appropriate*

Factor[†]	Examples
Renal insufficiency	Reduced excretion of digoxin, aminoglycoside antibiotics and lithium
Hepatic failure	Reduced elimination of theophylline, warfarin
Drug interactions	Reduced elimination of digoxin (verapamil, amiodarone) Reduced elimination of theophylline (erythromycin, fluoroquinolones) Reduced elimination of lithium (diuretics)
Thyroid dysfunction	Complex changes in the pharmacokinetics of digoxin
Diarrhoea	Altered absorption of lithium and ciclosporin; electrolyte imbalance causing retention of lithium
Factor[‡]	**Examples**
Electrolyte imbalance	Actions of digoxin and antiarrhythmic drugs enhanced by potassium depletion
Thyroid disease	Digoxin action enhanced (hypothyroidism) or decreased (hyperthyroidism)
Age	Actions of some drugs enhanced
Drug interactions	Increased action of warfarin (altered clotting factor synthesis) (tetracyclines) Increased ototoxicity of aminoglycoside antibiotics (loop diuretics)

Note: *Adapted from [2].

[†]Factors that can alter the pharmacokinetics of drugs, thereby altering the relation between the amount of drug in the body and the blood concentration.

[‡]Factors that can alter the pharmacodynamics of drugs, thereby altering the relation between the amount of drug at the site of action and the effect.

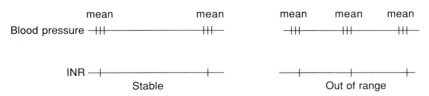

Figure 8.2 Measure variability and frequency of testing blood pressure and international normalized ratio (INR); each vertical line represents a single test (see text for discussion).

might otherwise be warranted, in anticipation of a lower rate of adherence to the schedule, but one that is within clinically appropriate values.

8.4. Cost-effectiveness

A detailed consideration of the basis of cost-effectiveness and cost-benefit calculations for different monitoring schedules is not within the scope of this chapter. However, several problems arise from attempts to introduce a systematic schedule for carrying out monitoring tests. Firstly, there can be increased costs from increasing the frequency of testing in order to increase the proportion of time the monitored measurements spent within the specified limits. Secondly, the introduction of external guidelines that lay out recommended testing intervals will both reduce the numbers of tests carried out by some individuals and increase the numbers of tests carried out by others. The latter is more common, with increased costs for health care. Consideration of the increased costs and the likely improvement in health gained from the changed schedule is needed, in order to judge the appropriateness of the revised schedules.

8.5. Further research and application of work on monitoring frequency

Further research in this area is likely to come from three strands. Firstly, there is a need for more descriptive work on the characteristics of tests; in particular, the ways in which tests are carried out in practice, the extent of biological variability and, in the case of self-monitoring tests, the extent to which analytical variability differs between individuals. Secondly, this work needs to be incorporated into modelling, in order to suggest different options for scheduling, taking into account disease and test characteristics. Thirdly, randomized controlled trials with different schedules for testing may help identify the extent to which different schedules offer advantages to health.

8.6. Conclusions

Judgements about the intervals at which tests are carried out are frequently made on the basis of expert judgements. Further work is required to systematize and apply available information about the test (e.g. its analytical variability). Knowledge of the pharmacological characteristics of the drug (e.g. its half-life) is essential, and the biological variability of the disease, the stage of the disease and its treatment, and the extent to which the test results are moving away from specified limits are also important in order to develop detailed guidance about follow-up intervals for use in general guidelines and to individualize monitoring schedules.

References

1 Glasziou P, Irwig L, Mant D. Monitoring in chronic disease: a rational approach. *BMJ* 2005; **330**: 644–8.

2 Grahame-Smith DG, Aronson JK. *The Oxford Textbook of Clinical Pharmacology and Drug Therapy*, 3rd edn. Oxford: Oxford University Press, 2002.

3 Stratton IM, Adler AI, Neil HA, et al. Association of glycaemia with macrovascular and microvascular complications of type 2 diabetes (UKPDS 35): prospective observational study. *BMJ* 2000; **321**: 405–12.

4 Tahara Y, Shima K. The response of GHb to stepwise plasma glucose change over time in diabetic patients. *Diabetes Care* 1993; **16**: 1313–4.

5 Hughes DA, Walley T. Predicting 'real world' effectiveness by integrating adherence with pharmacodynamic modeling. *Clin Pharmacol Ther* 2003; **74**: 1–8.

6 Stratton IM, Kohner EM, Aldington SJ, et al. UKPDS 50: risk factors for incidence and progression of retinopathy in type II diabetes over 6 years from diagnosis. *Diabetologia* 2004; **44**: 156–63.

CHAPTER 9

How should we adjust treatment?

Paul P. Glasziou

The usual purpose of monitoring is to detect when some change of management is needed and to make the appropriate adjustment. How much we adjust will depend on the degree of change. Chapters 6 and 7 examined how we can identify when a patient's monitoring measurement is within a desirable target range and how often we need to do this. In this chapter, I examine the next link in this chain—understanding the options for adjustment of treatment and how to make a reasonable choice between the options. The sequence to consider is

1 whether the cause of the change is explainable through non-adherence or another behavioural change;
2 whether to increase, add or switch therapies;
3 how much to increase (or decrease) therapy.

However, before we look at these it will be helpful to understand the problem of worsening control that can occur with poor adjustment of therapy.

9.1. The 'ping-pong' effect

A common error with adjustment of treatment is over-adjustment—changes in treatment that are either too frequent or too large can increase the variation in the monitored variable. The problem can be caused if clinicians respond too easily to random fluctuations, some of which can be quite large. This is easiest to understand when there is no true change in the patient's condition. In that case, variations in the measurements are merely random fluctuations. If we respond to some of these apparent fluctuations by changing treatment, this will lead to a change in measure, which in turn increases the likelihood of another change in treatment. This sequence of false alarms and inappropriate changes leads to increasing fluctuation and instability. Such a 'ping-pong' effect with subsequent overshoot has been observed when clinicians adjust the dose of warfarin in response to the international normalized ratio (INR) [1].

Evidence-based Medical Monitoring: from Principles to Practice. Edited by Paul Glasziou,
Les Irwig and Jeffrey K. Aronson. © 2008 Blackwell Publishing, ISBN: 978-1-4051-5399-7.

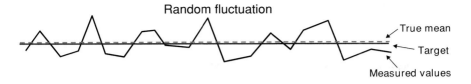

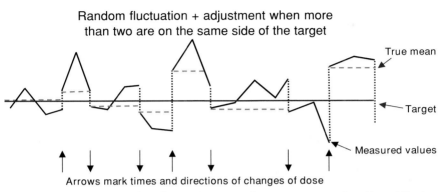

Arrows mark times and directions of changes of dose

Figure 9.1 Top panel: random fluctuation around a true concentration (dotted line), which is the same as the target (solid line). Bottom panel: increased variation from over-adjustment—each time two consecutive measurements are on the same side of the target the dose is altered (arrows); however, the true value on each occasion is shown as a dotted line, making it clear that the strategy is wrong.

   This is illustrated in Figure 9.1, which shows what happens when the 'rule' for changing treatment is to change it whenever two measurements are on one side of the target. (For several better rules, see Chapter 7.) As there is only random fluctuation, the adjustments cause an overshoot each time: the dotted line indicates the new true value. This unnecessary adjustment then increases the chance that the next two measures are on the same side, in turn leading to further adjustments.
   Hence the main messages of this chapter are as follows:
- Do not adjust if the measured variable is within the desirable ('control') limits.
- Make the adjustments small (but not too small).
I begin by looking at when and how therapy might be changed, then how much it should be changed, and finally when to recheck the impact of the change.

9.2. When and how should treatment be changed?

Some rules for reliably identifying when a patient's monitored variable has drifted beyond desirable limits were suggested in the discussion of control limits in Chapter 7. These rules usually consider a single extreme measure

Options in changing management

- Intensify/Stepped Care
  - —Titrate to maximum
    then add new agents

- Intensify then Switch
  - —Titrate and switch if insufficient

- Add low dose ('Polypill principle')
  - —Add new low-dose agents sequentially

Figure 9.2 Three generic options for adjusting therapy.

(such as one measure more than 3 standard deviations from target) or several measures that are consistently above or below target (for example, two measures that are 2 standard deviations above target) as indicating a likely drift from target. When such an alarm is triggered we need to consider several possibilities.

If the drift from target is real, there may be several causes. Firstly, the drift from target may be due to poor adherence. So patients should be sensitively questioned about their current treatment behaviour. Secondly, check other changes in the patient's behaviour, such as diet (e.g. grapefruit juice), other medications or changes that might cause poor absorption (such as timing or diarrhoea). For factors that can change the pharmacokinetics and pharmacodynamics of drugs, see Table 8.3. Once these causes have been excluded, we can consider whether we need further confirmation of the change in the patient's condition or whether an immediate change in management is appropriate.

9.2.1. Options in changing treatment

A control chart provides an indication of whether the monitored variable is above, within or below a desired set of limits. Some charts also indicate if the monitored variable is increasing or decreasing in an unacceptable manner. We face several fundamental choices in changing treatment. Our possible actions can be classified into three classes (see Figure 9.2):

1 Intensify or attenuate treatment; for example increase or decrease the dosage or change the hours of therapy.
2 Switch treatments; for example to another similar agent or a different class of therapy.
3 Add a different therapy; for example a low dose of an additional drug or another form of adjuvant therapy, or remove a therapy (if the current therapy has multiple components).

Different therapeutic arenas have tended to take on one or other of these paradigms. For example, in infectious diseases the usual response to treatment failure is to switch therapy (although sometimes an increased dosage or add-on therapy are used). In hypertension management, the classic regimen has been 'stepped care', whereby we intensify treatment to a maximum and then add on another therapy (though this has recently been questioned by approaches that test individual responses to a sequence of drugs or that suggest combined low-dose drugs). Let us look at some of the advantages and disadvantages of each.

9.2.1.1. Intensification

Intensification can be achieved by increasing the dosage or by reducing the dosage interval. If increasing the size of each dose could result in transient unwanted effects, then altering the dosage interval or using a modified-release formulation can help to smooth out the plasma concentration versus time curve, thereby reducing adverse fluctuations. Intensification is appropriate if it can increase therapeutic benefits without an excessive increase in adverse effects. As these can vary with the patient, individual titration can be used to tailor the dose to each patient's requirement, achieving different maximum plasma concentrations.

9.2.1.2. Switching

Instead of increasing the dose when the response is insufficient we can consider switching treatments, for example to another similar agent or a different class of therapy. This is particularly useful if there is variation in the individual response to different treatments; for example, some people with hypertension might respond better to an ACE inhibitor than to a beta-blocker or vice versa. For example, when new patients with hypertension were rotated through five different classes of antihypertensive drugs, there was a spread of which drug was 'best'; the average advantage of the 'best' in each case was 10 mmHg [2].

9.2.1.3. Combined low-dose therapy

Finally, if there is a partial but insufficient response it may be reasonable to add a different therapy, for example a low dose of an additional drug or another form of adjuvant therapy. This makes most sense when different drugs have different mechanisms of action; in that case each has a small beneficial effect and the beneficial effects are additive; however, the adverse effects of each are minimized, and for most of the adverse effects there is no additivity. An illustration of the use of this is a comparison of single agents with combined low-dose agents for hypertension, suggesting that the combined lower dosage may achieve better reduction of blood pressure with fewer adverse effects [3]. This is one of the principles of the Polypill, which would contain low doses of three antihypertensive drugs [4].

For most of the rest of this chapter, we shall assume that we are using the first strategy, that is, intensification of treatment.

9.2.2. By how much should you change?

An objective in changing treatment is to get the monitored variable into the desired target range as quickly as possible but without overshooting. As suggested in the introduction, the most common problem is an over-adjustment of treatment, because of an assumption that the apparent drift from target is entirely due to a true change in the patient's condition. For drug treatments, the exact adjustment can be difficult to calculate. The difficulties in calculating dosage changes are illustrated by a review of the recommendations for aminoglycoside dosage changes in 100 consecutive patients using three different methods: ALADDIN, DOSECALC and the Australian Antibiotic Guidelines nomogram. At least 25% of the recommendations differed by more than 80 mg [5].

The relation between drug dosage and serum concentrations will vary depending on a number of factors, such as adherence, absorption, the size of the individual and the rate of drug metabolism and excretion. The latter will vary with individual physiology and disease states, particularly renal and hepatic function. These factors are partly predictable, and hence helpful in guiding initial dosage, but the prediction will have some inaccuracy and serum concentration measurements may be required.

Adjusting for the drug concentration (pharmacokinetics) is relatively easy, because within the target range, for most drugs, there is an approximately linear relation between dose and concentration. We can use a proportional adjustment, namely,

$$\text{new dose} = \text{current dose} \times \frac{(\text{target concentration})}{(\text{measured concentration})}$$

However, there are two caveats to this approach. Firstly, it assumes that the concentration has been accurately measured; hence it is usually wise to use a smaller adjustment than predicted by the equation. For example, a single measure that is well beyond the target range (say 3 standard deviations) may be truly abnormal, but it is still likely to show some 'regression to the mean' on remeasurement without intervention. Such excessive dose adjustment has been seen in INR adjustment [1]. Secondly, for drugs with saturation kinetics in the therapeutic range of doses (e.g. phenytoin), the dose–concentration relation is non-linear [6] and hence this equation is inapplicable.

For most adjustments, we will not know the drug concentration (and even if we do, it is often not the most desirable guide; see Chapter 3). Hence, we need to consider the pharmacodynamics as well as the pharmacokinetics. Dose–response curves (more accurately called concentration–effect curves; see Chapter 3 for a more extensive discussion of the types of dose–response curve) are usually non-linear, although for some range of doses or concentrations they are log-linear. For drugs whose log concentration–effect curve is linear, each successive doubling of dosage results in the same incremental increase in response. For example, if a dose of X mg gives a 3 mmHg reduction in blood pressure, a dose of 2X mg will reduce the blood pressure by about 6 mmHg;

If you are taking 3 mg or less

Blood test result	Action	Next test
Over 5	⚠	As advised
3.1–4.9	Reduce dose by 0.5 mg	1 week
2.0–3.0	Take same dose	2 weeks
1.6–1.9	Reduce dose by 0.5 mg	1 week
Under 1.5	⚠	As advised

If you are taking more than 3 mg

Blood test result	Action	Next test
Over 5	⚠	As advised
3.1–4.9	Reduce dose by 1.0 mg	1 week
2.0–3.0	Take same dose	2 weeks
1.6–1.9	Reduce dose by 1.0 mg	1 week
Under 1.5	⚠	As advised

Figure 9.3 Example of a patient self-dosing adjustment chart for a target INR of 2.5 during warfarin therapy, with advice on the size of dose change needed and the timing of remeasurement. (Adapted from www.anticoagulation.org.uk)

however, non-linearity at higher doses leads to diminishing returns—a dose of 4X mg will only reduce the blood pressure by 9 mmHg. Even if the log-linear relation is maintained at higher doses, adverse effects will usually limit further dose increases.

For non-linear processes, many methods of varying complexity have been suggested, but head-to-head evaluations have not demonstrated a clearly superior method. For example, for warfarin dosing one study compared a complex Bayesian regression program with a simple nomogram. In the hands of the clinical pharmacist, the nomogram was the best at predicting the change in INR. Given simplicity and ease of access, it is generally wisest to use an empirically derived nomogram or chart for dose adjustment, unless a computer program has been clearly shown to be superior. An example of a simple chart [7] for patient self-adjustment of warfarin dosing for anticoagulation is shown in Figure 9.3 (self-monitoring of INR is more extensively discussed in Chapter 17).

For non-drug interventions, such as physiotherapy or psychotherapy, there are no simple principles for adjustment. However, the three suggestions considered above—intensification or attenuation, switching, and add-on or removal—are clearly still relevant.

9.3. When should we check for a response?

Sometimes we shall want to check whether there has been an adequate response to the change in therapy. This problem was introduced in the

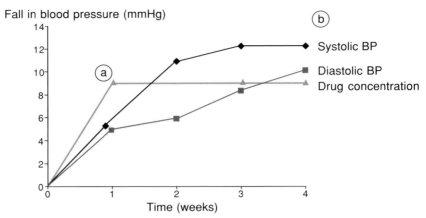

Figure 9.4 Changes in blood pressure after starting an ACE inhibitor: blood pressure (pharmacodynamic biomarker) becomes stable (point b) only weeks after the blood concentration (pharmacokinetic biomarker) has become stable (point a). (Data from [9].)

discussion, in Chapter 6, on checking for the initial response. We shall usually want to check earlier than the standard schedule of monitoring, and we may sometimes want to use a different measure.

The timing of remeasurement clearly depends on the delay between the change in treatment and the change in the measure we use. This will vary, depending on how far down the causal sequence the measure is. Hence, some-times we may want to switch from the usual low-term monitoring measure to a short-term measure.

For example, plasma amitriptyline concentrations generally reach a steady state within 7–10 days of changing treatment, but the full clinical benefit takes up to 4–6 weeks to be achieved [8]. This is because the therapeutic effect relies on an adaptive change, which takes longer to occur than it takes for the drug to accumulate at the site of action [9]; in other words, the pharmacokinetics and pharmacodynamics are dissociated.

The best understood timing is for pharmacokinetics, where knowledge of the half-life will usually predict how long it will take until a new steady state is reached (although active metabolites with long half-lives can complicate this process). Pharmacodynamic changes are generally more difficult to pre-dict, and will usually require an in vivo experiment to observe the time from initiation or change to the time of maximal effect. The difference between pharmacokinetic and pharmacodynamic responses is illustrated in Figure 9.4, which shows that the time for an ACE inhibitor to reach steady-state concen-trations was within a week, but that the full impact on blood pressure took almost a month to achieve [10].

9.4. Conclusions: summary of principles

Decisions about the need to change therapy, how much to change therapy, and when to recheck are beset with difficulties. Nevertheless, several general principles are suggested by the above discussion.

1 During the initiation of therapy, increase the dose slowly and monitor for both therapeutic and adverse effects.

2 During long-term therapy, monitor a single or a few target measures, but be sure that the measures are truly outside the target range before switching doses, as over-adjustment will only increase variability.

3 If there is an insufficient response or adverse effects occur, consider one of three options:

(a) change the dosage;

(b) switch to another drug;

(c) use a combination of (low-dose) drugs.

4 To check the impact of a change of dosage or therapy requires considering both pharmacokinetic and pharmacodynamic delays; in some cases the latter will be longer than the former.

Acknowledgements

Thanks to Martin Turner, Jeffrey Aronson and Les Irwig for helpful comments on this chapter.

References

1 Lassen JF, Kjeldsen J, Antonsen S, Hyltoft Petersen P, Brandslund I. Interpretation of serial measurements of international normalized ratio for prothrombin times in monitoring oral anticoagulant therapy. *Clin Chem* 1995; **41**: 1171–6.

2 Deary AJ, Schumann AL, Murfet H, Haydock SF, Foo RS, Brown MJ. Double-blind, placebo-controlled crossover comparison of five classes of antihypertensive drugs. *J Hypertens* 2002; **20**: 771–7.

3 Frishman WH, Hainer JW, Sugg J; M-FACT Study Group. A factorial study of combination hypertension treatment with metoprolol succinate extended release and felodipine extended release results of the Metoprolol Succinate–Felodipine Antihypertension Combination Trial (M-FACT). *Am J Hypertens* 2006; **19**: 388–95.

4 Wald NJ, Law MR. A strategy to reduce cardiovascular disease by more than 80%. *BMJ* 2003; **326**: 1419–21.

5 Paterson DL, Robson JM, Wagener MM, Peters M. Monitoring of serum aminoglycoside levels with once-daily dosing. *Pathology* 1998; **30**: 289–94.

6 Aronson JK, Hardman M, Reynolds DJ. ABC of monitoring drug therapy. Phenytoin. *BMJ* 1992; **305**: 1215–8.

7 Dalere GM, Coleman RW, Lum BL. A graphic nomogram for warfarin dosage adjustment. *Pharmacotherapy* 1999; **19**: 461–7.

8 Tharp R. Aminoglycoside dosing. Available from http://www.rxkinetics.com/ amino.html (last accessed on 3 May 2007).

9 Grahame-Smith DG. The Lilly Prize Lecture. 1996 keep on taking the tablets': pharmacological adaptation during long-term drug therapy. *Br J Clin Pharmacol* 1997; **44**: 227–38.

10 Smith DH, Matzek KM, Kempthorne-Rawson J. Dose response and safety of telmisartan in patients with mild to moderate hypertension. *J Clin Pharmacol* 2000; **40**: 1380–90.

CHAPTER 10

Monitoring as a learning and motivational tool

Susan Michie, Kirsten McCaffery, Carl Heneghan

'What people think, feel, and do about their health depends in great measure on how they interpret diagnostic information about it.' [1]

In this chapter, we describe the potential benefits that patients may obtain by being provided with systematic information over time so that they can monitor changes in key health or illness indicators. We consider ways in which information can motivate people to better understand and adhere to agreed treatment regimens, and to change their behaviour to improve their health. We present psychological explanations for these processes and discuss other benefits, such as providing a sense of control over symptoms and underlying health, and fostering a collaborative problem-solving approach to managing ill-health.

10.1. The importance of psychological factors in monitoring

Monitoring provides people with information, whether formally in a clinical encounter or informally by people outside the clinical context. Monitoring, especially self-monitoring of symptoms and behaviours, was developed as both an intervention technique and an assessment tool for problematic symptoms and behaviours in the 1970s and 1980s in the fields of behaviour analysis and behaviour therapy. Although psychological research into monitoring and self-monitoring has subsequently declined, it continues to be used in clinical settings for those with psychological problems, as well as physical ones. While there is little direct evidence about the psychological factors that influence clinical monitoring, there is much to draw on from theories and empirical findings in the areas of risk perception, judgment under uncertainty and behaviour change.

Evidence-based Medical Monitoring: from Principles to Practice. Edited by Paul Glasziou,
Les Irwig and Jeffrey K. Aronson. © 2008 Blackwell Publishing, ISBN: 978-1-4051-5399-7.

Increasing numbers of tests are available over the counter, for example for blood pressure, plasma glucose concentration and ovulation. In addition, self-monitoring by patients is becoming more common for several reasons:

- It provides motivation (e.g. home blood glucose measurement by people with non-insulin dependent diabetes)[1].
- It provides a clinician with information about measurements between visits (e.g. home blood pressure monitoring [2] or home glucose monitoring).
- It allows self-adjustment of therapy (e.g. peak flow rates to trigger actions in asthma patients [3] or self-monitored international normalized ratio (INR) measurements to adjust warfarin doses [4]).

In general, patients would like more information about their health and health care than they receive [5, 6]. Among the benefits of receiving such information are improved understanding, motivating adherence to treatment, giving more control over health and threats to health, reducing uncertainty and negative emotions, giving the advantage of warning time, preparing for self-protective responses that might reduce or avert the impact of the event and improving satisfaction with care and relationships with health professionals [7, 8]. On the other hand, monitoring can cause unnecessary worry and doubt. It is therefore important to understand the psychological processes at play in monitoring, in order to maximize the benefits and minimize the adverse effects of monitoring.

Monitoring may take place in a routine, preventive manner, for example measuring the blood pressure of someone whose hypertension is being successfully controlled. On the other hand, it may occur in circumstances that people find stressful, either because there is a perceived threat to their health or because the clinical setting and procedures engender anxiety. In these cases, there are individual differences in people's desire for information; some seek information about the threat ('monitors') and some try to avoid potentially threatening information ('blunters') [9]. Information seeking helps monitors cope with the threat by giving a greater sense of control over problems and by helping them manage their emotions [10, 11]. Context (or 'framing') also influences responses to monitored information. Clinical test results have been framed as a hypothesis-testing procedure; the result is judged relative to a hypothesis that the person is well or ill [12]. Patients who consider that the purpose of monitoring is to detect disease feel less confident about their test results and feel more vulnerable to the monitored disease than those who consider the purpose to be to detect wellness. There may, therefore, be psychological benefits for the patient in discussing health monitoring (e.g. for cholesterol, herpes, cancer remission) as checks for wellness rather than as temporary reprieves from eventual illness.

10.1.1. What is 'monitoring' from a psychological perspective?

Monitoring can serve as both an assessment tool and an intervention technique. To understand the process of monitoring, it is useful to analyse its component behaviours, of which there are up to four (Figure 10.1):

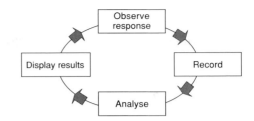

Figure 10.1 A schematic representation of the process of monitoring behaviours.

1 the target response must be observed or detected;
2 the occurrence must be recorded, along with any additional information relevant to the goals of the monitoring (e.g. intensity, antecedent stimuli);
3 analysis of the record may be required;
4 the results of the analysis should be displayed.

Whether or not these components are carried out may be influenced by different factors; for example, failure to notice monitored information may be influenced by competing demands for attention, while failure to record may be influenced by time pressure.

10.1.2. Adherence to monitoring

Several factors contribute to adherence [13]: the specific condition being treated, the health-care system and the team delivering the intervention, the social and economic conditions of the patient and setting, characteristics of the therapy itself and the contribution of the individual patient. With blood glucose self-monitoring, patients were more likely to continue to monitor if they felt more confident about testing blood sugar, thought it would improve their health and feeling well, and felt that their family and friends supported them in monitoring. The predictors of adherence in self-monitoring of blood glucose can be biological (e.g. the type of diabetes, the type of medication and the duration of the diabetes), environmental and psychological (e.g. self-efficacy [14], outcome expectations [15] and social support [16].)

Management can be improved by a monitoring strategy that best fits the factors that contribute to overall adherence. For instance, there is good evidence that particular elements of an asthma management plan improve patient self-management, through the use of monitoring asthma symptoms, seeking regular medical review and using a written asthma action plan. Clinical trials that have used these approaches have shown reductions in episodes of hospitalization, emergency department visits, unscheduled doctor visits and numbers of days lost from school because of asthma [17]. Presumably, the mechanism of improved asthma outcomes from these approaches to self-management is greater involvement, self-awareness of symptoms and behaviour and, hence, better adherence to the recommended health-care regimen [18]. Different approaches can be taken to help patients improve the management of their condition via self-monitoring; for instance, symptom monitoring through the use of diary records of medication use or assessment of airflow function (peak expiratory flow or spirometry). For young children, tailoring of the monitoring to symptoms is as effective as monitoring peak expiratory flow [19].

10.1.3. The nature of monitored information

The impact of monitoring varies according to how much information is given. For example, people may know that they are being monitored but receive no feedback, or they may receive feedback on its own or with a standard and information about the discrepancy between current and desired performance. The impact also varies with the nature of the information. While some results may be given in terms of a general statement (e.g. 'you are in the normal range'), much monitored information indicates probability rather than certainty. However, both health professionals and patients find probabilistic information difficult to understand [20] and may interpret it differently. For example, health professionals interpret risks of genetic conditions of 15–50% as 'high' or 'very high', whereas patients interpret the same probabilities as 'moderate' [21]. The way in which risk information is presented (e.g. words, frequencies, probabilities) affects understanding of the risk, the ways in which the information is processed, and decisions and actions taken as a result [22]. A further issue is that probabilistic information is processed most effectively if it can be extracted from perceived occurrences rather than from perceived non-occurrences [12]. This creates problems for negative test results, since 'good news' from clinical monitoring comes in the form of a non-event, which is perceived as being ambiguous. This 'uncertain wellness' can cause feelings of uncertainty, vulnerability, distress and concern about health; a desire for further testing in an effort to gain reassurance and a desire for further treatment. Thus, monitoring can increase the numbers of 'worried well', unnecessary and inappropriate health behaviours, and use of health-care resources. This has been documented in a variety of clinical circumstances [23, 24]. Since negative test results are unlikely to reassure, there is a danger in self-monitoring of setting up a vicious cycle of reassurance seeking.

10.1.4. The accuracy of monitoring

Like all measures of symptoms and behaviour, monitoring can be unreliable and inaccurate. If measures are not reliable, they will not be either clinically useful or trusted sufficiently to help people understand how to use the information or to adhere to recommended treatment. It is therefore important to establish the reliability of monitoring methods. An example is the development of the INR (see Chapter 17), which was undertaken by the World Health Organization because of problems associated with variability in prothrombin time measurements in different countries. An example of the problem was that for the same prothrombin time result a mean dose under 2 mg in Hong Kong was comparable with over 8 mg in North America [25].

Several factors influence accuracy when information is being monitored by people rather than machines [26]. Since recall may be inaccurate, recording should be as near as possible to the time of the observation. Observer load should be minimized: accuracy and reliability are inversely related to the number of different events being monitored [27, 28]. Poorly defined targets also lead to unreliable monitoring. These factors interact with the patient's state, such as tiredness, stress and competing demands. Accuracy is increased when monitors are made aware that their accuracy will be checked [29].

Several studies have shown that training improves the accuracy of monitored data [30]. With self-monitoring, suggestions for effective training include explicit definitions of targets for monitoring and explicit instructions for monitoring, demonstrations of how to do it and practice. Reinforcement, such as praise, which is contingent on accurate monitoring, increases its accuracy [29].

10.2. Psychological purposes of monitoring

10.2.1. Provision of information

For both patients and health professionals, information about biochemical and physiological indicators of health, symptoms and behaviours can affect thinking, emotional state and behaviour. It can affect thinking by helping pattern recognition, problem formulation and problem-solving (for example, how the target behaviour/indicator is associated with antecedents and consequences) and aiding decision-making. It can affect emotional state by increasing decision confidence and reducing anxiety. And it can change behaviour, since information can serve as a cue to action, motivate reduction in discrepancies observed between desired and current performance, and serve as a reward for past efforts.

10.2.2. Facilitation of communication and increased engagement with health care

Monitoring can both increase people's sense of control and reduce anxiety [31, 32]. For health professionals, monitoring can help engage them in thinking about the patient, which provides them with a sense of professional identity and satisfaction in circumstances that may offer little clarity or obvious ways forward. If monitoring is conducted by patients or monitoring information is shared with them, health care can become more patient centred. Patient-centred care is not just about health professionals taking the perspective of the patient; it is also about activating patients and engaging them in clinical decisions when they desire it, as in shared decision-making [33, 34]. A review of patient centredness in chronic illness showed that health-care consultations that actively engage patients in thinking about their care are more consistently associated with good physical health outcomes than consultations in which a more passive empathic approach was taken [35]. Such communication can facilitate both the quality of decisions and commitment to adhering to recommendations after those decisions.

10.2.3. Monitoring as a therapeutic intervention

The process and outcome of monitoring can serve as a motivator for change, since it engages people in 'doing something' (which can lead people to 'do more' to improve their health) and holds out the prospect that feedback will show a desired change. Monitoring is even more important when clinical indicators are invisible, for example cholesterol concentration and blood pressure. Monitoring can thus comprise a treatment itself, because of reactive effects on the behaviour being monitored [36] or on behaviours that influence the clinical indicator being monitored [37].

Reactive effects tend to occur in the therapeutically desired direction, desirable behaviours increasing and undesirable behaviours decreasing [38, 39], and are strongest when the person being monitored is motivated to change [29]. Self-monitoring is affected by factors related to characteristics of monitoring (e.g. schedule, timing of monitoring in relation to behaviour), the consequences of what is monitored (external consequences, standard, feedback) [40], the participant (intelligence, motivation to change, expectation, skills) and behaviour (type of behaviour, interactions with current behaviour).

However, self-monitoring alone does not always produce a reactive effect [41] and is therefore often used as part of a multicomponent intervention. For example, monitoring of weight, physical activity and dietary intake are important elements of weight reduction programmes [42, 43]. Self-monitoring is more effective when combined with perceived desirability of the behaviour [44], goal setting, feedback [45, 46], outcome expectancies [47] and reinforcement [48].

The schedule of monitoring (Chapter 8) is an important consideration. For example, the benefit of using continuous blood glucose monitoring equipment compared with self-monitoring of blood glucose shows mixed results; while some studies have equated continuous monitoring with better outcomes than self-monitoring [49], others have shown no significant difference [46]. Continuous monitoring is thought to be more reactive, but more intensive schedules place higher demands on the individual, as reflected in higher attrition rates [50].

There are several reasons for the effectiveness of monitoring to bring about behavioural change. When people notice a discrepancy between a desired and actual state, they become motivated to change their behaviour if the discrepancy is not too large and if the person feels a sense of control and has readily available strategies to put into action. Any observed reductions in discrepancy can also serve as a reinforcer for planned strategies and future monitoring. It may be the process of monitoring as well as its outcome that engenders change. For example, the act of monitoring can serve as a reminder of previously planned strategies for improvement. Monitoring is often a shared exercise (e.g. in 'Weight Watchers') that provides opportunities for support and advice, problem-solving and being rewarded for past efforts by others [51].

The usefulness of monitored information will depend on how much people trust the monitoring process and resulting information, whether their personal circumstances allow them to act constructively on the information, the social context and the individual's commitment to behaviour change.

10.3. Psychological theories that inform our understanding of monitoring

10.3.1. Self-regulation theory

Self-regulation theory provides a useful framework for considering the impact of monitoring on both patients' behaviours (e.g. becoming more physically active) and health professionals' behaviours (e.g. changing medication). The essence of this theory is that behaviour is goal driven and that people are active regulators of their own behaviour [52]. Monitoring is most likely to be effective in changing behaviour if there are clear goals, strong motivation to achieve the goals and an absence of conflicting goals. Effective regulation depends on having realistic, achievable goals, developing a method of reliably monitoring progress towards goals and acting on the basis of this feedback to reduce the discrepancy between current behaviour and goals. This theory explains why combining monitoring with goal setting and feedback leads to more change than monitoring on its own [46].

However, the way in which monitored information is presented can make a difference to subsequent behaviour. For example, if information emphasizes the size of the discrepancy and is not accompanied by information about a feasible way of reducing it, people may give up trying to achieve their goal. The beneficial impact of monitoring will therefore be assisted by having clear 'if–then' plans to put into operation after the feedback received from monitoring. The importance of people's confidence in their abilities to carry out these procedures ('self-efficacy') and their expectations of the outcomes of doing so ('anticipated outcomes') are also important predictors of behaviour change, as outlined in social cognitive theory [53].

The self-regulatory approach has been extended to understand the behavioural and emotional responses of those facing a threat, such as that posed by illness, as described in the common-sense model [54]. The ways in which people think about their illnesses, their diagnostic and monitoring tests, and their treatments influence their physical and psychological recovery [55]. The model has parallel cognitive and emotional pathways, which activate an individual's coping and appraisal responses when faced with illness. The cognitive pathway (also called 'illness representation') has six broad dimensions that people use to make sense of, and respond to, illness. These include beliefs about the illness identity (its symptoms and label), its coherence, its timeline (expectations of the duration of the illness), the cause (how or where the illness came from), its consequences (the perceived short-term and long-term effects of the illness) and controllability/cure (perceptions of how controllable or curable the illness is).

The extent to which people's illness representation is coherent with their diagnosed illness, the indicators being monitored and the recommended treatment affects their adherence to health advice and degrees of stress [55]. Both adherence and stress can have significant effects on disease prevention, course and recovery processes, and on health-care costs. An example of beliefs about how tests affect service uptake comes from studies of genetic testing for the bowel condition familial adenomatous polyposis [56, 57]. Many patients who receive low (population) risk results on genetic testing expressed a desire to continue with bowel screening, despite the fact that it carries a clinical risk, is experienced negatively, and is clinically unnecessary. This desire arose from the fact that people believe the result of bowel screening more than the result of a genetic test—the former was more coherent in that it was a concrete image of the 'at-risk' body part in real time. The genetic test consisted of blood taken from a body part not associated with the disease (the arm) and subjected to an unknown procedure, producing abstract results weeks later.

10.3.2. Learning ('operant') theory

Information gleaned as a result of monitoring can have a powerful influence on future behaviour. It can serve both as a trigger for health-care related behaviours and as a reinforcer for such behaviours, when monitoring shows progress towards a desired end-state. The influence of such 'antecedents' and 'consequences' of behaviour is explained by learning theory, specifically operant theory [58, 59], which accounts for the way in which behaviour changes as a result of changed environmental contingencies. By serving as a reminder and reinforcer of behaviour, monitoring can influence what, when, and how treatment is given, and adherence to health advice by patients. It can also influence future monitoring behaviours.

10.4. Clinician-led monitoring versus self-monitoring

In medical practice, monitoring is usually carried out by clinicians; however, there are several benefits associated with monitoring that is conducted by patients and/or family members.

10.4.1. Clinician-led monitoring

Clinicians are not always effective monitors; they may order tests when they are not necessary, not monitor when it would be useful to do so, or monitor the wrong things in the wrong ways. Estimates of inappropriate test usage range from 5 to 95% [60]. Inappropriate testing causes problems for patients in terms of inconvenience, anxiety and potentially unnecessary further investigations and treatments. For example, in a UK study before the new GP contract was implemented, only 14% of 21,024 patients with newly diagnosed hypertension had met the target blood pressure after 12 months [61]; among treated patients about 40% of INRs are outside target ranges, compared with the ideal of 5% [62].

Inappropriate monitoring also wastes health professionals' time and health service resources. Several studies have documented inconsistent monitoring of drugs with potential toxicity [63, 64]. Computerized alerts have been studied in a randomized controlled trial of 400,000 US health-plan members in the hope of increasing the percentage of patients receiving baseline laboratory monitoring at initiation of drug therapy [65]. The intervention involved the collaboration of researchers, physicians and pharmacists in agreeing a set of laboratory drug monitoring recommendations. Information about missing laboratory test results for 15 high-risk drugs were e-mailed to pharmacists who ordered tests or reminded patients to obtain the tests if they had already been ordered. In addition, various methods of improving clinical practice have been tried, such as audit and feedback, educational messages and reminding clinicians to monitor by stickers on medical records or beeping hand-held computers. However, they have had only small to modest effects, and there is little information about what works in what circumstances [66]. Effective monitoring may be led by nurses as well as pharmacists, for example in interventions to improve control of blood pressure in patients with hypertension [67].

10.4.2. Self-monitoring

Self-monitoring is the act of systematically observing and recording aspects of one's own behaviour, internal state (e.g. symptoms, clinical indicators) or external environmental events (e.g. contact with allergens) [26]. Self-monitoring can give information about symptoms, behaviours and events at the time and place of their occurrence, for example when the patient is at home or in other settings in which direct observation is not possible. It has the advantages of implicitly emphasizing the patient's control, providing continuous immediate feedback and giving a more complete record than can be obtained by other methods. Self-monitoring can provide information about the frequency and intensity of symptoms and document the disruption that symptoms can produce in different settings. Symptoms can be monitored at predetermined intervals or every time a particular symptom or intensity occurs.

Behaviour can also be monitored—accurate assessment of responses and their controlling variables is a cornerstone of behaviour therapy. When behaviour is part of someone's everyday life, for example smoking, monitoring may be easier and more accurate if performed by oneself than by others. Monitoring environmental events and circumstances, cognitions or emotional states that occur before and after behaviours can provide information about patterns of symptoms or behaviour, for example triggers or reinforcers. This can help inform the understanding of the initiation and maintenance of symptoms and behaviours, and thus the development of more effective interventions. Responses that are covert (e.g. symptoms, experience of clinical interventions, or private activity such as sexual behaviours) can only be monitored by the self.

Self-monitoring encompasses self-testing and referral to a clinician for advice, and self-testing and self-adjustment of treatment when appropriate, often referred to as self-management. It is important to recognize that self-monitoring is not suitable for all patients and that there may be circumstances in which patients prefer clinician-led monitoring. For example, in a study of attitudes towards self-monitoring for human papilloma virus (HPV) in prevention of cervical cancer, although women rated the ease, convenience and privacy of self-monitoring highly, they were concerned that they might carry out the test wrongly, and so stated that they would not feel reassured by, or confident in, a negative test result [68]. Clinician-led testing was preferred by most women.

Certain factors, such as manual dexterity and cognitive abilities, are relevant in determining patient suitability for self-monitoring; psychological traits may also predict and affect successful self-monitoring. However, little is known about how to assess patient suitability, and adherence to self-monitoring is poor. For instance, despite attempts by clinical pharmacists and physicians to assess patients' competence, compliance and willingness to self-manage their anticoagulation therapy [69], 29% of the intervention group discontinued self-monitoring compared with no drop-outs in the control group, who were not asked to self-monitor. Common reasons for dropping out included difficulty with monitoring, a preference for physician management and the availability of an alternative management strategy. Many patients who try to self-monitor oral anticoagulation have experience of, or know someone who has experience of, an alternative management strategy; they may prefer to go back to this system or to stay with it in the first place. Drop-out rates for anticoagulation self-monitoring range from 9 to 43%. However, in a randomized trial of patients with mechanical valves who were self-monitoring oral anticoagulation [70] and had no experience of usual management, drop-out rates were far less than average attrition rates in randomized trials. In diabetes mellitus, there is no alternative comparable testing strategy to self-monitoring of blood glucose, apart from urine testing. In a small trial of 30 self-monitoring individuals who compared blood glucose with urine glucose [71] most patients preferred urine testing (71%) and one-third dropped out of the intervention group.

What to monitor will partly be determined by the nature of the condition. For stable conditions, such as asthma, it is appropriate to monitor symptoms that signal the need for intervention. In other conditions, such as non-insulin dependent diabetes, the need for monitoring of blood glucose is less well established, although the practice is increasing [72]. Possible explanations for the lack of an effect of self-monitoring of blood glucoses include the following:
- patients receive little or no feedback on their results;
- patients are not taught the self-management skills required to lower the measured glucose values;
- the actual timing of blood glucose monitoring may affect the educational component of testing.

Measuring the fasting blood glucose concentration (when an individual wakes in the morning) or pre-prandially (before meals), rather than post-prandially (after meals), serves neither to educate (there is no information on the effect of meal composition or size) nor to motivate the individual effectively (post-prandial values are much higher) [73].

In contrast to self-monitoring of blood glucose, self-monitoring of oral anticoagulation, which is less widely adopted, clearly reduces the risk of thromboembolism and mortality [4]. Several factors account for this apparent improvement. Patients receive constant feedback about whether they are within the narrow control limits that occur when measuring the INR (see Chapter 17) and receive frequent dosage adjustments in response to monitoring, demonstrating the value of self-monitoring. This feedback also has the potential to educate patients about what factors may or may not affect fluctuations in the INR. Self-regulators may also benefit from this feedback, learning when to adjust appropriately or not adjust, and they can relate this to the magnitude of the deviance from the INR range.

One problem in experimentally assessing the impact of self-monitoring as a procedure is that the self-monitoring group receives intensive training at the outset, which is often absent from control groups. To allow for this confounding factor, one trial of self-monitoring of oral anticoagulation gave self-monitoring training to all participants and then randomized individuals to self-monitoring or control. This showed the benefits of self-monitoring—patients in the self-monitoring group reported higher treatment satisfaction, less distress and less strain on their social networks than those in the control group [74].

A clear distinction needs to be made between the different purposes of self-monitoring, for example, to increase medication adherence or adjust dosages, to use as an educational tool to help self-regulation, or to change a targeted behaviour. If self-monitoring is used to change behaviour, it is important to monitor behaviour rather than symptoms. This has been shown in a controlled trial of asthma self-management [75]. Those who were assigned to self-monitoring peak expiratory flow rate (PEFR) performed better than those who were assigned to symptom monitoring, in that they took appropriate action (e.g. use of medication), as required by their management plans. The data collected by PEFR monitoring can be charted and statistically analysed to identify significant changes, reasons for changes, and those at risk, allowing for decision-making and care to be provided in an anticipatory manner [76].

Monitoring allows assessment of the acceptability and effectiveness of medication or other interventions in individuals. This can be done using rigorous scientific designs, by comparing them with a placebo or alternative interventions in multiple crossover trials with people serving as their own controls. These have been referred to as 'within-person randomized controlled trials', 'n-of-1' trials and 'personalized treatment assessments' (PTAs) [77–81]. This approach has the advantages of recognizing individual variation in response to medical and other health interventions and of facilitating patients' involvement in treatment decisions [12]. Individual differences and generalizability across person and setting can be assessed by multiple n-of-1 trials.

Within-person randomized controlled trials can also be used to investigate causal associations between variables, such as symptoms, behaviours, internal states such as pain or stress, and environmental events [77, 82]. Theories of change can be tested, an important step for guiding effective interventions.

10.5. Conclusions

Monitoring provides a wealth of information in and out of the clinical context. We know that patients want more information about their disease; monitoring allows them to receive feedback about their health status. Monitoring involves giving health professionals and/or patients systematic information over time so that they can ascertain whether there is an improvement, a deterioration or no change in key health or illness indicators. Monitoring can be considered as both an assessment tool and an intervention technique. It has the potential to motivate people to adhere to treatment regimens and to provide information about possible extrinsic and intrinsic factors that influence health, which may suggest improvements in the management plan. Monitoring provides a sense of control over symptoms and underlying health and fosters a collaborative problem-solving approach to managing ill-health.

These advantages must be considered in parallel with the possible worry and doubt that monitoring can cause. For example, patients who see the purpose of monitoring to detect disease feel less confident about their results and feel more vulnerable to the monitored disease than those who consider the purpose to be to detect wellness. The way in which monitored information is provided to patients can affect its impact on their behaviour, for example giving categorical rather than probabilistic information, framing the process as detecting signs of progress towards a health goal rather than avoiding illness and engendering confidence in the monitoring tests. Individuals also vary in their responses to monitoring; some find it reassuring and others become more anxious.

Thus, while monitoring is a potentially powerful technique in delivering effective health care, clinicians should also monitor its impact on individual patients and adjust their practices to maximize the benefits of monitoring and minimize its adverse effects.

Acknowledgements

This work was supported in part by an Australian National Health and Medical Research Council (NHMRC) grant 211205 to the Screening and Test Evaluation Program. We thank Aimee Hadert for providing us with references to evidence about the effectiveness of self-monitoring. Susan Michie is supported by the MRC Health Services Research Collaboration.

References

1 Lowy C. A memorable patient. Home glucose monitoring, who started it? *BMJ* 1998; **316**: 1467.

2 Cappuccio FP, Kerry SM, Forbes L, Donald A. Blood pressure control by home monitoring: meta-analysis of randomised trials. *BMJ* 2004; **329**: 145–8.

3 Thoonen BP, Schermer TR, Van Den Boom G, et al. Self-management of asthma in general practice, asthma control and quality of life: a randomised controlled trial. *Thorax* 2003; **58**: 30–6.

4 Heneghan C, Alonso-Coello P, Garcia-Alamino JM, Perera R, Meats E, Glasziou P. Self-monitoring of oral anticoagulation: a systematic review and meta-analysis. *Lancet* 2006; **367**: 404–11.

5 Coulter A. Patient information and shared decision-making in cancer care. *Br J Cancer* 2003; **89** (Suppl): S15–S16.

6 Davey HM, Barratt AL, Davey E, et al. Medical tests: women's reported and preferred decision-making roles and preferences for information on benefits, side-effects and false results. *Health Expect* 2002; **5**: 330–40.

7 Feldman-Stewart D, Brundage MD, Hayter C, et al. What questions do patients with curable prostate cancer want answered? *Med Decis Making* 2000; **20**: 7–19.

8 Krohne HW. The concept of coping modes: relating cognitive person variables to actual coping behaviour. *Adv Behav Res Ther* 1989; **11**: 235–48.

9 Miller SM. To see or not to see. Cognitive informational styles in the coping process. In: Rosenbaum M (ed), *Learned Resourcefulness*. New York: Springer, 1991, pp. 95–126.

10 Lazarus RS, Folkman S. *Stress, Appraisal and Coping*. New York: Springer, 1984.

11 Shiloh S, Orgler-Shoob M. Monitoring: a dual process coping style. *J Pers* 2006; **74**: 457–78.

12 Cioffi D. Asymmetry of doubt in medical self-diagnosis: the ambiguity of 'uncertain wellness'. *J Pers Soc Psychol* 1991; **61**: 969–80.

13 World Health Organization. Adherence to long-term therapies. In: *Evidence for Action*. Geneva: World Health Organization, 2003.

14 Wilson W, Ary DV, Biglan A, Glasgow RE, Toobert DJ, Campbell DR. Psychosocial predictors of self-care behaviors (compliance) and glycemic control in non-insulin dependent diabetes mellitus. *Diabetes Care* 1986; **9**: 614–22.

15 Wagner JA, Schnoll RA, Gipson MT. Development of a scale to measure adherence to self-monitoring of blood glucose with latent variable measurement. *Diabetes Care* 1998; **21**: 1046–51.

16 Glasgow RE, Toobert DJ, Riddle M, Donnelly J, Mitchell DL, Calder D. Diabetes-specific social learning variables and self-care behaviors among persons with type II diabetes. *Health Psychol* 1989; **8**: 285–303.

17 Gibson PG, Powell H, Coughlan J, et al. Self-management education and regular practitioner review for adults with asthma. *Cochrane Database Syst Rev* 2003; (1): CD001117.

18 Sawyer SM. Action plans, self-monitoring and adherence: changing behaviour to promote better self-management. *Med J Aust* 2002; **177**:S72–S74.

19 Wensley D, Silverman M. Peak flow monitoring for guided self-management in childhood asthma: a randomized controlled trial. *Am J Respir Crit Care Med* 2004; **170**: 606–12.

20 Gigerenzer G. *Reckoning with Risk*. London: Penguin, 2002.

21 Wertz DC, Sorenson JC, Heeren TR. Clients' interpretations of risks provided in genetic counselling. *Am J Hum Genet* 1986; **39**: 253–64.

22 Michie S, Lester K, Pinto J, Marteau TM. Communicating risk information in genetic counseling: an observational study. *Health Educ Res* 2005; **32**: 589–98.

23 Channer KS, James MA, Papouchado M, Rees JR. Failure of a negative exercise test to reassure patients with chest pain. *Q J Med* 1987; **63**: 315–22.

24 Lucock MP, White C, Peake MD, Morley S. Biased perception and recall of reassurance in medical patients. *Br J Health Psychol* 1998; **3**: 237–43.

25 Fitzmaurice DA, Hobbs RD, Murray JA. Monitoring oral anticoagulation in primary care. *BMJ* 1996; **312**: 1431–2.

26 Korotitsch WJ, Nelson-Gray RO. An overview of self-monitoring research in assessment and treatment. *Psychol Assess* 1999; **11**: 415–25.

27 Hayes SC, Cavior N. Multiple tracking and the reactivity of self-monitoring: I. Negative behaviours. *Behav Ther* 1977; **8**: 819–31.

28 Hayes SC, Cavior N. Multiple tracking and the reactivity of self-monitoring: II. Positive behaviours. *Behav Assess* 1980; **2**: 283–96.

29 Lipinski DP, Black JL, Nelson RO, Ciminero AR. The influence of motivational variables on the reactivity and the reliability of self-recording. *J Consult Clin Psychol* 1975; **43**: 637–46.

30 Mahoney MJ. Some applied issues in self-monitoring. In: Cone CD, Hawkins RP (eds), *Behavioral Assessment: New Directions in Clinical Psychology*. New York: Brunner/Mazel, 1977, pp. 241–54.

31 Waller J, McCaffery KJ, Kitchener H, Nazroo JN, Wardle J. Women's experiences of repeated HPV testing in the context of cervical screening: a qualitative study. *Psychooncology* 2007; **16**: 196–204.

32 Jones MH, Singer A, Jenkins D. The mildly abnormal cervical smear: patient anxiety and choice of management. *J R Soc Med* 1996; **89**: 257–60.

33 Charles C, Gafni A, Whelan T. Shared decision-making in the medical encounter: what does it mean? (Or it takes at least two to tango). *Soc Sci Med* 1997; **44**: 681–92.

34 Whitney SN, McGuire AL, McCullough LB. A typology of shared decision making, informed consent, and simple consent. *Ann Intern Med* 2004; **140**: 54–9.

35 Michie S, Miles J, Weinman J. Patient-centredness in chronic illness: what is it and does it matter? *Patient Educ Couns* 2003; **51**: 197–206.

36 Guerci B, Drouin P, Grange V, et al.; ASIA Group. Self-monitoring of blood glucose significantly improves metabolic control in patients with type 2 diabetes mellitus: the Auto-Surveillance Intervention Active (ASIA) study. *Diabetes Metab* 2003; **29**: 587–94.

37 Lavery LA, Higgins KR, Lanctôt DR, et al. Home monitoring of foot skin temperatures to prevent ulceration. *Diabetes Care* 2004; **27**: 2642–7.

38 Craig KE. Self-observation in natural environments: reactive effects of behavior desirability and goal-setting. *Cogn Ther Res* 1978; **2**: 39–56.

39 Kazdin AE. Reactive self-monitoring: the effects of response desirability, goal setting, and feedback. *J Consult Clin Psychol* 1974; **42**: 704–16.

40 Fremouw WJ, Brown JP, Jr. The reactivity of addictive behaviors to self-monitoring: a functional analysis. *Addict Behav* 1980; **5**: 209–17.

41 Sieck WA, McFall RM. Some determinants of self-monitoring effects. *J Consult Clin Psychol* 1976; **44**: 958–65.

42 Kruger J, Blanck HM, Gillespie C. Dietary and physical activity behaviors among adults successful at weight loss maintenance. *Int J Behav Nutr Phys Act* 2006; **3**: 17.

43 Labib M. The investigation and management of obesity. *J Clin Pathol* 2003; **56** (1): 17–25.

44 Sieck WA, McFall RM. Some determinants of self-monitoring effects. *J Consult Clin Psychol* 1976 December; **44** (6): 958–65.

45 Halme L, Vesalainen R, Kaaja M, Kantola I. Self-monitoring of blood pressure promotes achievement of blood pressure target in primary health care. *Am J Hypertens* 2005; **18**: 1415–20.

46 Febbraro GAR, Clum GA. Meta-analytic investigation of the effectiveness of self-regulatory components in the treatment of adult problems behaviors. *Clin Psychol Rev* 1998; **18**: 143–61.

47 Steven AH, Dennis LW, Gail AH. Effects of expectancy of outcome on the reactivity of self-monitoring. *J Psychopathol Behav Assess* 1979; **1**: 281–8.

48 Mace FC, Shapiro ES, West BJ, Campbell C, Altman J. The role of reinforcement in reactive self-monitoring. *Appl Res Ment Retard* 1986; **7**: 315–27.

49 Lagarde WH, Barrows FP, Davenport ML, Kang M, Guess HA, Calikoglu AS. Continuous subcutaneous glucose monitoring in children with type 1 diabetes mellitus: a single-blind, randomized, controlled trial. *Pediatr Diabetes* 2006; **7**: 159–64.

50 Frederiksen L-W, Epstein L-H, Kosevsky B-P. Reliability and controlling effects of three procedures for self-monitoring smoking. *Psychol Rec* 1963; **25**: 255–63.

51 Labib M. The investigation and management of obesity. *J Clin Pathol* 2003; **56**: 17–25.

52 Scheier MF, Carver CS. Goals and confidence as self-regulatory elements underlying health and illness behaviour. In: Cameron LD, Leventhal H (eds), *The Self-Regulation of Health and Illness Behaviour*. London: Taylor Francis, 2003.

53 Bandura A. Health promotion from the perspective of social cognitive theory. In: Norman P, Abraham C, Conner M (eds), *Understanding and Changing Behaviour*. Amsterdam: Harwood Academic, 2000.

54 Leventhal H, Brissette I, Leventhal EA. The common-sense model of self-regulation of health and illness. In: Cameron LD, Leventhal H (eds), *The Self-Regulation of Health and Illness Behaviour*. London: Routledge, 2003.

55 Kaptein AA, Scharloo M, Helder DI, Kleijn WC, van Korlaar IM, Woertman M. Representations of chronic illness. In: Cameron LD, Leventhal H (eds), *The Self-Regulation of Health and Illness Behaviour*. London: Routledge, 2003.

56 Michie S, Weinman J, Miller J, Colins V, Halliday J, Marteau TM. Predictive genetic testing: high risk expectations in the face of low risk information. *J Behav Med* 2002; **25**: 33–50.

57 Michie S, Smith J, Senior B, Marteau TM. Understanding why negative test results sometimes fail to reassure. *Am J Med Genet* 2003; **119A**: 340–7.

58 Skinner BF. *Science of Human Behavior*. New York: Free Press, 1953.

59 Nemeroff CJ, Karoly P. Operant methods. In: Kanfer FH, Goldstein AP (eds), *Helping People Change: A Textbook of Methods*. London: Allyn and Bacon, 1991.

60 Van Walraven C, Naylor CD. Do we know what inappropriate laboratory utilization is? A systematic review of laboratory clinical audits. *JAMA* 1998; **280**: 550–8.

61 Walley T, Duggan AK, Haycox AR, Niziol CJ. Treatment for newly diagnosed hypertension: patterns of prescribing and antihypertensive effectiveness in the UK. *J R Soc Med* 2003; **96**: 525–31.

62 Sterne JA, Juni P, Schulz KF, Altman DG, Bartlett C, Egger M. Statistical methods for assessing the influence of study characteristics on treatment effects in 'meta-epidemiological' research. *Stat Med* 2002; **21**: 1513–24.

63 Kahan BD, Keown P, Levy GA, Johnston A. Therapeutic drug monitoring of immunosuppressant drugs in clinical practice. *Clin Ther* 2002; **24**: 330–50.

64 Preskorn SH, Jerkovich GS. Central nervous system toxicity of tricyclic antidepressants: phenomenology, course risk factors, and the role of therapeutic drug monitoring. *J Clin Psychopharmacol* 1991; **10**: 88–95.

65 Raebel MA, Lyons EE, Chester EA, et al. Improving laboratory monitoring at initiation of drug therapy in ambulatory care: a randomized trial. *Arch Intern Med* 2005; **165**: 2395–401.

66 Grimshaw JM, Thomas RE, MacLennan G, et al. Effectiveness and efficiency of guideline dissemination and implementation strategies. *Health Technol Assess* 2004; **8**: 1–72.

67 Fahey T, Schroeder K, Ebrahim S. Interventions used to improve control of blood pressure in patients with hypertension. *Cochrane Database Syst Rev* 2006; **19** (2): CD005182.

68 Forrest S, McCaffery KJ, Waller J, Desai M, Swarewski A, Wardle J. Attitudes to self-sampling among Indian, Pakistani, African Caribbean and White British women in Manchester. *J Med Screen* 2004; **11**: 85–8.

69 Sunderji R, Gin K, Shalansky K, et al. A randomized control trial of patient self-managed versus physical-managed oral anticoagulation. *Can J Cardiol* 2004; **20**: 1117–23.

70 Horstkotte D, Piper C, Wiemer M. Optimal frequency of patient monitoring and intensity of oral anticoagulation therapy in valvular heart disease. *J Thromb Thrombolysis* 1998; **3** (Suppl 1): 19–24.

71 Gallichan MJ. Self-monitoring by patients receiving oral hypoglycaemic agents: a survey and a comparative trial. *Pract Diabetes* 1994; **11**: 28–30.

72 The Diabetes Control and Complications Trial Research Group. The effect of intensive treatment of diabetes on the development and progression of long-term complications in insulin-dependent diabetes mellitus. *N Engl J Med* 1993; **329**: 977–86.

73 Davidson MB. Counterpoint. Self-monitoring of blood glucose in type 2 diabetes patients not receiving insulin: a waste of money. *Diabetes Care* 2005; **28**: 1531–3.

74 Gadisseur AP, Kaptein AA, Breukink-Engbers WG, van der Meer FJ, Rosendaal FR. Patient self-management of oral anticoagulant care vs. management by specialized anticoagulation clinics: positive effects on quality of life. *J Thromb Haemost* 2004; **2**: 584–91.

75 Bheekie A, Syce JA, Weinberg EG. Peak expiratory flow rate and symptom self-monitoring of asthma initiated from community pharmacies. *J Clin Pharm Ther* 2001; **26**: 287–96.

76 Boggs PB, Wheeler D, Washburne WF, Hayati F. Peak expiratory flow rate control chart in asthma care: chart construction and use in asthma care. *Ann Allergy Asthma Immunol* 1998; **81**: 552–62.

77 March L, Irwig L, Schwartz J, Simpson J, Chock C, Brooks P. N of 1 trials comparing a non-steroidal anti-inflammatory drug with paracetamol in osteoarthritis. *BMJ* 1994; **309**: 1041–5.

78 Sheather-Reid RB, Cohen ML. Psychophysical evidence for a neuropathic component of chronic neck pain. *Pain* 1998; **75**: 341–7.

79 Haines DR, Gaines SP. N of 1 randomized controlled trials of oral ketamine in patients with chronic pain. *Pain* 1999; **83**: 283–7.

80 Wegman AC, van der Windt DA, de Haan M, Deville WL, Fo CT, de Vries TP. Switching from NSAIDs to paracetamol: a series of n of 1 trials for individual patients with osteoarthritis. *Ann Rheum Dis* 2003; **62**: 1156–61.

81 Woodfield R, Goodyear-Smith F, Arroll B. N of 1 trials of quinine efficacy in skeletal muscle cramps of the leg. *Br J Gen Pract* 2005; **55**: 181–5.

82 Nikles CJ, Glasziou PP, Del Mar CB, Duggan CM, Clavarino A, Yelland MJ. Preliminary experiences with a single-patient trials service in general practice. *Med J Aust* 2000; **173**: 100–3.

CHAPTER 11

Monitoring from the patient's perspective: the social and psychological implications

Kirsten McCaffery, Susan Michie

In this chapter, we describe the social and psychological factors that influence the patient through the process of monitoring and identify areas in which further research is needed. We discuss some of the social and psychological benefits and harms of monitoring, patients' preferences for different monitoring regimens, and the application of shared decision-making and decision-support tools in this area. We also consider approaches to optimize adherence to agreed monitoring strategies and methods of measuring social and psychological outcomes.

11.1. The social and psychological effects of monitoring

11.1.1. What is meant by social and psychological outcomes?

Social and psychological outcomes cover a range of factors relating to the everyday well-being of the patient. Social outcomes relate to the individual's position and functioning within social settings, such as family, work environment and community. This includes social relationships, social roles and factors such as social stigma and identity. Psychological outcomes include patients' individual cognitions about their health and well-being, such as their attitudes, beliefs, perceptions and values about events or outcomes. They include patients' emotional responses, such as anxiety, depression, fear or happiness. Patient behaviour is also included under psychological outcomes. Behaviour may be directly related to the monitoring condition (e.g. dietary practices among diabetics) but may also include behaviours that appear to be unrelated to the medical condition being monitored; for example, women may exercise more after an abnormal Pap smear result. Behaviour includes adherence to recommended health advice and the monitoring schedule itself, for example

Evidence-based Medical Monitoring: from Principles to Practice. Edited by Paul Glasziou, Les Irwig and Jeffrey K. Aronson. © 2008 Blackwell Publishing, ISBN: 978-1-4051-5399-7.

attendance for repeated tests or following a recommended dosage regimen
[1]. Quality of life (QOL) is often included in monitoring studies. Although its
definition varies, it generally incorporates social and emotional constructs in
addition to physical function and somatic sensations [1, 2].

11.1.2. Characteristics of monitoring and the role of social and psychological factors

Monitoring strategies for different chronic conditions vary enormously. Some
strategies may be entirely clinician led with little responsibility or control given
to the patient. In other conditions, patients can take total responsibility for
their own testing or assessment (self-monitoring) and can adjust medication
or therapy according to their results without direct input from a clinician.

Monitoring is made up of different phases, which may have different psychological and social implications for the patient. Initiating monitoring involves the establishment of the monitoring schedule. It includes decisions
between the patient and the clinician about whether to monitor and how to
monitor, identifying patient preferences, acquiring knowledge and skills, and
adapting to a new regimen, which may have both positive and negative social
and psychological effects. Maintaining monitoring involves incorporating repeated assessment into an individual's lifestyle and requires them to sustain
complex behaviours over time. This may require important long-term social
and psychological changes.

Applying monitoring schedules that fail to meet the social and psychological
needs of patients can lead to poor adherence to health advice. Such behaviour
can have a substantial impact on patient health and QOL [3], which benefits
neither the patient nor the provider.

11.2. Social and psychological benefits and harms of monitoring

Monitoring strategies have different benefits and harms for the patient. Often these may be diverse and difficult to predict and may appear to be only
indirectly related to the monitoring strategy and primary illness. Individual
patients will also value the same benefits and harms differently.

11.2.1. Benefits and harms of monitoring

A wide range of benefits and harms have been associated with different monitoring regimens, but there appears to be little consistent pattern—the effects
vary, depending on the condition being monitored and the monitoring technique. A systematic review is needed for a more thorough understanding and
to determine whether there are underlying similarities across conditions and
monitoring regimens. The most convincing studies have used randomized designs. Other studies have been observational, cross-sectional or qualitative and
provide valuable insights for understanding monitoring but require further

Table 11.1 Some benefits and harms associated with monitoring

Effects of monitoring	Condition
Benefits	
Increased self-efficacy	*Self-management + counselling in patients with diabetes mellitus [4]
Reassurance	HPV testing in cervical screening [5]
Motivation	Weight management/obesity [6]
Reduced depression	*Self-management + counselling in patients with diabetes [4]
Increased QOL	*Meal-related self-monitoring in patients with diabetes [7]
Increased satisfaction	*Self-management of oral anticoagulant care [8]
Reduced distress	*Self-management of oral anticoagulant care [8]
Reduced strain on social networks	*Self-management of oral anticoagulant care [8]
Harms	
Increased absence from work	Blood pressure measurement for hypertension [9]
Stigma	HIV [12], HPV testing in cervical screening [5, 10–11]
Anxiety	HPV testing in cervical screening [5, 10, 11]
Reduced self-esteem	*Weight management/obesity [13, 14]
Negative impact on mood/affect	*Weight management/obesity [13, 14]
Body dissatisfaction	Weight management/obesity [15]
Fear about disclosing illness to others, being identified as ill or being infected by others	HIV [12], HPV testing in cervical screening [11]
Negative impact on sexual relationships	HPV testing in cervical screening [10, 11]
Desire to continue unnecessary monitoring	Familial adenomatous polyposis [17], cervical screening [16]
Increased discomfort, sleep disturbance	*Ambulatory blood pressure monitoring for hypertension [18, 19]
Reduced motivation after negative results	Weight management/obesity, diabetes [20, 21]

Note: *Randomized controlled trials.

testing to determine their exact role. Some of these findings are highlighted below and are summarized in Table 11.1.

Benefits associated with self-monitoring compared with clinician-led regimens include enhancing the patient's sense of self-efficacy and control [4, 7]. Increased satisfaction and well-being, reduced distress, depression and strain on social networks have also been associated with self-monitoring compared with controls [4, 7]. Some self-monitoring techniques are perceived as being more convenient, less hassle, more hygienic, and more private than their alternatives [22, 23]. For example, self-management programmes for oral anticoagulant care increase QOL and reduce depression [8].

Repeated testing or measurement can provide patients with additional reassurance, and give information about progress or decline to provide feedback to motivate and support behaviour change [24]. In weight management/obesity, frequent weight monitoring is the most successful strategy for weight loss and is recommended for dieters, in order to motivate and maintain behaviour change [6, 25]. Monitoring can also bring benefits by providing an opportunity for patients to obtain further information, advice and clarification from the clinician, and can impart a sense of reassurance, safety and support [5].

Research on the potential harms of monitoring has assessed its impact on the labelling of people as being unwell, with the suggestion that it can lead to illness behaviours, such as increased GP visits and absence from work, and to diagnoses of other illness. However, the findings have been conflicting: one study showed an increase in absenteeism after the detection of hypertension [3], while other studies have shown no effects on sick leave or other illness behaviours [26, 27].

The frequency of monitoring has been examined in the area of obesity/weight management, and more frequent weight monitoring (daily weighing versus weekly weighing) is linked to negative mood, reduced self-esteem and body dissatisfaction [13]. When weight measurement results were 'bad news' for chronic dieters (those who dieted for long periods), the negative impact on mood and self-worth was greatest, and this group was at highest risk of attrition [20, 21]. This research provides insights into the psychological and behavioural effects of monitoring when frequent negative results can dishearten and demotivate the patient [15].

Monitoring can lead to high degrees of anxiety, with the repeated experience of uncertainty and distress about testing and waiting for results [5]. There can be stigma from the persistent labelling of infection and the need for repeated attendance for medical checks [10–12]. Some forms of monitoring and medical management act as unwanted reminders of illness and elicit fears among patients that their illness status will be revealed to others [28–30]. Similarly, repeated testing can increase the pressure to disclose test results or illness status to others, when it is undesired [5, 28–30]. Monitoring of cervical abnormalities using human papilloma virus (HPV) testing negatively affects patients' relationships with their partners and family by reminding them that they are infected, enhancing feelings of anxiety, guilt and shame [5, 10–12]. Further negative effects of monitoring include the desire to continue unnecessary monitoring despite evidence of a lack of benefit [16, 17, 31]. Monitoring when it is not required can cause patients unnecessary discomfort, expose them to risks of further investigation and treatments, and waste patient and provider resources.

Psychological processes can mediate how benefits and harms are interpreted and managed by the patient. The process of minimization is a common response for adapting and coping with threatening health information. It can help to manage anxiety and other negative emotional responses in the short term but can result in subsequent failure to respond appropriately to a health threat [32]. Similarly, emotion-focused coping strategies, such as avoidance or denial [33], can help to reduce initial negative psychological effects but can be detrimental if they prevent engagement in risk-reducing health behaviours in the long term.

11.2.2. The functions of monitoring as perceived by the patient

Understanding the broad range of perceived functions that monitoring can serve patients is important in developing monitoring schedules that are clinically appropriate and meet patients' needs. Patients actively seek to make sense of their conditions and to understand the best way to manage them, and their views may or may not fit with the medical approach to management.

Research among patients with hypertension showed that monitoring was used by patients to test the efficacy of their medication [30, 34]. Similarly, patients with HIV infection discarded monitoring results and medical advice that did not match their own subjective experiences. Patients with improved T cell counts or viral loads discounted test results when subjectively they felt worse [35–38]. This phenomenon has been described as 'naive scientist' behaviour [35, 38], whereby patients form hypotheses about their illness, medication and management, and find means to test them.

Monitoring can also serve functions that can be difficult to predict and identify. For example, a qualitative study of adults at high risk of colorectal cancer undergoing annual colonoscopy screening showed that testing served a social function, bringing family members closer together to experience a shared event, which was highly valued by some adults [39]. In the same study, patients were found to distrust negative genetic test results and favoured repeated colonoscopy, since this method of monitoring was perceived as being more understandable and concrete for the detection of polyps and the prevention of colorectal cancer. In another study, some women's strong preference for annual Pap testing, despite recommendations for biennial testing, was explained by the desire to use the Pap smear as an opportunity to obtain an annual internal examination and gynaecological check [16]. People may choose or prefer certain monitoring regimens for reasons that are unrelated to the primary aim of the clinical management.

11.3. Adopting a shared decision-making approach in monitoring

The need to involve patients in decisions about their health care is now widely recognized [40–42]. For chronic conditions that require repeated testing and sustained behaviour change, it may be particularly important. Quality care involves giving patients evidence-based information about the different options that are available, identifying their values and preferences, and incorporating them into decision-making [43]. This has been termed shared decision-making and is similar to the concept of patient-centred care. Patients have a strong desire to be involved in health-care decisions [44, 45]. A shared approach can lead to better outcomes for the patient, including increased knowledge of the options, more realistic expectations of outcomes, reduced uncertainty about decision-making, greater satisfaction and in some cases better adherence to management [46–49].

Shared decision-making recognizes that patients have different preferences. Some may be willing to tolerate a lot of adverse effects for a relatively small benefit whereas others only tolerate minimal adverse effects for a large potential gain. Some value early monitoring or increased frequency of monitoring over less intensive assessment schedules. Determining the patient's individual preference for monitoring and eliciting their values of the benefits and harms is an important part of deciding when and how to monitor. Clinicians are poor at predicting their patient's preference and there is evidence that patients and clinicians value treatment outcomes differently [50, 51].

11.3.1. Identifying patient preferences and incorporating them into monitoring decisions

Patient preferences for the type or frequency of monitoring can be guided by overall preferences collected among a representative sample or, when possible, by giving individual patients a choice and matching their care to their preference.

Patients' perceptions of and preferences for monitoring are embedded within their understanding of and attitudes towards their chronic condition. For monitoring abnormalities found on Pap smears, anxiety levels were higher in women who were randomized to colposcopy follow-up than in those randomized to repeat Pap testing [52]; however, 70% of women in each arm stated that they would prefer colposcopy. Similar findings were reported among women with persistent HPV infection [5]. Women favoured immediate colposcopy, which was explained by a strong preference for early resolution and treatment in preference to an anxious wait for 12 months for repeat testing. Preference for early management was also related to beliefs about HPV and cervical cancer, including an exaggerated perception of cancer risk and rate of progression, and a lack of understanding of the high probability that HPV would regress over time.

Few studies have elicited patient preferences for monitoring and matched patients to their preferred approach. In one trial, women who were matched to their preference for either immediate colposcopy or repeated Pap testing were compared with women who had been randomly allocated to either management [53]. There was more anxiety at baseline among the women who selected colposcopy, which suggests that the option to choose earlier management may have short-term beneficial effects in very anxious women. There were no differences in psychological well-being at follow-up. However, measures were taken at 12 months only, and given that psychological effects of most testing/screening procedures disappear after 6 months, this finding is not surprising [54]. It is not known whether matching patients to their preferences confers any psychological benefits.

11.3.2. Strategies to involve patients in decisions about monitoring

Decision aids are tools that have been developed to involve patients in the decision process and to support shared decision-making. A decision aid provides evidence-based information on the clinical options and outcomes that are relevant to a person's health. They are explicit about choices and encourage patients to express their clinical preferences [55]. Although decision aids vary, there is general consensus [56] that tools should be

- explicitly evidence-based in content, format and design;
- balanced in presentation of options and information;
- evaluated by experts for methodology;
- evaluated with patients for efficacy.

A systematic review of over 30 decision aids [46] has suggested that they increase patient knowledge, involvement in the decision-making process, and agreement between values and choice; they create more realistic expectations and reduce uncertainty in decision-making (decisional conflict). To date no published decision aids have been developed and tested explicitly for use in monitoring. A decision aid trial among women at high risk of ovarian cancer offered them a choice of different management options, including annual surveillance, watchful waiting, medication or prophylactic surgery, supported by a decision aid or usual care information [57]. There was no difference in the choice of management between the two groups and psychological outcomes (anxiety and depression) were also similar. However, the women in the decision aid arm had greater knowledge and lower decisional conflict than the controls.

Giving patients clear evidence-based information on the benefits and harms of different monitoring schedules and supporting them in selecting their preferred approach should lead to the use of monitoring strategies that are better matched to patients' needs, which may translate into better outcomes.

11.4. Patient adherence to agreed monitoring regimens and health-care advice

Poor adherence to beneficial therapy is associated with poor health outcomes [3]. This can be particularly significant for surveillance and management of chronic conditions. Poor adherence has been cited as the 'primary reason for suboptimal clinical benefit', causing the patient 'medical (and) psychosocial complications' [58]. Problems of adherence have been demonstrated repeatedly across many disease types, management regimens and population groups [59]. In a review of chronic life-threatening conditions, it was estimated that mean adherence was around 50% [60] with even lower estimates for developing countries [58].

11.4.1. Understanding adherence

Adherence has been defined as the extent to which the patient follows medical instructions [61]. Concordance, a relatively new term, acknowledges the need for an agreement about management between the patient and the practitioner [62]. This concept incorporates the principles of shared decision-making and patient-centred care. In this chapter, we use the term 'adherence' with the understanding that it reflects a patient's ability to follow medical advice once agreement has been reached. Decision aids, as discussed above, are tools that can support this process.

Adherence to monitoring regimens is often complex and demanding for the patient, since it requires repeated behaviours over an extended period of time, sometimes with little immediately perceptible reward. A range of factors influence patient adherence to health advice. Adherence is more difficult when an illness is asymptomatic or characterized by episodic or recurrent symptoms. It is also lower when a medication regimen is complex or time intensive or requires substantial change in behaviour [29, 63].

Reasons for poor adherence can be highly specific to the clinical context and require an understanding of how people perceive their illness and therapy and their emotional responses to both. Patients form their own implicit model of their illness, referred to as 'illness perceptions' or 'illness representations', which guide their responses, for example whether and how they take prescribed medications and whether they adhere to medical advice, as described in self-regulation theory [64] (see Chapter 10). This 'common-sense model' includes both cognitive and emotional dimensions. The cognitive component incorporates the patient's perception of the seriousness of the disease, interpretation of symptoms, its likely duration, the personal consequences and its potential for control or cure. The emotional component incorporates emotional responses to illness, such as fear, anxiety or depression.

A standardized measure to assess illness perceptions across a range of illnesses has been developed. The original questionnaire, the Illness Perceptions Questionnaire (IPQ) [65], has been superseded by the revised IPQ-R [66], which includes additional dimensions of and emotion. More recently, a brief nine-item version of the questionnaire has been developed [67]. Perceptions of illness as measured by the IPQ have been related to adherence behaviour in a range of chronic illnesses, including hypertension [68], diabetes [69] and HIV infection [70]. Patients have similar perceptions about medications, and these have also been associated with adherence behaviour in chronic disease [71–74]

11.4.2. Variation in adherence

Reviews of adherence behaviour suggest that most non-adherence is due to omissions of doses, rather than additional doses or delays in the timing of doses [75, 76]. Patients also commonly have better adherence in the 5 days before and after an appointment with their health-care provider than 30 days after; this is known as 'white coat adherence' [77, 78]. Patients' sociodemographic characteristics, such as age, sex and ethnicity, have been inconsistently associated with adherence. However, poor literacy is linked to poor adherence and poor health outcomes in diabetes and asthma [79–81]. Patients with poor literacy often find it difficult to understand the language used by health providers, to follow written instructions and to use reminders. They often fail to report reading difficulties owing to embarrassment, shame and stigma. Patients with psychiatric illnesses are also particularly poor at adhering to medical regimens: 50% of patients with major depression are non-adherent to their medication within 3 months of starting therapy [82]. Monitoring these groups can therefore be particularly difficult and require intensive strategies to maintain adherence.

Clinicians contribute to poor adherence by prescribing complex regimens, failing to explain the benefits and adverse effects of medications adequately, ignoring the patient's lifestyle and costs of medications, and having a poor therapeutic relationship with their patients [59].

11.4.3. Strategies used to increasing adherence

Recent high-quality reviews include a Cochrane review of trials to increase adherence to medication [61] and a WHO publication on adherence to long-term therapies [58]. Their findings have applications for use in monitoring research and practice. The various strategies used to increase adherence can be considered in four general categories [59]:

- patient education;
- improved dosing schedules;
- increased access to the clinic and health-care provider (e.g. increased clinic opening hours and shorter waiting times);
- improved communication between patient and provider.

Successful methods of improving adherence are multifactorial, involving complex combinations of behavioural interventions, increasing the convenience of care, and providing education about the patient's condition, the recommended treatment and regimen to be followed [61, 83]. The diversity and complexity of interventions used to increase adherence make generalization difficult and even the best interventions do not lead to large improvements [61]. However, the following general factors are effective in improving patient adherence in practice:

- the use of simpler treatment regimens;
- recalling patients who miss appointments;
- the use of complex strategies to increase adherence, including combinations of
  - more thorough patient instructions,
  - provision of patient counselling,
  - reminders, and
  - close follow-up of patients.

In a more detailed review of studies in chronic illnesses (including asthma, hypertension, hyperlipidemia and HIV infection), interventions that reduced or simplified the dosages consistently improved adherence, with a large effect size (0.89–1.20) [83]. Although none of these particular studies included monitoring regimens per se, it is plausible that simplifying monitoring regimens may lead to similar improvements in adherence. The reviewers also found that the combination of monitoring and feedback was effective in improving medication adherence. Three studies combined self-monitoring with tailored feedback (either reinforcement or rewards) and showed significant improvements in adherence [83]. One study, which used monitoring strategies alone, did not report any impact on adherence to treatment [83], suggesting that feedback may be critical.

Despite a large body of literature, there is no magic bullet that improves adherence. This will present a continuing challenge in monitoring. Using alternative approaches to understanding patients' perspectives and drawing on different disciplines may be the best way forward [61]. Recent developments in the synthesis of qualitative findings look promising [84] and offer insights into patient behaviour that traditional quantitative research alone often cannot provide. Including patients in the development of interventions and tailoring techniques to individual needs may also provide more successful and sustainable strategies to improve adherence.

11.5. Measuring social and psychological outcomes of monitoring

We have outlined a range of social and psychological factors that can influence the patient during monitoring. However, data to inform a thorough understanding of this area are lacking, and as monitoring technologies develop and change, the need for research will continue to grow. Important social and psychological factors will need to be identified, measured, quantified and compared with alternative strategies.

11.5.1. Using qualitative methods to identify important social and psychological outcomes

Including qualitative methods of research is essential to understand the patient's perspective [85]. Interviews and focus groups can identify both outcomes and mediators, including cognitions that might influence well-being and adherence to monitoring schedules. In this formative research, it is important to include a wide range of people with respect to clinical characteristics, age, sex, ethnicity, social position and degree of adherence. This will enable a broad range of patients' perspectives to be elicited, which may be used to guide further quantitative or in-depth qualitative research [86]. Depending on the key areas identified, existing validated measures may be used for further quantitative assessment or new measures may need to be developed and validated.

11.5.2. Use of QOL measures

QOL measures have often been used in monitoring trials. The best known and validated generic measure designed to be applicable to patients with all medical conditions is the Medical Outcomes Survey Short Form (SF36) [1]. Although generic measures enable comparison of outcomes across different medical conditions, they may be unresponsive to small but important changes specific to certain conditions [87, 88]. They may also fail to capture the individual's sense of QOL because they are constrained to pre-selected domains.

To counteract some of these problems, disease-specific measures have been developed to incorporate the social, emotional and physical outcomes that are most important to the patient [83, 89, 90]. Individualized patient-generated measures have been developed to capture aspects of QOL that are most important to the individual at a given time (the patient-generated index [91, 92]), and may be more responsive to change than generic measures [98].

For QOL and other self-reported measures, a response shift can occur if patients adapt and reconceptualize the constructs they are rating or the metrics used to rate them [94–97]. An assessment of response shift may therefore be needed to obtain a valid and sensitive assessment of change over time, and methods to assess response shift have now been developed [96, 98, 99].

11.5.3. Measuring self-reported health and behavioural outcomes

It is common in monitoring research and practice to include self-reported measures of patient behaviour or physical health and function. In many cases this is the only way to assess certain outcomes, for example in chronic pain. The patient's psychological state influences self-reported monitoring outcomes [29]. In addition, self-reported outcomes can vary according to the patient's emotional state; for example, depression has been associated with higher pain ratings [100] and satisfaction influences the reporting of some behaviours [101].

There are also self-presentation biases, which influence self-reporting. If patients have a strong desire to be viewed positively they may alter self-reports, minimize symptoms and fail to report undesirable behaviours. Behaviour can be under-reported or over-reported, depending on the value associated with the behaviour [102]. If patients with pain believe that reduced reporting of symptoms will be rewarded, they report less pain [103]. Whenever possible, it is best to verify self-reported measures against objective measures. Options include the use of electronic counting devices, prescription refill rates and the use of physiological markers and biochemical measurements.

11.6. Conclusions: future directions

Social and psychological factors are important in making decisions about which monitoring strategies to use and will affect the success of any monitoring programme for the patient and the provider. Monitoring strategies should aim to minimize the psychological and social burden to the patient, and providers should seek to involve patients in decision-making whenever possible. Both patients and providers should seek ways to maximize adherence once a monitoring strategy has been agreed upon.

Further research that is needed includes the following:
- Identification of the social and psychological benefits and harms of monitoring and developing ways to quantify diverse effects. This will require the use of both qualitative and quantitative methods.
- Systematic reviews of the social and psychological effects of monitoring and the influence of various characteristics of monitoring (e.g. mode and frequency) on outcomes.
- Randomized comparisons of the social and psychological burdens of different monitoring strategies over the short, medium and long term.
- Developing ways to support shared decision-making in monitoring and comparisons of outcomes when patients are matched or not matched to their preferred monitoring strategy.
- Developing and testing strategies to maximize adherence to monitoring in partnership with patients.

Consideration of the broader context of monitoring is crucial to develop an effective approach. This requires understanding the patient's social, cognitive and emotional responses, not only to the monitoring regimen itself but to the condition and its therapy. The relations between these will affect the overall success of any monitoring strategy.

Acknowledgements

We should like to thank Dr Carl Heneghan, Professor Patrick Bossuyt and Dr Andrew Farmer for reading and commenting on earlier drafts of this chapter. This work was supported in part by an Australian National Health and Medical Research Council (NHMRC) grant 402764 to the Screening and Test Evaluation Program. Kirsten McCaffery is supported by an NHMRC Career Development Award Fellowship (no: 402836). Susan Michie is supported by the MRC Health Services Research Collaboration.

References

1 Ware JE, Jr, Sherbourne CD. The MOS 36-item short-form health survey (SF-36). I. Conceptual framework and item selection. *Med Care* 1992; **30**: 473–83.
2 Schipper H, Clinch J, Powell V. Definitions and conceptual issues. In: Spilker B (ed), *Quality of Life and Pharmacoeconomics in Clinical Trials*. Philadelphia: Lippincott-Raven, 1996, pp. 11–23.
3 Haynes RB, Dantes R. Patient compliance and the conduct and interpretation of therapeutic trials. *Control Clin Trials* 1987; **8**: 12–19.
4 Siebolds M, Gaedeke O, Schwedes U. Self-monitoring of blood glucose—psychological aspects relevant to changes in HbA1c in type 2 diabetic patients treated with diet or diet plus oral antidiabetic medication. *Patient Educ Couns* 2006; **62**: 104–10.

5 Waller J, McCaffery K, Kitchener H, Nazroo J, Wardle J. Women's experiences of repeated HPV testing in the context of cervical cancer screening: a qualitative study. *Psychooncology* 2007; **16**: 196–204.

6 Heinberg LJ, Thompson J, Matzon JL. Body image dissatisfaction as a motivator for healthy lifestyle change: is some distress beneficial? In: Striegel-Moore, Ruth H, Smolak L (eds), *Eating Disorders. Innovative Directions in Research and Practice*. Washington, DC: American Psychological Association, 2001, pp. 215–32.

7 Schwedes U, Siebolds M, Mertes G. Meal-related structured self-monitoring of blood glucose: effect on diabetes control in non-insulin-treated type 2 diabetic patients. *Diabetes Care* 2002; **25**: 1928–32.

8 Gadisseur AP, Kaptein AA, Breukink-Engbers WG, van der Meer FJ, Rosendaal FR. Patient self-management of oral anticoagulant care vs. management by specialized anticoagulation clinics: positive effects on quality of life. *J Thromb Haemost* 2004; **2**: 584–91.

9 Haynes RB, Sackett DL, Taylor DW, Gibson ES, Johnson AL. Increased absenteeism from work after detection and labeling of hypertensive patients. *N Engl J Med* 1978; **299**: 741–4.

10 McCaffery K, Waller J, Forrest S, Cadman L, Szarewski A, Wardle J. Testing positive for human papillomavirus in routine cervical screening: examination of psychosocial impact. *BJOG* 2004; **111**: 1437–43.

11 McCaffery K, Waller J, Nazroo J, Wardle J. Social and psychological impact of HPV testing in cervical screening: a qualitative study. *Sex Transm Infect* 2006; **82**: 169–74.

12 Safren SA, Kumarasamy N, Hosseinipour M, et al. Perceptions about the acceptability of assessments of HIV medication adherence in Lilongwe, Malawi and Chennai, India. *AIDS Behav* 2006; **10**: 443–50.

13 Ogden J, Evans C. The problem with weighing: effects on mood, self-esteem and body image. *Int J Obes Relat Metab Disord* 1996; **20**: 272–7.

14 Ogden J, Whyman C. The effect of repeated weighing on psychological state. *Eur Eat Disord Rev* 1997; **5**: 121–30.

15 Dionne MM, Yeudall F. Monitoring of weight in weight loss programs: a double-edged sword? *J Nutr Educ Behav* 2005; **37**: 315–8.

16 Sirovich BE, Woloshin S, Schwartz LM. Screening for cervical cancer: will women accept less? *Am J Med* 2005; **118**: 151–8.

17 Michie S, McDonald V, Marteau T. Understanding responses to predictive genetic testing: a grounded theory approach. *Psychol Health* 1996; **11**: 455–70.

18 Beltman FW, Heesen WF, Smit AJ, May JF, Lie KI, Meyboom-de Jong B. Acceptance and side effects of ambulatory blood pressure monitoring: evaluation of a new technology. *J Hum Hypertens* 1996; **10** (Suppl 3): S39–S42.

19 Little P, Barnett J, Barnsley L, Marjoram J, Fitzgerald-Barron A, Mant D. Comparison of acceptability of and preferences for different methods of measuring blood pressure in primary care. *BMJ* 2002; **325**: 258–9.

20 Teixeira PJ, Going SB, Houtkooper LB, et al. Weight loss readiness in middle-aged women: psychosocial predictors of success for behavioral weight reduction. *J Behav Med* 2002; **25**: 499–523.

21 Teixeira PJ, Going SB, Houtkooper LB, et al. Pretreatment predictors of attrition and successful weight management in women. *Int J Obes Relat Metab Disord* 2004; **28**: 1124–33.

22 Forrest S, McCaffery K, Waller J, et al. Attitudes to self-sampling for HPV among Indian, Pakistani, African-Caribbean and white British women in Manchester, UK. *J Med Screen* 2004; **11**: 85–8.

23 Lawton J, Peel E, Douglas M, Parry O. 'Urine testing is a waste of time': newly diagnosed type 2 diabetes patients' perceptions of self-monitoring. *Diabetic Med* 2004; **21**: 1045–8.

24 Renard E. Monitoring glycemic control: the importance of self-monitoring of blood glucose. *Am J Med* 2005; **118**(Suppl 9A): 12S–19S.

25 Wing RR, Hill JO. Successful weight loss maintenance. *Annu Rev Nutr* 2001; **21**: 323–41.

26 Stone DH, Crisp AH. The effect of multiphasic screening on aspects of psychiatric status in middle age: results of a controlled trial in general practice. *Int J Epidemiol* 1978; **7**: 331–4.

27 Van Weel C. Does labelling and treatment for hypertension increase illness behaviour? *Fam Pract* 1985; **2**: 147–50.

28 Adams S, Pill R, Jones A. Medication, chronic illness and identity: the perspective of people with asthma. *Soc Sci Med* 1997; **45**: 189–201.

29 Barton KA, Blanchard EB, Veazey C. Self monitoring as an assessment strategy in behavioural medicine. *Psychol Assess* 1999; **11**: 490–7.

30 Johnson MJ, Williams M, Marshall ES. Adherent and nonadherent medication-taking in elderly hypertensive patients. *Clin Nurs Res* 1999; **8**: 318–35.

31 Sirovich BE, Welch HG. The frequency of Pap smear screening in the United States. *J Gen Intern Med* 2004; **19**: 243–50.

32 Croyle RT, Hunt JR. Coping with health threat: social influence processes in reactions to medical test results. *J Pers Soc Psychol* 1991; **60**: 382–9.

33 Lazarus RS, Folkman S. *Stress Appraisal and Coping*. New York: Springer, 1984.

34 Van Wissen K, Litchfield M, Maling T. Living with high blood pressure. *J Adv Nurs* 1998; **27**: 567–74.

35 Siegel K, Schrimshaw E, Raveis V. Accounts for non-adherence to antiviral combination therapies among older HIV-infected adults. *Psychol Health Med* 2000; **5**: 29–42.

36 Siegel K, Schrimshaw EW, Dean L. Symptom interpretation and medication adherence among late middle-age and older HIV-infected adults. *J Health Psychol* 1999; **4**: 247–57.

37 McDonald K, Bartos M, Rosenthal D. Australian women living with HIV/AIDS are more sceptical than men about antiretroviral treatment. *AIDS Care* 2001; **13**: 15–26.

38 Siegel K, Schrimshaw E, Dean L. Symptom interpretation: Implications for delay in HIV testing and care among HIV-infected late middle-aged and older adults. *AIDS Care* 1999; **11**: 525–35.

39 Michie S, Smith JA, Senior V, Marteau TM. Understanding why negative genetic test results sometimes fail to reassure. *Am J Med Genet A* 2003; **119**: 340–7.

40 Eddy DM. Clinical decision making: from theory to practice. A collection of essays from the Journal of the American Medical Association. *JAMA* 1996; **275**: 650–7.

41 Mazur DJ. *Shared Decision Making the Patient Physician Relationship*. Tampa: Hillsboro Printing Company, 2001.

42 Whitney SN, McGuire AL, McCullough LB. A typology of shared decision making, informed consent, and simple consent. *Ann Intern Med* 2004; **140**: 54–9.

43 Haynes RB, Devereaux PJ, Guyatt GH. Physicians' and patients' choices in evidence based practice. *BMJ* 2002; **324**: 1350.

44 Coulter A, Jenkinson C. European patients' views on the responsiveness of health systems and healthcare providers 10.1093/eurpub/cki004. *Eur J Public Health* 2005; **15**: 355–60.

45 Davey HM, Lim J, Butow PN, Barratt AL, Redman S. Women's preferences for and views on decision-making for diagnostic tests. *Soc Sci Med* 2004; **58**: 1699–707.

46 O'Connor AM, Stacey D, Entwistle V, et al. Decision aids for people facing health treatment or screening decisions. *Cochrane Database Syst Rev* 2003; (2): CD001431.

47 Greenfield S, Kaplan S, Ware JE, Jr. Expanding patient involvement in care. Effects on patient outcomes. *Ann Intern Med* 1985; **102**: 520–8.

48 Kaplan SH, Greenfield S, Ware JE, Jr. Assessing the effects of physician–patient interactions on the outcomes of chronic disease. *Med Care* 1989; **27** (Suppl 3): S110–S127.

49 Michie S, Miles J, Weinman J. Patient-centredness in chronic illness: what is it and does it matter? *Patient Educ Couns* 2003; **51**: 197–206.

50 Gordon K, MacSween J, Dooley J, Camfield C, Camfield P, Smith B. Families are content to discontinue antiepileptic drugs at different risks than their physicians. *Epilepsia* 1996; **37**: 557–62.

51 Protheroe J, Fahey T, Montgomery AA, Peters TJ. The impact of patients' preferences on the treatment of atrial fibrillation: observational study of patient based decision analysis. *BMJ* 2000; **320**: 1380–4.

52 Jones MH, Singer A, Jenkins D. The mildly abnormal cervical smear: patient anxiety and choice of management. *J R Soc Med* 1996; **89**: 257–60.

53 Kitchener HC, Burns S, Nelson L, et al. A randomised controlled trial of cytological surveillance versus patient choice between surveillance and colposcopy in managing mildly abnormal cervical smears. *BJOG* 2004; **111**: 63–70.

54 Shaw C, Abrams K, Marteau TM. Psychological impact of predicting individuals' risks of illness: a systematic review. *Soc Sci Med* 1999; **49**: 1571–98.

55 O'Connor AM, Rostom A, Fiset V, et al. Decision aids for patients facing health treatment or screening decisions: systematic review. *BMJ* 1999; **319**: 731–4.

56 IPDAS: International Patient Decision Aid Standards, 2006.

57 Tiller K, Meiser B, Gaff C, et al. A randomized controlled trial of a decision aid for women at increased risk of ovarian cancer. *Med Decis Making* 2006; **26**: 360–72.

58 Sabate E. *Adherence to Long-Term Therapies, Evidence for Action*. Geneva: World Health Organization, 2003.

59 Osterberg L, Blaschke T. Adherence to medication. *N Engl J Med* 2005; **353**: 487–97.

60 Sackett DL, Snow JC. *The Magnitude of Adherence and Non Adherence*. Baltimore: John Hopkins University Press, 1979.

61 Haynes RB, Yao X, Degani A, Kripalani S, Garg A, McDonald HP. Interventions to enhance medication adherence. *Cochrane Database Syst Rev* 2005; (4): CD000011.

62 Marinker M, Blenkinsopp A, Bond C, et al. *From Compliance to Concordance. Achieving Shared Goals in Medicine Taking*. London: Royal Pharmaceutical Society of Great Britain, 1997.

63 Claxton AJ, Cramer J, Pierce C. A systematic review of the associations between dose regimens and medication compliance. *Clin Ther* 2001; **23**: 1296–310.

64 Leventhal H, Brissette I, Leventhal EA. The common-sense model of self-regulation of health and illness. In: Cameron LD, Leventhal H (eds), *The Self-Regulation of Health and Illness Behaviour*. London: Routledge, 2003.

65 Weinman J, Petrie KJ, Moss-Morris R, Horne R. The Illness Perception Questionnaire: a new method for assessing the cognitive representation of illness. *Psychol Health* 1996; **11**: 431–45.

66 Moss-Morris R, Weinman J, Petrie KJ, Horne R, Cameron LD, Buick D. The revised Illness Perception Questionnaire (IPQ-R). *Psychol Health* 2002; **17**: 1–16.

67 Broadbent E, Petrie KJ, Main J, Weinman J. The Brief Illness Perception Questionnaire. *J Psychosom Res* 2006; **60**: 631–7.

68 Meyer D, Leventhal H, Gutmann M. Common-sense models of illness: the example of hypertension. *Health Psychol* 1985; **4**: 115–35.

69 Gonder-Frederik LA, Cox DJ. Symptom perception, symptom beliefs and blood glucose, discrimination in the self-treatment of insulin dependent diabetes. In: Skelton JA, Croyle RT (eds), *Mental Representation in Health and Illness*. New York: Springer, 1991, pp. 220–46.

70 Petrie KJ, Broadbent E, Meechan G. Self-regulatory interventions for improving the management of chronic illness. In: Cameron LD, Leventhal H (eds), *The Self-Regulation of Health and Illness Behaviour*. London: Routledge, 2003, pp. 257–77.

71 Horne R, Weinman J. Patients' beliefs about prescribed medicines and their role in adherence to treatment in chronic physical illness. *J Psychosom Res* 1999; **47**: 555–67.

72 Joos SK, Hickam DH, Gordon GH, Baker LH. Effects of a physician communication intervention on patient care outcomes. *J Gen Intern Med* 1996; **11**: 147–55.

73 Poppa A, Davidson O, Deutsch J, et al. British HIV Association (BHIVA)/British Association for Sexual Health and HIV (BASHH) guidelines on provision of adherence support to individuals receiving antiretroviral therapy (2003). *HIV Med* 2004; **5** (Suppl 2): 46–60.

74 Butler JA, Peveler RC, Roderick P, Smith PW, Horne R, Mason JC. Modifiable risk factors for non-adherence to immunosuppressants in renal transplant recipients: a cross-sectional study. *Nephrol Dial Transplant* 2004; **19**: 3144–9.

75 Burnier M. Long-term compliance with antihypertensive therapy: another facet of chronotherapeutics in hypertension. *Blood Press Monit* 2000; 5 (Suppl 1): S31–S34.

76 Paes AH, Bakker A, Soe-Agnie CJ. Impact of dosage frequency on patient compliance. *Diabetes Care* 1997; **20**: 1512–7.

77 Cramer JA, Scheyer RD, Mattson RH. Compliance declines between clinic visits. *Arch Intern Med* 1990; **150**: 1509–10.

78 Feinstein AR. On white-coat effects and the electronic monitoring of compliance. *Arch Intern Med* 1990; **150**: 1377–8.

79 Dewalt DA, Berkman ND, Sheridan S, Lohr KN, Pignone MP. Literacy and health outcomes: a systematic review of the literature. *J Gen Intern Med* 2004; **19**: 1228–39.

80 Schillinger D, Barton LR, Karter AJ, Wang F, Adler N. Does literacy mediate the relationship between education and health outcomes? A study of a low-income population with diabetes. *Public Health Rep* 2006; **121**: 245–54.

81 Williams MV, Baker DW, Honig EG, Lee TM, Nowlan A. Inadequate literacy is a barrier to asthma knowledge and self-care. *Chest* 1998; **114**: 1008–15.

82 Vergouwen AC, Bakker A. Patient adherence with antidepressant treatment. *Br J Psychiatry* 2002; **181**: 78–9.

83 Burke LE, Dunbar-Jacob JM, Hill MN. Compliance with cardiovascular disease prevention strategies: a review of the research. *Ann Behav Med* 1997; **19**: 239–63.

84 Pound P, Britten N, Morgan M, et al. Resisting medicines: a synthesis of qualitative studies of medicine taking. *Soc Sci Med* 2005; **61**: 133–55.

85 Blaxter M, Britten N. Lay beliefs about drugs and medicines and the implications for community pharmacy. Pharmacy Practice Research Resource Centre, University of Manchester, 1996.

86 Ritchie J, Spencer L, O'Connor W. Carrying out qualitative analysis. In: Ritchie J, Spencer L (eds), *Qualitative Research Practice: A Guide for Social Science Students and Researchers*. London: Sage, 2003, pp. 219–62.

87 Juniper EF, Guyatt GH, Ferrie PJ, Griffith LE. Measuring quality of life in asthma. *Am Rev Respir Dis* 1993; **147**: 832–8.

88 Rutten-van Molken MP, Custers F, van Doorslaer EK, et al. Comparison of performance of four instruments in evaluating the effects of salmeterol on asthma quality of life. *Eur Respir J* 1995; **8**: 888–98.

89 Juniper EF, Buist AS, Cox FM, Ferrie PJ, King DR. Validation of a standardized version of the Asthma Quality of Life Questionnaire. *Chest* 1999; **115**: 1265–70.

90 Juniper EF, Guyatt GH, Cox FM, Ferrie PJ, King DR. Development and validation of the Mini Asthma Quality of Life Questionnaire. *Eur Respir J* 1999; **14**: 32–8.

91 Ruta DA, Garratt AM, Leng M, Russell IT, MacDonald LM. A new approach to the measurement of quality of life. The patient-generated index. *Med Care* 1994; **32**: 1109–26.

92 Ruta DA, Garratt AM, Russell IT. Patient centred assessment of quality of life for patients with four common conditions. *Qual Health Care* 1999; **8**: 22–9.

93 Camilleri-Brennan J, Ruta DA, Steele RJ. Patient generated index: new instrument for measuring quality of life in patients with rectal cancer. *World J Surg* 2002; **26**: 1354–9.

94 Schwartz CE, Sprangers MA. Methodological approaches for assessing response shift in longitudinal health-related quality-of-life research. *Soc Sci Med* 1999; **48**: 1531–48.

95 Sprangers MA, Schwartz CE. The challenge of response shift for quality-of-life-based clinical oncology research. *Ann Oncol* 1999; **10**: 747–9.

96 Sprangers MA, Schwartz CE. Integrating response shift into health-related quality of life research: a theoretical model. *Soc Sci Med* 1999; **48**: 1507–15.

97 Wilson IB. Clinical understanding and clinical implications of response shift. *Soc Sci Med* 1999; **48**: 1577–88.

98 Lenert LA, Treadwell JR, Schwartz CE. Associations between health status and utilities: indirect evidence for response shift. In: Schwartz CE, Sprangers MAG (eds), *Adaptation to Changing Health: Response Shift in Quality of Life Research*. Washington, DC: American Psychological Association, 2000, pp. 255–67.

99 O'Boyle CA, McGee HM, Browne JP. Measuring response shift using the schedule for evaluation of individual quality of life. In: Schwartz CE, Sprangers MAG (eds), *Adaptation to Changing Health: Response Shift in Quality of Life Research*. Washington, DC: American Psychological Association, 2000, pp. 201–9.

100 Parmelee PA, Katz IR, Lawton MP. The relation of pain to depression among institutionalized aged. *J Gerontol* 1991; **46**: P15–P21.

101 Jacobson NS, Moore D. Spouses as observers of the events in their relationship. *J Consult Clin Psychol* 1981; **49**: 269–77.

102 Catania JA, Gibson DR, Chitwood DD, Coates TJ. Methodological problems in AIDS behavioral research: influences on measurement error and participation bias in studies of sexual behavior. *Psychol Bull* 1990; **108**: 339–62.

103 Kremer EF, Block A, Atkinson JH. Assessment of pain behaviour: factors that distort self report. In: Melzack R (ed), *Pain Measurement and Assessment*. New York: Raven Press, 1983, pp. 165–72.

CHAPTER 12

Evaluating the effectiveness and costs of monitoring

Patrick M.M. Bossuyt

In an era of evidence-based medicine and increasing scrutiny of the use of health-care resources, decisions about monitoring should ultimately be based on solid evidence of its effectiveness and cost-effectiveness. A specific monitoring strategy should not be used in practice unless there is evidence that it improves or maintains patients' health, and that this gain in health outcome is in reasonable balance with the additional resources needed. If several approaches to monitoring are possible, one should identify and select the one with the most attractive balance between effectiveness and cost.

In this chapter I shall briefly outline general concepts for evaluating the effectiveness and costs of monitoring. In the second part I shall discuss the advantages and disadvantages of randomized clinical trials for evaluating monitoring strategies. In the third part I shall introduce modelling as an alternative paradigm for looking at the costs and consequences of alternative approaches to monitoring. In the final section I offer elements for a staged evaluation of monitoring, using different designs at each stage.

12.1. Elements of evaluation

In any evaluation of monitoring, the following items should be addressed:
- The monitoring strategy
- Comparators
- Health outcomes
- Effectiveness
- Costs
- Perspective.

12.1.1. The monitoring strategy
Whenever we evaluate the effectiveness of monitoring, we assess more than the monitoring test itself. To find out whether patients get better from

Evidence-based Medical Monitoring: from Principles to Practice. Edited by Paul Glasziou,
Les Irwig and Jeffrey K. Aronson. © 2008 Blackwell Publishing, ISBN: 978-1-4051-5399-7.

Table 12.1 Elements of a staged evaluation for the development of monitoring strategies and the evaluation of their effectiveness and costs

Phase	Aim	Design	Study objectives
Phase 1	Collect evidence to build monitoring strategies	Various	Document variability of condition; association with downstream health outcomes; test characteristics; effectiveness of further actions
Phase 2	Identify the most effective monitoring strategy and its competitors	Modelling	Evaluate, compare, optimize projected effectiveness of monitoring strategies
Phase 3	Determine empirical estimates of effectiveness (and costs) of monitoring strategy	RCT	Compare estimated effectiveness of monitoring strategies versus comparator strategy
Phase 4	Control quality of monitoring	Surveillance	Document outcomes of implemented monitoring strategy

monitoring, we have to consider the monitoring test and procedure, as well as all other actions based on monitoring. It means that what we evaluate is not the act of monitoring itself, but a specific monitoring strategy, including a protocol for repeated testing, action thresholds and the actions to be taken if any of the thresholds is reached.

12.1.2. Comparators

An informative evaluation of the effectiveness of a monitoring strategy should also specify a comparator. With what shall we compare the monitoring strategy? For any particular monitoring strategy, the comparator could be either no monitoring at all (is any monitoring effective?) or a different monitoring strategy (which strategy is best?), one that differs in one or more features from the monitoring strategy that is evaluated—in the test, the action thresholds, the testing interval or the actions to be taken. The comparator should be defined with a level of detail that is comparable to that of the monitoring strategy under evaluation. Denominating 'usual care' as the comparator, for example, may not be very informative, as what constitutes usual monitoring care may vary across practices and across countries.

12.1.3. Health outcomes

Many evaluations of medical technology have relied primarily on biomedical measures, such as laboratory test results, to determine whether a health intervention is useful. More recently, it has been argued that these measures are not always the outcomes that matter most to patients, who may be more interested in functional status, and mental and social health [1]. Depending on the type of problem, monitoring may be expected to prevent death, reduce morbidity, improve functioning or meet a patient's other health needs. Other aspects may also be relevant to patients and practitioners, ranging from the desire to know and to learn, the need to control or be controlled, or anxiety and the need for reassurance. Some of these elements have been discussed in the chapter on social and psychological outcomes (Chapter 11).

It may not always be possible or feasible to measure the actual health outcomes, and researchers may turn to surrogate outcome measures (Chapter 4). A surrogate marker is intended to substitute for the final health outcome of interest. Surrogate outcome measures are generally chosen because they can be measured earlier than the actual health outcome.

12.1.4. Effectiveness
To document whether patients are better off with a monitoring strategy relative to its comparator, a measure has to be selected to express the changes in health outcome. Most often, descriptive summary measures of health outcome are used. In some evaluations, researchers rely on valued outcomes, such as utilities or quality-adjusted life years (QALYs). In such studies, the health outcomes receive a quantitative expression of a valuation.

12.1.5. Costs
Societal concerns about the rate of increase in cost of medical care have led to intense interest in evaluating procedure-specific or treatment-specific costs. To find out to what extent additional resources are needed to achieve the health gains through monitoring, relative to the comparator, we have to calculate the difference in costs from switching from the comparator to the monitoring strategy. This is usually measured by counting volumes of resources used and calculating unit prices. The resources will include not only the monitoring tests themselves, but any knock-on costs in additional or reduced treatments, and changes in events such as hospitalizations or procedures.

A distinction must be made between financial and economic concepts of cost. Financial costs relate to monetary payments associated with the price of an item or service traded in the market place. Economic costs relate to the wider concept of resource consumption, irrespective of whether such resources are traded. For example, the time spent by patients in a hospital waiting room represents a real cost to them, despite the fact that no financial payment arises.

12.1.6. Perspective
Before an economic evaluation can begin, the perspective of the study should be determined [2]. Costs and effects can be evaluated from the perspective of the health service, the third-party insurer or society. In the latter, sectors other than the health service that may incur costs or benefits as a result of health-care interventions are included in the evaluation.

12.2. Randomized designs

Some interventions achieve dramatic results. For many others there are doubts about their effectiveness: some patients seem to improve, some do not, and some worsen; one can question whether alternative measures would have led to better results. To evaluate the overall benefits of such interventions, randomized controlled trials (RCTs) can be used.

RCTs have become the cornerstone of evidence of medical effectiveness. The central features of an RCT are strict eligibility criteria, random allocation of participants to the strategies that are to be compared, the ceteris paribus principle (all other features of management being equal), the use of predefined measures of outcomes and effectiveness, and the inclusion of all randomized patients in the final analyses.

Randomization means that the participants are randomly allocated to the monitoring strategy and the comparator. If done properly, although the two groups of participants may differ in age, sex distribution or other relevant factors, these differences are all generated by chance. In that case, any differences in outcome beyond those that can be expected based on chance can be attributed to the difference in strategy.

RCTs of monitoring have some characteristics in common that set them apart from trials of other types of interventions. In many RCTs in health care, the participants and their clinicians are 'blinded' or 'masked', i.e. they are unaware of the strategy they have been allocated to. Sometimes placebo drugs or sham treatments are used to achieve blinding, which is helpful for achieving the ceteris paribus principle, for making sure that the non-specific features in each intervention arm are equal. Blinding is difficult, though not impossible, to achieve in trials of monitoring. Some trialists have resorted to alternatives to blinding to monitoring itself, such as randomly generated results from tests [3].

RCTs of monitoring will always be trials of monitoring strategies. This makes them similar to RCTs of diagnostic tests, which evaluate diagnostic test strategies, not just tests [4]. It means that what is evaluated in a monitoring RCT is a strategy, a planned and organized system of repeated assessments and subsequent decisions about additional interventions, such as starting, stopping or modifying treatment. If the trial results are to be interpreted properly, all elements of the monitoring strategy must be specified in advance: the protocol for repeated testing, the intervals, the decision limits and the nature and extent of subsequent interventions.

For example, in a study of whether blood pressure control in primary care could be improved with the use of patient-held targets and self-monitoring, 441 participants with hypertension who were taking treatment but whose blood pressure was not controlled below the target of 140/85 mmHg were included [5]. The blood pressure of the participants in the comparator strategy arm was monitored by their doctors. The trialists compared the change in systolic blood pressure and costs at 6 months and 1 year in both intervention and control groups. They also documented changes in health behaviour, anxiety and prescribed antihypertensive drugs, and they evaluated patients' preferences. Systolic blood pressure in the intervention group fell significantly after 6 months but not after 1 year. Overall, self-monitoring did not cost significantly more than usual care (£251 versus £240).

When conventional treatment was compared with a continuous glucose monitoring system in a medical intensive care unit (maintenance of blood glucose concentration at 80–110 mg/dl; 4.44–6.11 mmol/l), the study was terminated early after 1548 patients had been randomized [6]. Intensive insulin therapy reduced mortality during intensive care from 8% with conventional therapy to 4.6%. Patients who received intensive therapy were also less likely to require prolonged mechanical ventilation and intensive care. In a separate paper, the same researchers reported the costs of both monitoring strategies [7]. The total cost of intensive monitoring and treatment was €144 per patient versus €72 per patient with the conventional strategy. The excess cost of intensive insulin therapy was €72 per patient. The total hospitalization cost in the intensive treatment group was 7931 per patient versus €10,569 per patient in the conventional treatment group. These intensive care unit benefits were not offset by additional costs for care on regular wards.

Because of interactions between tests, repeated tests, test results and the decisions based on these results, monitoring RCTs will usually require large sample sizes. Any difference in aggregated outcome between groups allocated to a monitoring strategy and its comparator will be generated by the subgroup with results that require a change in intervention. For example, in a comparison of monitoring for early signs of adverse effects of treatment versus no monitoring, the only subgroup that will contribute to a difference in outcome beyond chance is the group of patients with test results that point to adverse effects. The alternative group—the one without such test results—will be managed similarly in the monitoring strategy and in the no-monitoring comparator strategy, as no change in intervention is required.

RCTs of monitoring strategies provide several other challenges and disadvantages. One of them is that RCTs are usually limited to comparisons of two or three monitoring strategies, whereas in many circumstances an enormous number of monitoring strategies can be developed, differing in the type of assessment, the people who are doing the assessments, the timing, the decision limits and the changes in interventions. Because of these limitations, modelling may be a useful alternative for evaluating monitoring strategies [2].

12.3. Modelling

With modelling, researchers intend to support decisions about monitoring by building a decision analytical model. In this process, they look at a hypothetical cohort of patients and try to estimate the change in health outcome relative to a comparator, by implementing one or more monitoring approaches. In the model, pieces of evidence from a variety of study designs are incorporated to estimate the final health outcomes. These pieces of evidence may include the natural course of the condition that is being monitored, the accuracy of the monitoring tests, and the effectiveness and risks of treatment.

An example of such a model is a study of postoperative annual surveillance with chest computed tomography (CT) in patients who had undergone resection of non-small cell lung cancers [8]. The authors compared the survival and costs with those in a similar group of patients who did not undergo annual surveillance with CT (control group), using a Markov model, in which patients transition from one health state to another annually. The effectiveness of CT monitoring was expressed as a gain in QALYs. They used published data on survival after surgery, on the annual incidence of second primary lung cancer, on the sensitivity of surveillance CT, on survival after resection of second primary lung cancer and a variety of other sources. They estimated that the cost of surveillance CT was $47,676 per QALY.

Kimmel and colleagues also used modelling to determine the optimal CD4 cell count and HIV RNA monitoring frequency in HIV-infected patients before the start of antiretroviral therapy [9]. They compared CD4 cell count and HIV RNA monitoring at frequencies of 2–24 months before antiretroviral therapy and accelerated monitoring frequencies as CD4 cell counts approached a specified treatment threshold. They concluded that monitoring HIV-infected patients every 12 months until the CD4 count was 100×10^6/l, followed by more frequent monitoring every 2 or 3 months until the start of antiretroviral therapy, would be both more effective and more cost-effective than the current standard of care, which recommends a monitoring interval of 2–6 months.

Unlike RCTs, the number of alternative monitoring strategies that can be evaluated in decision analysis is virtually unlimited. Different monitoring schedules, test sequences and various detection limits can all be evaluated. Monte Carlo approaches allow exploration of the distributions of risk factors and incidence patterns, to accommodate between-patient variability in the natural course of the condition that is monitored and heterogeneity in the response to treatment.

12.4. A staged evaluation

Despite its attractions, modelling is not intended as a replacement for RCTs. The quality of the model is determined by the validity of the parameters that it relies on, and also by the quality of the structure of the model. Difficult structures and complex conditions may be very hard to capture in a valid model, and it may be challenging to define all the relations, associations and possible events a priori.

Modelling should therefore not be seen as a substitute for properly designed trials, but as complementary. Modelling will usually precede trials, as it allows the identification of the set of approaches to monitoring that are most likely to be effective.

There are several reasons to make a plea for a staged evaluation, not very dissimilar from similar approaches that have been proposed and developed for the evaluation of pharmaceuticals and medical tests.

In the first stage, researchers would try to collect evidence about the key components of the monitoring strategy. These include the variability and predictability of the condition that is to be monitored. How variable is it over time? What key factors—related to patients or other interventions—predict the changes in the conditions? Other components relate to the characteristics of the test or procedure considered as a monitoring tool. What do we know about their reliability? Yet another component is made up of the additional actions that can be taken as part of a monitoring strategy. Are they effective in changing the condition or its association with health outcomes in the middle or long run? How rapidly can we expect the changes in the condition that is monitored to occur?

A variety of study designs have to be used in this early phase of the development and evaluation of a monitoring strategy. It is conceivable that evidence collected in the early stages of evaluation points convincingly to the ineffectiveness of any monitoring strategy, for example because of the absence of a reliable test or a lack of effective interventions.

If there is evidence that monitoring can change health outcomes, a second stage should be directed at the development and identification of monitoring strategies that are most likely to be effective. Because of the infinite possibilities, modelling is an essential tool at this stage.

Once effective strategies have been discovered, they should be empirically evaluated in clinical trials. This step, although not easy, will be essential in any demonstration of the effectiveness of a monitoring strategy, as models cannot substitute for empirical studies.

Trials are sometimes designed and conducted in circumstances that do not reflect daily practice. They can include selected patients and usually involve the dedicated attention of well-trained and highly motivated health-care professionals. These factors make it necessary to monitor the outcomes of monitoring itself, once such a strategy has been introduced in daily practice.

Evaluation of monitoring is not easy. In a sense, monitoring strategies qualify as complex interventions [10]. But even complex interventions should be carefully evaluated, to prevent the persistence of ineffective routines and encourage the introduction of optimal procedures into present day health care.

References

1 Sherbourne CD, Sturm R, Wells KB. What outcomes matter to patients? *J Gen Intern Med* 1999; **14**: 357–63.
2 Gold MR, Siegel JE, Russell LB, Weinstein MC. *Cost-Effectiveness in Health and Medicine*. New York: Oxford University Press, 1996.

3 Anticoagulants in the Secondary Prevention of Events in Coronary Thrombosis Research Group. Effect of long-term oral anticoagulant treatment on mortality and cardiovascular morbidity after myocardial infarction. *Lancet* 1994; **343**: 499–503.

4 Bossuyt PM, Lijmer JG, Mol BW. Randomised comparisons of medical tests: sometimes invalid, not always efficient. *Lancet* 2000; **356**: 1844–7.

5 McManus RJ, Mant J, Roalfe A, et al. Targets and self monitoring in hypertension: randomised controlled trial and cost effectiveness analysis. *BMJ* 2005; **331**: 493.

6 Van den Berghe G, Wouters P, Weekers F, et al. Intensive insulin therapy in critically ill patients. *N Engl J Med* 2001; **345**: 1359–67.

7 Van den Berghe G, Wouters PJ, Kesteloot K, Hilleman DE. Analysis of healthcare resource utilization with intensive insulin therapy in critically ill patients. *Crit Care Med* 2006; **34**: 612–6.

8 Kent MS, Korn P, Port JL, Lee PC, Altorki NK, Korst RJ. Cost effectiveness of chest computed tomography after lung cancer resection: a decision analysis model. *Ann Thorac Surg* 2005; **80**: 1215–22.

9 Kimmel AD, Goldie SJ, Walensky RP, et al.; Cost-Effectiveness of Preventing AIDS Complications Investigators. Optimal frequency of CD4 cell count and HIV RNA monitoring prior to initiation of antiretroviral therapy in HIV-infected patients. *Antivir Ther* 2005; **10**: 41–52.

10 Medical Research Council. *A Framework for Development and Evaluation of RCTs for Complex Interventions to Improve Health*. London: Medical Research Council, 2000.

CHAPTER 13

Good practice in delivering laboratory monitoring

W. Stuart A. Smellie

In this chapter, I shall describe a framework for delivering monitoring tests by a laboratory and consider some of the problems raised by central laboratory analysis. I shall specifically cover those monitoring tests that require the presence of a patient to give a biological sample, which can be provided either directly by the patient (e.g. urine) or taken by a member of the care team (e.g. blood by phlebotomy). Unlike physiological measurements, such as blood pressure or peak flow, for which point-of-care testing relies almost exclusively on the practicality and performance of near-patient testing instruments, these tests introduce the additional circuit of sample transport and result delivery, and therefore have a large potential impact on the organization of the care process. In part of this chapter I shall therefore examine the two opposing or complementary paradigms of the use of centralized laboratory testing (CLT) and point-of-care testing (POCT)—the latter is considered in detail in Chapter 14.

It is unlikely that there is a single ideal model for delivering a monitoring test service, and the decision to adopt one or the other, or a combination of both, will take account of the health and social insurance care system of the region in question, technological advancement, geographical distribution and means of transport available to patients, sample collection, information technology requirements, the cost perspective (user, provider, health-care system patient or community; see Chapter 12), and the place where the clinical review visit will occur.

I shall first examine a description of the sample cycle, and then use this to look at alternative models and standards for delivering laboratory-based monitoring tests.

Evidence-based Medical Monitoring: from Principles to Practice. Edited by Paul Glasziou, Les Irwig and Jeffrey K. Aronson. © 2008 Blackwell Publishing, ISBN: 978-1-4051-5399-7.

Pre-analytical	Analytical	Post-analytical
• Specimen collection	• Analysis on instrument	• Result validation
• Transport	• Result confirmation	• Result communication
• Laboratory processing	• Choice of instrument/method	• Archiving
• Number of sites; transport needs	• Dedicated space	• Result interpretation
• Sample registration/ recording: IT and personnel requirements	• Operating personnel	• Method-specific idiosyncrasies-exceptions
	• Maintenance/ troubleshooting	• Infrastructure for result archiving
• Sample handling: health and safety requirements	• Backup in event of failure	• Hazardous waste disposal
• Continued infrastructure needed to support testing not done by point-of-care testing (more complex tests, acute care services)	• Internal/external quality assurance subscription and administration	• External access to results: interfacing with local secondary care providers:
	• Unit test cost	
	• Stock control	• Retrospective investigation of systematic bias or error:
	• Error recognition	
	• Test activity per site compatible with doing the test	• Result comparability between different methods
	• Repertoire availability	

Figure 13.1 Simplified laboratory turnaround cycle with main contributory processes (dark blue); 'hidden factors' to be considered when setting up a point-of-care system (light blue).

13.1. The sample cycle

Historically, laboratories have dedicated much of their resources to the analytical stages of the sample cycle (see Figure 13.1) and have had varying degrees of control over stages outside the laboratory. As a large and increasing proportion of monitoring testing takes place outside the hospital or unit that houses the testing laboratory, the pre- and post-analytical phases of the sample cycle take on increasing importance in delivering a seamless clinical service. Any model that is designed to deliver a monitoring service must pay particular attention to these phases of the cycle. While it has been conventional to consider the sample cycle as distinct from the patient cycle, monitoring is a continuous and iterative process, and it is important to include the patient in the cycle.

13.1.1. The pre-analytical phase

The pre-analytical phase is the period between obtaining the sample and the start of its analysis in the laboratory. However, this could reasonably be extended to begin at the time when the patient begins the journey to provide a biological sample. This can be broken down into several individual stages:

1 Patient journey to the sampling site.
2 Sampling process (e.g. phlebotomy).
3 Sample processing—completion of the request form, packaging, awaiting transport.
4 Transport to point of testing.
5 Pre-analytical processing (e.g. centrifugation) at the site of testing before analysis.

Depending on the perspective, the pre-analytical time has conventionally been calculated as the time from obtaining the sample to the time of its analysis in the laboratory (total pre-analytical time) or as the time from receipt of the sample in the laboratory until its analysis (laboratory pre-analytical time). The transport cost and opportunity cost to a patient attending to give a sample are significant and can contain variable proportions of direct and indirect costs to the patient, society, the employer and the health-care system. These costs will vary depending on the heath-care and social insurance regimes of the country in question. This raises accounting difficulties, as the overall cost of delivering a monitoring service will vary greatly, depending on the perspective from which the costs are assessed. It will also influence patient compliance, as high cost and loss of earnings will have the greatest effect on the poorest patients, which includes many of those for whom poor attendance at clinics and compliance with monitoring already poses a problem.

13.1.2. The analytical phase

Although it takes the shortest time, the analytical phase is the period that has traditionally received most attention from laboratories. As centralized laboratory monitoring tests are often planned and conducted in advance of the clinical review, outside of the acute hospital, the laboratory analytical time conventionally has limited impact on the overall sample processing time. It takes on greater significance with increasing community clinical care [1, 2], POCT and 'one-stop' patient visits, particularly in a specialized clinic when large numbers of patients are being reviewed (such as a diabetes clinic), when the time needed to analyse sample under 'real-time conditions' may introduce delays into the patient's visit.

The main problem of the analytical phase of the sample cycle lies in the validity of the test result: this is determined by its accuracy (the right result), precision (the variability in the results obtained), both within and between laboratory analyser runs, error recognition (identifying potentially erroneous results and the use of quality-control material to demonstrate that the method is performing satisfactorily) and validation of the result in the clinical context. As monitoring compares the results of tests across time, a key problem is the requirement of a consistent method. If methods or laboratories are changed, clinicians may be misled into believing that there has been a change in the patient rather than the method. Hence, communication of changes of method is vital for monitoring tests.

13.1.3. The post-analytical phase

The post-analytical phase is conventionally the phase from production of a valid result at the analyser to the receipt of the result at the point of request. From the user's perspective, it also incorporates the time taken from receipt of the result at the point of request to the availability of the result to the clinician (for example, being filed in records or available in a patient's computerized record).

Awareness of all these phases of the sample cycle is important when evaluating and choosing monitoring tests. While the test itself is clearly important, the organization and speed of the other phases will influence the impact, convenience and costs of monitoring tests.

13.1.4. Accreditation

A detailed review of accreditation is outside the scope of this chapter. Briefly, the standards set by accreditation bodies are designed to ensure suitable and documented procedures for receiving, storing, analysing and reporting laboratory results in the choice and operation of the analytical methods used, under acceptable quality conditions. This area is of particular relevance when samples are analysed outside laboratories in a point-of-care setting.

There are various national and international generic [2] and laboratory-specific [3–8] quality systems of accreditation. There are also specific proposals for POCT [9, 10]. In the UK, where most testing is conducted in the National Health Service, laboratories are required to be registered with the national accreditation body (Clinical Pathology Accreditation UK Ltd) [8].

13.2. Two paradigms: POCT and CLT—opposing or complementary?

Services that deliver monitoring tests will, as discussed above, vary depending on national health-care and social insurance regimes. Cost and cost-effectiveness are inescapable central components of a monitoring service, and create difficulties, as these are conventionally measured from the perspective of the health-care provider, whose accounting methods do not recognize the direct and opportunity costs to patients individually and to society in general.

In the UK, the organization of the health-care system is such that most primary-care biological testing has conventionally been performed in laboratories on samples obtained either in hospital or in primary care (i.e. in general practitioners' surgeries). Samples are then transported to the laboratory for analysis. The funding of this system has not supported the development of independent testing laboratories, other than to serve the relatively smaller private sector, for which a significant proportion of work is still processed in National Health Service Laboratories. Tests are initiated by a medical practitioner or on the practitioner's behalf by a nurse or another care worker. The patient is called to attend for a test, the sample is sent to a laboratory, usually via a local collection service organized by or on behalf of the laboratory, samples are analysed, and the results are either returned in paper form or sent electronically to the point of request. The patient is then seen for the clinical review process.

Health service reforms in the UK [1, 2] are increasingly challenging this approach, leading laboratories and users to examine alternative paradigms, notably allowing the sample to be analysed at the point of care. However, a centralized laboratory service offers a number of distinct advantages:

- *Consistent accredited analysis.* Centralized laboratories have dedicated laboratory computing services set up to record and keep patient records, results and audit trails under conditions that should, when correctly followed, lead to a minimum of errors, mechanisms for identifying and processing errors that occur, documented accuracy and variability (precision) of the results that they produce, and validation of the results in the clinical context.
- *Economies of scale.* By performing large numbers of tests, the costs of the materials required to analyse the sample are generally reduced, although a central laboratory infrastructure is required to support analyses. This means that smaller laboratories cost proportionately more and this has led to debates in laboratory medicine about ways in which increasing economies of scale can be obtained, either by centralizing smaller laboratory facilities on to a single geographical site or by combining infrastructure resources between disciplines to create multidisciplinary laboratories. Technological advances are further influencing this debate, with increasing availability of laboratory robotics, reducing the staff needed to process high volumes of samples routinely.
- *Trained and experienced personnel.* Staff who perform or supervise the tests and review the test results are professional laboratory personnel trained to monitor the performance of the test, identify potential errors, and provide clinical interpretation of results. Clinical interpretation may be of less importance in uncomplicated cases but becomes increasingly important in the cases of clinically relevant abnormal results and when abnormal or spurious results are obtained.

POCT (discussed in more detail in Chapter 14) allows tests to be performed at the point of clinical contact and therefore offers the potential for 'one-stop' clinical services, in which the monitoring measurements and clinical review can be performed at the same visit. The timeliness of POCT has clear advantages for clinical decision-making. However, it requires equipment (instruments or materials such as test strips) that can be used by non-specialist staff to provide results of comparable quality to those conducted on a laboratory analyser. It does not require the infrastructure of a laboratory, although to be used safely and correctly an analogous infrastructure is needed at each site.

In addition to convenience for practitioners and patients, POCT is often perceived as cost-saving compared with CLT, although this can be deceptive.

Much of the cost (typically 70% of the cost of a thyroid test and 95% of a serum electrolyte test) is made up of the fixed overheads of the laboratory (principally staffing) or host institution (principally organizational buildings and administrative staffing overheads). Typically, POCT instruments are perceived to avoid these laboratory overheads, which are associated with a far higher unit test cost than the cost of the materials used in the machine to produce the result. However, as discussed elsewhere, the costing of a POCT service cannot ignore other elements: the need for staff to be trained and approved in the use of a POCT machine, the time taken to perform the tests, the need for suitable premises, and the necessary information technology (IT) and other infrastructure, which must be available to support suitable record keeping and traceability (see Figure 13.1).

Opposing drivers are influencing the delivery of laboratory tests. Robotics, laboratory centralization and a desire to improve efficiency of processing support the use of centralized laboratories. Conversely, drivers of patient choice and convenience and delivery of services from primary care are fuelling a move towards POCT. It is likely that both paradigms offer opportunities, but that the opportunities will vary depending on the population and geography in question: remoteness of clinical services, population density, etc. However, in terms of the absolute cost of delivering tests, a mixed central laboratory POCT arrangement will tend, irrespective of convenience, to increase overall cost, as the marginal (test reagent) cost of most POCT far exceeds that of the corresponding laboratory test at present.

13.3. Standards for delivering a monitoring test service

In addition to conventional parameters of test performance, a monitoring service must seek to optimize the clinical review process, providing timely and reliable results to the clinical practitioner, in order to minimize the time and effort required in recovering results during the clinical review. These can be summarized as follows.

13.3.1. Obtaining samples
The service must support sample collection. Facilities must be available to allow patients to provide biological samples close to their home or place of work, with minimum professional involvement and rapid transport of the sample to the point of analysis, sufficiently quickly to avoid sample deterioration and safely to protect those transporting the sample.

A range of options are available to achieve this aim. The choice of facilities to be made available will depend largely on cost and convenience. These range from personal visits to a patient's home to obtain a sample, through a spectrum of community sample collection points, to a single central sampling point. Clearly these are simplified for POCT analysis, when the sample is obtained at the point where a patient attends before clinical review or when the patient is self-monitoring. The centralized laboratory service model therefore requires a significant infrastructure cost to support a sample delivery service, which increases with the number and geographical spread of the sampling points. Sample deterioration over time and safety do not currently make the use of a postal service a suitable option for the delivery of large numbers of most routine samples.

13.3.2. Data records

Suitable support must be available to record the relevant demographic and clinical information about the patient, the tests requested, and the results once the sample has been received. An audit trail must be available. Suitable means must be available to convert this information into a format accessible both by the service performing the test and by clinical users

The existing IT infrastructure in centralized laboratories is designed to provide this, although, as for the transport infrastructure for centralized laboratories, the complexity of the systems required increases with the number of testing points and users. While individual analysers can incorporate detailed facilities to record patients' demographic information, these data are held in the instrument unless it is linked (interfaced) to a wider informatics network, to allow access from clinical users.

13.3.3. Clinical support in method choice

Clinical support must be available to guide the correct choice of test and test interval

The choice of test is protocol led. Establishing the right monitoring test and the optimal monitoring interval depending on clinical context are described in Chapters 5 and 8. The clinical use of tests by practitioners is extremely variable [11]: this variability is not explained by demographic differences between practices or by socioeconomic factors (such as deprivation index) and appears to be due to differences in clinical decision-making [12]. The UK is currently embarking on a model to encourage practitioners to standardize use of monitoring tests, by incorporating a number of standards into the general practitioners' contract of service [13, 14]. This is one mechanism of driving use of testing, but it clearly depends on the correct decisions being taken in setting the tests and testing intervals.

Until recently, the knowledge bases for using tests to monitor diseases have been fragmented, and the stimulus to testing appears to have been mostly clinical culture and habit. Increasingly in the UK the development of National Service Frameworks [15] and the Primary Care Contract are introducing direct standards and guidance. Whether the patient sample is tested in a central laboratory or peripherally using POCT, strengthening the clinical decision-making process will remain an essential component of care, as it is recognized that guideline production alone has limited success in implementing change [16, 17] and enabling mechanisms are required.

13.3.4. Validity of chosen method
The test method used must produce results consistent with the methods that are used to validate the choice of monitoring test; when methods are different, a detailed relation of results between methods must be known, together with the factors that produce different results with different methods (e.g. matrix effects, haematocrit)

While it may appear obvious that a wide range of different instruments and methods used to perform a test may have particular impact on POCT, the same applies to centralized laboratory services. Much of the instrumentation provided by manufacturers is supplied by a limited number of large providers, and there are significant differences between methods used, both between manufacturers of 'closed' methods, which are specific to the instrument supplied, and 'open' methods, which can be used on a range of analysers. This is exemplified by laboratory measurement of creatinine, and therefore estimation of glomerular filtration rate, which is significantly influenced by the choice of method used [18]. Some of the difficulties associated with method variation can be addressed by harmonizing results and methods against a reference method, as occurred with the DCCT alignment of glycated haemoglobin (Hb_{A1c}) results [19], adopted as UK national standards [20], although inherent differences will remain. This has, for example, reduced several of the earlier problems associated with Hb_{A1c} measurement [21].

13.3.5. Performance of chosen method
The performance of the method must be compatible with its use as a monitoring test in terms of accuracy, imprecision, limit of detection and quantification and interfering factors

These analytical factors should be taken into account when deciding on a monitoring test method (see Chapter 5). This recommendation may be made at a national or international level, although it should also contain guidance on the choice of specific methods for performing the same test, as local choice may govern the selection of test provider, whether for a central laboratory or POCT. The scope for adopting different methods is clearly greater for POCT, and hence the need for coordinated introduction of any such service through an appropriate POCT committee. Centralization of test methods does not remove problems relating to method accuracy and imprecision. Imprecision or bias at clinical decision thresholds are of particular importance. Current practice in most laboratories is to report a result, which is then compared against a population reference or clinical action value. The user must be made aware of the intrinsic variability of the result [22]. This is particularly so when interpreting sequential monitoring tests. Interpretation of the significance of two different sequential monitoring tests does not currently form part of the routine interpretation offered by most laboratories or POCT providers, but is of great importance when monitoring leads to a change in active management, such as alteration of the dose of insulin based on glycated haemoglobin (Hb_{A1c}). The imprecision of a test directly influences the probability that two sequential results will be statistically significantly different (95% probability of significant difference for a difference of 2.8 times the standard deviation of the result, incorporating both test and biological variability [23]). The interpretation of variability in sequential tests is perhaps best captured by the use of control charts, which are still underused in clinical care (see Chapter 7 for more details).

A particular trap can occur with 'shared care' clinical models, in which patients may attend for different types of clinical review (e.g. periodic community monitoring and programmed annual hospital visits), when samples may be analysed on different instruments with different methods, producing greater intrinsic variability of results.

13.3.6. Quality control
Appropriate internal and external quality-control procedures must be followed at recommended intervals to monitor assay performance and a record of results held

This forms an integral part of CLT and provides an indication (but not a guarantee) that the test is being performed consistently at the test site and that the results it produces are compatible with a target value for all sites that perform the test. These are requirements, for example, of the UK CPA standards [8], for which all laboratories in the UK must currently be registered.

13.3.7. Training
The test must only be performed by a person trained and approved to perform it

This should form an integral part of CLT, although changes in working practices may lead to increasing numbers of technically less qualified laboratory assistants playing increasing roles in some laboratories. It raises greater questions in POCT, and requires suitable thought to be given when designing work rosters to ensure that the necessary trained staff are available to service the testing needed. Operation of POCT instruments is becoming increasingly simple, although training must include knowledge of the relevant quality-control and documentation processes.

13.3.8. Accuracy of recording
Appropriate facilities must be available to record and archive results with minimal error

The infrastructure requirements for this are similar to standard 2, and potentially increase in complexity with the number of testing sites. While results and information can be entered manually into health-care IT systems, from an analyser this carries a human error rate that is greatly reduced by computerized result transfer.

13.3.9. Availability of results
Results must be available to be transmitted to or consulted by the clinical user and any other testing service to which monitoring results are to be sent as part of the patient's care, within a timescale compatible with the clinical review process

In a fully integrated IT network between laboratory or POCT and the clinical user, this should be limited only by system limitations in the frequency with which results can be updated. This process can be bypassed with POCT, by providing patients with printouts of their own results to take to a clinical consultation, but does not remove the need for POCT to be linked to patient management IT, to reduce human input errors and to create accessible records and an audit trail. It is of major importance for a centralized laboratory service, and the timing of sampling must be organized to allow sufficient time to ensure that results are available to clinical users when needed. However, information transfer systems are not infallible, and suitable backup facilities must be available to transmit results should the system fail.

13.3.10. Ongoing clinical support
Clinical support must be available to provide interpretation of unexpected results and results inconsistent with the clinical circumstances and advice on further testing required in the cases of unexpected results

Information support has historically been the role of the laboratory specialist and can be provided in several ways: through manual addition of comments to laboratory reports, comments added via automated flow pathways written into laboratory IT systems, and direct contact between laboratory specialist and user, initiated by either side. It should act as a safety filter to detect potential errors, unusual clinical circumstances or major changes in a patient's condition.

Suitable operating procedures for analysers will include a non-exhaustive list of common problems that can arise in erroneous results and can be incorporated into policies for POCT, although the decision to seek specialist advice is in this case shifted solely to the user, unless POCT systems are interfaced to laboratory computing systems.

13.4. Addressing the disadvantages of CLT

Some of the standards proposed above would appear to be intrinsically more compatible with a strategy of CLT, whereas others favour POCT. CLT in a suitably accredited laboratory should provide the necessary information technology infrastructure and laboratory expertise to optimize data registration audit, analytical performance and clinical interpretation. On the other hand, the point-of-care paradigm potentially allows the test result to be obtained and clinical review performed at the same patient visit, if the throughput of testing is compatible with the length of the visit. Blood samples may be obtained by finger prick more easily and more quickly than by phlebotomy, which is needed to perform the analyses required on most current large laboratory instruments. A transport infrastructure is needed to deliver samples to a laboratory, to avoid the costs and practical difficulties associated with large-scale carriage by post. While POCT is frequently put forward as being convenient to patients and an alternative to 'expensive' central laboratory testing, correct use carries with it several implications (see Figure 13.1). Many of these form part of laboratory accreditation systems, to which central laboratories subscribe, and may not be immediately apparent to non-laboratory specialists proposing to set up POCT services.

The balance of the decision between CLT and POCT can be influenced by, for example, geographical factors in remote communities, in which a disseminated peripheral collection system for samples may prove expensive. Conversely, in dense communities, flexible availability of phlebotomy services would minimize patient cost, inconvenience and lost opportunity cost. Locating phlebotomy services or POCT facilities, through a wide range of providers (e.g. pharmacies) would optimize patient access, but must be balanced against the infrastructure requirements. Within the primary-care network in the UK, general practice surgeries, the increasing development of walk-in centres and laboratory providers, linked by a transport system, add to an existing network in which local arrangements may have been made, for example to transport samples from a small branch surgery to a main surgery, to minimize the need for a transport system serving a very large number of low-volume sites. The principal weaknesses of this type of service appear to have been more the availability of staff time to take phlebotomy samples and the inconvenience and difficulty some patients have experienced in obtaining an appointment to give a sample. As phlebotomy can readily be taught as a specific clinical skill, expansion in the numbers and range of people able to take phlebotomy samples would, even through the existing network of general practice surgeries, greatly improve patient access.

Similarly, when patient access to sampling services is improved, the need for tests to be performed in the same clinical visit, to ensure that they are available, should become less important. This requires patient involvement and a willingness on the part of the patient to attend to provide a sample some days before the clinical visit. This organizational approach, in my experience, has a low non-compliance rate. Most reasons given for failing to have a sample taken are either forgetfulness or lack of availability of an appointment to have a blood sample taken. Increased use of electronic reminders and widening the availability of phlebotomy would resolve both of these problems, subject to a compromise between fragmenting the sample collection facilities and the complexity of the POCT or sample transport facilities needed to service the increased level of fragmentation.

13.5. Conclusions

Regardless of how a monitoring service for laboratory is delivered, it plays a central role in the management of chronic disease. Inaccurate results can lead to incorrect clinical decisions, and lost or delayed results create clinical waste, delay the patient episode, and add considerable cost to overall patient management. In order to establish a monitoring service that provides reliable results to allow correct clinical decision-making, a number of essential quality criteria must be met. However, they must also be combined with cost-effectiveness criteria, so that the service is sustainable within a health-care system that does not have limitless resources. One difficulty in achieving this is the different components of cost in a monitoring service, from patient opportunity cost to the marginal cost of the test being performed. The ideal choice will inevitably vary according to the cost perspective used, and care must be taken that in designing a service the result is not improved cost-effectiveness of clinical care but a diversion of cost to an alternative sector. These different cost centres will vary according to the health-care and social insurance systems in different countries, and it is important that all relevant factors are taken into account in delivering a quality monitoring service.

References

1 Department of Health. *Our Health, Our Care, Our Say. A New Direction for Community Services*. London: The Stationery Office, 2006, p. 230.
2 Department of Health. Supporting people with long term conditions to self care: a guide to developing local strategies and good practice. Available from http://www. dh.gov.uk/PublicationsAndStatistics/Publications/PublicationsPolicyAndGuidance/ PublicationsPolicyAndGuidanceArticle/fs/en?CONTENT_ID=4130725&chk= o9VokD (last accessed 2 May 2007).
3 International Organization for Standardization. Quality Management Systems. Requirements (ISO 9001:2000). Available from www.ISO.org (last accessed 2 May 2007).
4 International Organization for Standardization. Medical laboratories. Particular Requirements for Quality and Competence (ISO 15189:2003).Available from www.ISO-15189.com (last accessed 2 May 2007).
5 International Organization for Standardization. General Requirements for the Competence of Testing and Calibration Laboratories (ISO/IEC 17025:1999). Available from www.iso.org (last accessed 2 May 2007).
6 European Communities Confederation of Clinical Chemistry. Essential criteria for quality systems of medical laboratories. *Eur J Clin Chem Clin Biochem* 1997; **35**: 121–32.
7 European Communities Confederation of Clinical Chemistry. Additional essential criteria for quality systems of medical laboratories. *Eur J Clin Chem Clin Biochem* 1998; **36**: 249–52.

8 Clinical Pathology Accreditation (UK). Standards for the Medical Laboratory. CPA-UK.co.uk, November 2004.

9 Burnett D. Accreditation and point-of-care testing. *Ann Clin Biochem* 2000; **37**: 241–3.

10 Ehrmeyer SS, Laessig RH. Regulation, accreditation and education for point-of-care testing. In: Kost G (ed), *Principles and Practice of Point-of-Care Testing*. Philadelphia: Lippincott Williams and Wilkins, 2002, pp. 434–43.

11 Smellie WSA, Galloway MJ, Chinn D. Benchmarking general practice use of pathology services: a model for monitoring change. *J Clin Pathol* 2000; **53**: 476–80.

12 Smellie WSA, Galloway MJ, Chinn D. Is clinical practice variability the major reason for differences in pathology requesting patterns in general practice? *J Clin Pathol* 2002; **55**: 312–4.

13 General Medical Services Contract. Available from www.nhsconfed.org/docs/contract.pdf (last accessed 25 May 2006).

14 Revisions to the GMS contract 2006/7. Delivering investment in general practice. Available from http://www.nhsemployers.org/primary/primary-902.cfm#NHS-28159–1.

15 National; Service frameworks. Available from http://www.dh.gov.uk/Policy-AndGuidance/HealthAndSocialCareTopics/HealthAndSocialCareArticle/fs/en?CONTENT_ID=4070951&chk=W3ar/W (last accessed 2 May 2007).

16 Van Walraven C, Goel V, Chan B. Effect of population-based interventions on laboratory utilization. *JAMA* 1998; **280**: 2028–33.

17 Solomon DH, Hideki H, Daltroy L, Liang MH. Techniques to improve physicians' use of diagnostic tests. *JAMA* 1998; **280**: 2020–7.

18 Lamb EJ, Tomson CRV, Roderick PJ. Estimating kidney function in adults using formulae. *Ann Clin Biochem* 2005; **42**: 321–45.

19 Marshall SM, Barth JH. Standardisation of Hb_{A1c} measurements—a consensus statement. *Diabetic Med* 2000; **17**: 5–6.

20 National Institute for Clinical Excellence. Management of type 2 diabetes. Managing blood glucose levels (Guideline G.). September 2002. Available from http://www.nice.org.uk/page.aspx?o=36737 (last accessed 2 May 2007).

21 Kilpatrick ES. Problems in the assessment of glycaemic control in diabetes mellitus. *Diabetic Med* 1997; **14**: 819–31.

22 Fraser CG, Petersen PH. The importance of imprecision. *Ann Clin Biochem* 1991; **28** (Pt 3): 207–11.

23 Jones RG, Payne RB. *Clinical Investigation and Statistics in Laboratory Medicine*. London: ACB Venture Publications, 1997, p. 196.

CHAPTER 14
Point-of-care testing in monitoring

Christopher P. Price

Historically, diagnostic tests were undertaken close to the patient, integrating the information gained with the physician's observation of the patient's current symptoms and history [1]. These early tests were probably used for making a diagnosis rather than for monitoring. Early reports of diagnostic tests described the observation of urine at the bedside, which initially evolved with the aid of very basic chemical tests. The history of medicine, and indeed of laboratory medicine, demonstrates the evolution of care—and of early diagnostic testing—away from the bedside in the home. As patients began to be cared for in the early hospitals, these tests moved away from the bedside into some form of side room, and effectively the concept of a laboratory was born. As care moved increasingly away from the home, so the performance of the test moved further away from the bedside. Interestingly, and perhaps more specifically in the management of long-term diseases, we are now beginning to see a reversal of this trend, with care moving away from the hospital and back into the community and home [2], and a high proportion of tests are required for monitoring.

The development of hospitals and laboratories, and technological innovation across the breadth of health care, has led to a paradigm shift from the physician attending the patient to the reverse. This has led to a shift from a patient-centred approach to care, with a lengthening of the decision-making process, sometimes to unacceptable degrees, when a rapid intervention may be required. As the process of care becomes more complex there is an increased risk of fragmentation of care and a reduced quality of care. Thus, several recent reviews of the quality of care in specific health-care systems have pointed out the problems with fragmented services, making reference to problems associated with delay in receiving test results [3–5] as well as patients' results not being recorded [6]. A systems engineering perspective recognizes that as the number of steps in a process increases so does the risk of errors [7]. The place of the test in a care pathway (Figure 14.1) and the steps involved in

---

Evidence-based Medical Monitoring: from Principles to Practice. Edited by Paul Glasziou, Les Irwig and Jeffrey K. Aronson. © 2008 Blackwell Publishing, ISBN: 978-1-4051-5399-7.

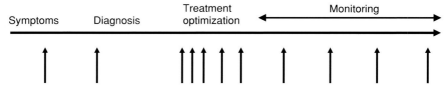

Figure 14.1 A schematic representation of a patient's journey through a disease or illness and the points at which a test might be requested (↑).

obtaining each test result (Figure 14.2) illustrate the opportunity for errors to be made.

The concept of point-of-care testing (POCT) is therefore appealing from a number of perspectives. POCT was born when the first tests were made on the urine, and it has evolved with the development of new tests and testing technology. It is now firmly established in meeting clinical needs and patient preferences, as well as facilitating alternatives to the ways in which health care can be provided. In particular, POCT has become popular in a number of areas of monitoring, including self-monitoring of blood glucose in diabetes, international normalized ratio (INR) monitoring for patients on warfarin, home blood pressure monitoring and home peak flow monitoring in asthma, together with POCT in a number of clinic and ward settings. In this chapter, I

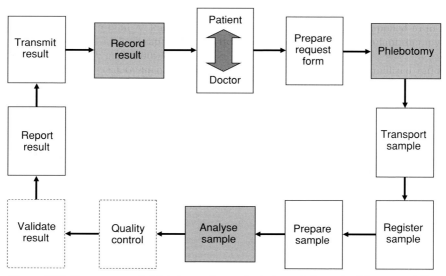

Figure 14.2 The process of obtaining a diagnostic test result from the laboratory (all boxes), compared with the reduced number of steps associated with POCT (shaded boxes only); only a subset of samples are subjected to quality control and validation (dashed boxes).

shall first look at some characteristics of POCT, describe some case studies to illustrate why it is important in monitoring, and give guidance for its safe and effective use.

14.1. What is POCT?

POCT can be defined as 'the performance of a test at the time at which the test result enables a decision to be made and an action taken that can lead to an improved health outcome' [1]. The term 'point' has both physical and temporal implications, but the ability to provide a result quickly, at the time when the need for the test is recognized, is the over-riding criterion. However, this simple definition does not adequately reflect all the potential benefits from POCT, and the importance of being able to provide a patient-centred approach to care has to be recognized, as well as acknowledging the benefits that this approach will bring. Other names given to this form of testing have included 'bed side' [8], 'near patient' [9], 'physician's office' [10], 'extra-laboratory' [11], 'decentralized' [12], and 'off-site', 'ancillary' and 'alternative site' [13, 14] testing.

The evaluation of point-of-care tests should consider the need to make an immediate decision, and whether that might improve the outcome. In the context of monitoring, that decision will broadly comprise an evaluation of the current disease status and the possible need to modify the disease management strategy. The health outcome can be viewed from the perspective of a number of stakeholders: that of the patient and the carer, the manager responsible for the provision of care and the purchaser of that care. The perspective of the patient and clinician will primarily consider the opportunity for an improved clinical outcome. The managers' and the purchasers' perspectives will also consider operational and economic outcomes.

14.2. Where is POCT performed?

POCT has been described in a number of settings, from the home to the intensive care unit, all of which can include monitoring applications. The most common form of testing performed in the home, in the workplace and in the leisure place is self-monitoring of blood glucose in the management of diabetes mellitus [15]. There is also now a trend to undertake anticoagulation monitoring, although the frequency of testing is much lower [16]. In primary care, POCT can be performed at the health centre, at the pharmacy or at a so-called diagnostic and treatment centre. Some of this testing may be opportunistic, for example on the part of the pharmacist, or it may be part of a strategy by the local health-care provider organization to improve access to care in the community, especially in the management of long-term diseases [17]. The provision of monitoring to support the management of diabetes using POCT in the community has been described, as well as anticoagulation testing [16, 18] and cholesterol testing [19]. In hospitals, point-of-care tests may be provided in the ambulatory care (out-patient) clinic, in the emergency department, on the ward, and in a number of intensive care settings, including the operating room. Thus, in the diabetes clinic one can test for Hb_{A1c} and urine albumin [20]; in the emergency department the reasons for using POCT are rapid diagnosis of life-threatening conditions (e.g. hypoglycaemia), establishing and monitoring the status of critical variables (e.g. potassium and blood gases), and rapid triage [21]; in intensive care, the predominant use is in monitoring critical physiological variables (e.g. potassium, blood gases, ionized calcium), with a view to maintaining them within acceptable limits [22]. The benefits of all of these applications can be measured in clinical, operational and economic outcomes [23, 24].

14.3. Why choose POCT for monitoring?

The application of POCT to monitoring can be beneficial in three main areas:
  (i) self-monitoring;
 (ii) in the monitoring of long-term diseases;
(iii) in the monitoring of acute interventions.
These can be illustrated in a few brief case studies.

14.3.1. Self-monitoring of blood glucose concentration in diabetes

Randomized controlled trials have shown reductions in the Hb_{A1c}, although the data are more controversial in type 2 diabetes [15, 25, 26]. Importantly, feedback of test results to the patients appears to produce greater improvement [27], which illustrates the value of monitoring using POCT, as it involves (empowers) the patient in the management of the condition. This field is now being enhanced with the aid of tele-healthcare [28], although its additional benefits are still unclear.

14.3.2. Self-monitoring of the INR

Empowering patients to change the warfarin dosage on the basis of INR self-testing is supported by data from randomized controlled trials [16, 18, 29]. Specific benefits include a longer time in the target range, fewer dosage changes, fewer bleeding episodes and fewer clinic visits. Previously, patients would have had to attend out-patient clinics, with the problems associated with transport, taking time off work, long clinic waits, freedom to travel, etc. POCT therefore provides greater convenience for patients, many of whom are older and less mobile.

14.3.3. Monitoring glycated haemoglobin (Hb_{A1c}) in the clinic

Randomized controlled trials in both out-patient and primary-care settings have suggested that there is improved lowering of the Hb_{A1c} compared with using a laboratory service [20, 30–33]. The benefit is to both patient and caregiver, as it enables the current Hb_{A1c} concentration to be discussed and any treatment change advised immediately. It also ensures that the patient is aware of the Hb_{A1c} result, which in itself is beneficial [34]. There are also economic benefits, with a reduction in clinic visits and the opportunity to transfer more care into the community.

14.3.4. Monitoring glycaemic control in intensive care

Randomized controlled trials have shown that using the blood glucose concentration to guide insulin dosage in intensive care units, in order to maintain the blood glucose within tight limits, there is a reduction in infection rates and length of stay, with improved mortality [35, 36].

14.3.5. Optimization of therapy in the clinic

One small 'before and after' study has suggested that quicker optimization of drug concentrations may be possible when there is a practical measure of efficacy available [37]. In patients with newly diagnosed epilepsy there was a significant reduction in the number of weeks needed to achieve optimal drug concentrations, in the number of clinic visits, and the number of drug assays required when using POCT to optimize phenytoin therapy. The implication from this small study is that the frequency of testing will be greater in the 'optimization' phase than in the 'monitoring of compliance' phase. Overall this approach greatly improves both patient and care-giver satisfaction.

14.3.6. Monitoring coagulation status in the operating room

Monitoring of coagulation status during cardiopulmonary bypass has been shown in 'before and after' studies to reduce the use of blood products, as well as requirements for postoperative care [38, 39]. Similarly, monitoring the ionized calcium concentration during liver transplantation reduces the risks associated with the complications of giving citrated blood [40].

14.3.7. Monitoring in the operating room during parathyroidectomy

Measuring the circulating parathyroid hormone concentration after removal of malignant tissue helped to assess the efficacy of the procedure in a 'before and after' study. This led to a reduction in the re-operation rate, and, in combination with imaging, the transfer of the procedure to a day-case unit, with obvious benefits to patient, clinician and provider organization [41, 42].

14.4. Ensuring quality in point-of-care monitoring

Most diagnostic tests are initially established using a laboratory service, but the need for a more rapid response, necessitating POCT, can become clear when one takes an overarching view of the patient-care pathway. Thus, the introduction of a POCT service requires a risk assessment that takes into account the following checklist elements:

- the robustness of the POCT device;
- the quality of the results produced, for example accuracy and precision;
- the training and competence required of the operator of the device;
- the process for transmission of the results to the care-giver;
- the ability of the patient and care-giver to interpret the results provided;
- the procedures to ensure that an accurate record of the results is kept;
- the identification of what management changes may have to be made in order to deliver the benefits that have been identified, including reallocation of resources;
- how the patients or staff will be retrained, if and when appropriate;
- how the changes in practice will be implemented, for example integration of POCT into clinic visits.

A good approach to error reduction is to use a multidisciplinary POCT co-ordinating committee, together with an organization-wide POCT policy. For a primary-care organization, this may simply involve one person taking responsibility for POCT, working with professionals in other organizations, for example the local laboratory service.

14.4.1. POCT coordinating committees

A coordinating committee for POCT should be charged with managing the whole process of delivering a high-quality POCT service. Membership should include doctors, nurses, the local laboratory, those involved in the use of other diagnostic and therapy equipment close to the patient (e.g. respiratory measurement technologists), the organization's management team, preferably a person from the quality management team, and possibly a patient. The group should be chosen to represent as widely as possible the locations where POCT might be used.

14.4.2. POCT policy and accountability

Organizations that use POCT should have a policy that sets out the procedures required to ensure a high-quality service, together with a definition of the lines of responsibility and accountability for all staff associated with it. This may be part of the organization's total quality management system, and may also be part of the clinical governance policy [43], as well as for accreditation [44]. The elements of a POCT policy are set out in Table 14.1 [45].

14.4.3. Equipment procurement and introduction

The procurement of POCT equipment should involve the identification of the tests required, the desired analytical performance (accuracy and precision), the turnaround time (in order to define the time-to-result required of the equipment), the requirements made of the operator, together with expectations of the system in relation to the stability of the system and any consumables, calibration and quality-control requirements, obtaining information on the systems available and independent evaluation reports (for example those performed by agencies such as the Medicines and Healthcare products Regulatory

Table 14.1 Sample outline of an organization's POCT policy

Documentation information
- Review time......
- Approved by......
- Original distribution......
- Related policies......
- Further information......
- Policy replaces......

Introduction
- Background
- Definition
- Accreditation of services
- Audit of services

Laboratory services in the organization
- Location
- Logistics
- Policy on diagnostic testing

Management of POCT
- Committee and accountability
- Officers
- Committee members
- Terms of reference
- Responsibilities
- Meetings

Procurement of equipment and consumables
- Criteria for procurement
- Process of procurement

Standard operating procedures
Training and certification of staff
- Training
- Certification
- Re-certification

Quality control and quality assurance
- Procedures
- Documentation and review

Health and safety procedures

Bibliography

Agency (MHRA) in the UK and reports in the peer-reviewed literature), and an economic assessment of the equipment, including the costs of consumables and servicing.

When a system has been chosen it is always helpful if the laboratory professional undertakes a short evaluation of the equipment in order to become familiar with the system. Such an evaluation should also document the concordance between results generated with the device and those provided by the laboratory.

14.4.4. Training and certification

Confidence in a POCT device depends heavily on the robustness of the device and the competence of the operator, given that it has already been shown to meet the analytical needs of the clinical setting. Many of the agencies involved in the regulation of health-care delivery now require that all personnel associated with the delivery of diagnostic results demonstrate their competence through a process of regulation, and this applies equally to POCT.

A training programme should cover the context in which the test is used, the preparation of the patient and the sample, operation of the device (and its safe disposal) and understanding of the significance of the result, and the action required.

14.4.5. Quality control, quality assurance and audit

Quality control and assurance programmes provide a formal means of monitoring the quality of a service. The internal quality-control programme is a relatively short-term, real-time means of assessing the quality of an analytical system. It typically compares current performance with that of the last time an analysis was performed. External quality assurance on the other hand takes a longer term view and compares the testing performance of different sites and/or different pieces of equipment or methods. Audit is a more retrospective form of analysis of performance and can take an overarching view of the whole process. However, the foundation to ensuring good quality remains a successful training and certification scheme.

14.4.6. Internal quality control

Internal quality control involves the analysis of a sample for which the analyte concentration is known, with the mean and range of results quoted for the method used. For analysers that involve re-useable technology (e.g. blood gas sensor systems), at least one quality-control sample should be analysed a minimum of once per shift for a reliable machine, i.e. three times a day. For a single measurement, disposable devices are commonly used in POCT, for example glucose strips; this strategy has less logic, as each unit should be quality controlled, but the same approach is generally recommended.

14.4.7. External quality assurance

External quality assurance or proficiency testing involves analysing samples sent from a scheme organizer. In this case, the operator has no knowledge of the analyte concentration and is thus closer to real life. The results are sent back to the scheme organizer and a performance report is then sent out a few days later. The report will identify the range of results obtained for the complete cohort of participants, and may be broken down according to the different methods used by participants in the scheme. The scheme may encompass both laboratory and POCT users, which gives an opportunity to compare results with laboratory-based methods.

14.4.8. Documentation

The recording of all aspects of POCT has been a major problem for many years, compounded by the fact that until recently the storage of data in laboratory and hospital information systems has been limited and often inconsistent. It is therefore important at an absolute minimum to keep an accurate record of the test request, the result and the action taken. Some problems have been resolved with the advent of the electronic patient record, electronic requesting, and the connectivity of POCT instrumentation to information systems that link to the patient record. In addition to the patient's results, the documentation should extend to the standard operating procedure for the POCT system, records of training and certification of operators, internal quality control and quality assurance, and error logs and corrective actions taken.

14.4.9. Accreditation and regulation of POCT

The features of the organization and the management of POCT described above are all embodied in systems designed for the accreditation of diagnostic services, both delivered from a central laboratory and by POCT [44, 46]. Accreditation of POCT can be part of the overall accreditation of laboratory medicine services, or indeed part of the accreditation of the full clinical service, as has been the case in the USA and the UK for a number of years. Thus, the 1988 Clinical Laboratory Improvement Amendments (CLIA) legislation in the USA stipulates that all POCT must meet certain minimum standards [47]. The Centres for Medicare and Medicaid Services, the Joint Commission on Accreditation of Healthcare Organizations and the College of American Pathologists assume responsibility for inspecting sites and each is committed to ensuring compliance with testing regulations for POCT [47].

14.5. The case for point-of-care monitoring

The key questions when introducing POCT relate to (i) the analytical performance required of the POCT device, (ii) the potential benefits and problems, (iii) the cost of POCT, (iv) the changes in clinical practice, delivery of care and resource allocation required to deliver POCT.

Table 14.2 Some examples of reference intervals and action points

Parameter	Use	Example
Reference interval	Screening	Cholesterol and cardiovascular risk
	Screening	Phenylalanine and phenylketonuria
	Diagnosis	Blood glucose and diabetes
Action limit	Diagnosis	Troponin and myocardial infarction
	Diagnosis	Paracetamol and antidote
	Monitoring	Blood glucose and insulin dosage
	Monitoring	Hb_{A1c} and diabetes care
	Monitoring	INR and warfarin dosage
	Monitoring	Phenytoin dosage

14.5.1. Analytical performance requirements

The basic characteristics of the assay will include the analytical range of the assay, the accuracy (trueness) across that range and the precision across that range. The interpretation of the result will be made by comparison with established decision points or ranges, the biological variation for that analyte [48] and assessment of a statistically significant change in the result [49]. These decision points include reference ranges established in a healthy population and decision or action limits established in the clinical population for which the test is going to be used; examples are illustrated in Table 14.2.

The POCT device should usually be calibrated against the same reference point as is used for calibrating its laboratory equivalent. However, any POCT device should give results that are concordant with the local laboratory, as the patient is likely to be managed on the basis of results from both systems. The accuracy of any test is usually established against a reference method that has been calibrated against a defined international reference material. However, these are not available for all analytes, especially the more complex ones, such as micro-organisms.

The day-to-day precision of the simple laboratory tests that might be used in monitoring, i.e. well-defined molecules measured on automated systems (e.g. potassium, glucose, cholesterol, TSH, Hb_{A1c}), will typically be within the range of 3–5%; an example is illustrated by the evaluation of Hb_{A1c} POCT devices by nurses [50]. In the case of more complex molecules this can rise to 10%, and higher in the case of less commonly performed tests using manual techniques. Knowledge of the degree of analytical precision can help to define an analytically significant difference. However, it should be combined with the intra-individual (biological) variation to determine the true value of a statistically significant difference. If this has been established for the analytes of interest, it is possible to assess the potential usefulness of the POCT device by knowing its day-to-day analytical precision. However, for many tests the total precision requirement is not stated, and there are few studies of the impact of precision on diagnostic performance, especially in the case of monitoring tests.

Table 14.3 Examples of the benefits of POCT for monitoring; all will result in a reduced cost of care

Test	Setting	Clinical benefit	Operational benefit
Blood glucose concentration	Home	Improved glycaemic control	Fewer hospital admissions
INR	Primary care	More time in control	Fewer out-patient visits
Hb$_{A1c}$	Primary care	Lower Hb$_{A1c}$	Fewer hospital visits
Blood gases	Intensive therapy unit	Improved mortality	Shorter stay
Parathormone	Operating room	Lower re-operation rate	Move to day-case surgery
Prothrombin time	Operating room	Reduced risk of bleeding	Less blood required

One example of the influence of precision on clinical decision-making is glucose testing systems, in which a Monte Carlo simulation was used to assess the impact of precision on decisions to change insulin dosages [51]. At a total analytical error of 5% the insulin dosage errors were 8–23%, and when the total analytical precision rose to 10% the errors rose to 16–45%. To ensure that 95% of the intended insulin dosages were correct, the total precision of the glucose measurement had to be between <1% and <2%, depending on the blood glucose concentration. In a comparison of glucose analysers with different degrees of analytical performance for use in the tight management of glycaemic control in an intensive care unit, the more precise system resulted in more reliable clinical decisions [52].

14.5.2. Benefits of POCT

POCT allows clinical decisions to be made and action to be taken at the time of the patient consultation. The benefits can be expressed in clinical, operational and economic terms. Examples of the clinical and economic benefits are given in Table 14.3; most will generate an economic benefit, although this may be outside of the 'testing silo budget' and will require changes to the way in which care is organized and resources reallocated. In practical terms, many of the benefits accrue from a reduction in the number of patient–clinician inter-actions, as well as clinic visits, bringing convenience and increased satisfaction to both parties.

14.5.3. Risks of POCT

The risks associated with using POCT are primarily those involving the pro-duction of inaccurate results and the incorrect use of those results, especially when using self-monitoring. Therefore, attention to the operating procedures for producing good-quality results and regular audit of outcomes are important management considerations.

14.5.4. Costs of POCT

When viewed in terms of cost per test, POCT is invariably more expensive than laboratory-based testing, owing to the cost of the more complex technology used and the loss of the economies of scale associated with a central laboratory service. However, if one takes a broader view and looks at the cost per episode, or the annual cost of care, POCT can bring considerable benefits. The reduced cost of saved clinical visits or hospital admissions can far outweigh the higher costs of testing [20]. For example, savings made by introducing intraoperative measurement of parathyroid hormone used to monitor the effectiveness of parathyroidectomy allowed the transition of this procedure to day-case surgery [42]. These cost-savings can only be realized if the savings in clinic visits and hospital stay etc. can be realized (e.g. staff costs and bed costs).

14.5.5. Changes in practice

It is clear that POCT prompts the need to consider service redesign and reconfiguration of the care pathway. This will include training of staff to use POCT, unless laboratory personnel are going to be seconded to the clinic, as happens in some cases, [20] and reorganization of patient flow through the clinical department (ED, OR, out-patients, health centre), in order to enable test results to be available at the right time.

   Experience suggests that it is the challenge of resource allocation that is going to give the greatest problems. In countries where there is reimbursement for tests it may be possible to effect this change, although there is little evidence of differential reimbursement to accommodate the shift towards POCT.

14.6. Conclusions

When monitoring a long-term disease, or in monitoring acute interventions, POCT can facilitate faster and earlier decision-making, thereby providing more efficient and effective health care, either in the home or the hospital, to support the dialogue between patient and carer. However, there are challenges to the successful implementation of POCT:
  (i) the availability of robust POCT devices;
 (ii) ensuring that reliable results can be delivered;
(iii) changing the care pathways to integrate POCT in such a way that a benefit is achieved;
(iv) reallocating resources in order to enable POCT to be undertaken and resource savings captured.
The technological challenges have been overcome and so the opportunities to exploit POCT successfully lie in how POCT can be best integrated into the process of care, and the willingness of health-care professionals to adapt to its

requirements. If rapid delivery of results improves health outcomes POCT is to be preferred to laboratory-based testing.

References

1 Price CP, St John A, Hicks JM (eds). *Point-of-Care Testing*, 2nd edn. Washington, DC: AACC Press, 2004, p. 488.
2 Department of Health. *Our Health, Our Care, Our Say. A New Direction for Community Services*. London: The Stationery Office, 2006, p. 230.
3 Institute of Medicine. In: Kohn LT, Corrigan JM, Donaldson MS (eds), *To Err is Human: Building a Safer Health System*. Washington, DC: National Academies Press, 2000, p. 287.
4 Institute of Medicine. *Crossing the Quality Chasm: A National Health System for the 21st Century*. Washington, DC: National Academies Press, 2001, p. 383.
5 Davis K. Mirror, mirror on the wall. An update on the quality of American health care through the patient's lens. The Commonwealth Fund. April 2006. Available from www.cmwf.org (last accessed on 9 May 2006).
6 Peters AL, Legorreta AP, Ossorio RC, Davidson MB. Quality of outpatient care provided to diabetic patients. A health maintenance organization experience. *Diabetes Care* 1996; **19**: 601–6.
7 Price CP, St John A. *Point-of-Care Testing for Managers and Policymakers*. Washington, DC: AACC Press, 2006, p. 120.
8 Oliver G. *On Bedside Urine Testing*. London: HK Lewis, 1884.
9 Marks V, Alberti KGMM (eds). *Clinical Biochemistry Nearer the Patient*. Edinburgh, UK: Churchill Livingstone, 1988, p. 240.
10 Mass D. Consulting to physician office laboratories. In: Snyder JR, Wilkinson DS (eds), *Management in Laboratory Medicine*, 3rd edn. New York: Lippincott, 1998, pp. 443–50.
11 Price CP. Quality assurance of extra-laboratory analyses. In: Marks V, Alberti KGMM (eds), *Clinical Biochemistry Nearer the Patient II*. London: Baillière Tindall, 1987, pp. 166–78.
12 Ashby JP (ed). *The Patient and Decentralized Testing*. Lancaster: MTP Press, 1988, p. 128.
13 Handorf CR. College of American Pathologists Conference XXVIII on alternate site testing: introduction. *Pathol Lab Med* 1995; **119**: 867–71.
14 O'Leary D. Global view of how alternate site testing fits in with medical care. *Arch Pathol Lab Med* 1995; **119**: 877–80.
15 Coster S, Gulliford MC, Seed PT, Powrie JK, Swaminathan R. Monitoring blood glucose in diabetes mellitus: a systematic review. *Health Technol Assess* 2000; **4**: 1–93.
16 Heneghan C, Alonso-Coello P, Garcia-Alamino JM, Perera R, Meats E, Glasziou P. Self-monitoring of oral anticoagulation: a systematic review and meta-analysis. *Lancet* 2006; **367**: 404–11.
17 Price CP, St John A. Diabetes management in the community. *Point of Care Test* 2006; **5**: 52–7.
18 Murray ET, Fitzmaurice DA, McCahon D. Point of care testing for INR monitoring: where are we now? *Br J Haematol* 2004; **127**: 373–8.
19 Taylor JR, Lopez LM. Cholesterol: point-of-care testing. *Ann Pharmacother* 2004; **38**: 1252–7.

20 Grieve R, Beech R, Vincent J, Mazurkiewicz J. Near patient testing in diabetes clinics: appraising the costs and outcomes. *Health Technol Assess* 1999; **3**: 1–74.

21 Lee-Lewandrowski E, Corboy D, Lewandrowski K, Sinclair J, McDermot S, Benzer TI. Implementation of a point-of-care satellite laboratory in the emergency department of an academic medical center. Impact on test turnaround time and patient emergency department length of stay. *Arch Pathol Lab Med* 2003; **127**: 456–60.

22 Halpern MT, Palmer CS, Simpson KN, et al. The economic and clinical efficiency of point-of-care testing for critically ill patients: a decision–analysis model. *Am J Med Qual* 1998; **13**: 3–12.

23 Price CP. Point of care testing. Potential for tracking disease management outcomes. *Dis Manage Health Outcomes* 2002; **10**: 749–61.

24 Price CP. Point-of-care testing. *BMJ* 2001; **322**: 1285–88.

25 Welschen LM, Bloemendal E, Nijpels G, et al. Self-monitoring of blood glucose in patients with type 2 diabetes who are not using insulin: a systematic review. *Diabetes Care* 2005; **28**: 1510–7.

26 Davidson MB. Counterpoint. Self-monitoring of blood glucose in type 2 diabetic patients not receiving insulin: a waste of money. *Diabetes Care* 2005; **28**: 1531–3.

27 Jansen JP. Self-monitoring of glucose in type 2 diabetes mellitus: a Bayesian meta-analysis of direct and indirect comparisons. *Curr Med Res Opin* 2006; **22**: 671–81.

28 Farmer A, Gibson OJ, Tarassenko L, Neil A. A systematic review of telemedicine interventions to support blood glucose self-monitoring in diabetes. *Diabetic Med* 2005; **22**: 1372–8.

29 Fitzmaurice DA, Hobbs FD, Murray ET, Holder RL, Allan TF, Rose PE. Oral anticoagulation management in primary care with the use of computerized decision support and near-patient testing: a randomized, controlled trial. *Arch Intern Med* 2000; **160**: 2343–8.

30 Cagliero E, Levina E, Nathan D. Immediate feedback of Hb_{A1c} levels improves glycemic control in type 1 and insulin-treated type 2 diabetic patients. *Diabetes Care* 1999; **22**: 1785–9.

31 Thaler LM, Ziemer DC, Gallina DL, et al. Diabetes in urban African-Americans. XVII. Availability of rapid Hb_{A1c} measurements enhances clinical decision-making. *Diabetes Care* 1999; **22**: 1415–21.

32 Miller CD, Barnes CS, Phillips LS, et al. Rapid A1c availability improves clinical decision-making in an urban primary care clinic. *Diabetes Care* 2003; **26**: 1158–63.

33 Kennedy L, Herman WH, Strange P, Harris A; GOAL AIC Team. Impact of active versus usual algorithmic titration of basal insulin and point-of-care versus laboratory measurement of Hb_{A1c} on glycemic control in patients with type 2 diabetes: the Glycemic Optimization with Algorithms and Labs at Point of Care (GOAL A1C) trial. *Diabetes Care* 2006; **29**: 1–8.

34 Levetan CS, Dawn KR, Robbins DC, Ratner RE. Impact of computer-generated personalized goals on HbA(1c). *Diabetes Care* 2002; **25**: 2–8.

35 Van den Berghe G, Wouters PJ, Bouillon R, et al. Outcome benefit of intensive insulin therapy in the critically ill: insulin dose versus glycemic control. *Crit Care Med* 2003; **31**: 359–66.

36 Plank J, Blaha J, Cordingley J, et al. Multicentric, randomized, controlled trial to evaluate blood glucose control by the model predictive control algorithm versus routine glucose management protocols in intensive care unit patients. *Diabetes Care* 2006; **29**: 271–6.

37 Patsalos PN, Sander JWAS, Oxley J. Immediate anticonvulsive drug monitoring in management of epilepsy. *Lancet* 1987; **2**: 39.

38 Despotis GJ, Joist JH, Hogue CW, Jr, et al. The impact of heparin concentration and activated clotting time monitoring on blood conservation: a prospective, randomized evaluation in patients undergoing cardiac operations. *J Thorac Cardiovasc Surg* 1995; **110**: 46–54.

39 Despotis GJ, Joist JH, Goodnough LT. Monitoring of hemostasis in cardiac surgical patients: impact of point-of-care testing on blood loss and transfusion outcomes. *Clin Chem* 1997; **43**: 1684–96.

40 Wu AH, Bracey A, Bryan-Brown CW, Harper JV, Burritt MF. Ionized calcium monitoring during liver transplantation. *Arch Pathol Lab Med* 1987; **111**: 935–8.

41 Irvin GL, Solorzano CC, Carneiro DM. Quick intraoperative parathyroid hormone assay: surgical adjunct to allow limited parathyroidectomy, improve success rate, and predict outcome. *World J Surg* 2004; **28**: 1287–92.

42 Chen H, Sokoll LJ, Udelsman R. Outpatient minimally invasive parathyroidectomy: a combination of sestamibi-SPECT localization, cervical block anesthesia, and intraoperative parathyroid hormone assay. *Surgery* 1999; **126**: 1016–22.

43 Freedman DB. Clinical governance—bridging management and clinical approaches to quality in the UK. *Clin Chim Acta* 2002; **319**: 133–41.

44 Burnett D. Accreditation and point-of-care testing. *Ann Clin Biochem* 2000; **37**: 241–3.

45 Price CP, St John A. Point-of-care testing. In: Burtis CA, Ashwood ER, Bruns DE (eds), *Tietz' Textbook of Clinical Chemistry and Molecular Diagnostics*. St Louis, MO: Elsevier Saunders, 2006, pp. 299–320.

46 Burnett D. *A Practical Guide to Accreditation in Laboratory Medicine*. London: ACB Venture, 2002, p. 314.

47 Ehrmeyer SS, Laessig RH. Regulation, accreditation and education for point-of-care testing. In: Kost G (ed), *Principles and Practice of Point-of-Care Testing*. Philadelphia: Lippincott, Williams and Wilkins, 2002, pp. 434–43.

48 Fraser CG. *Biological Variation: From Principles to Practice*. Washington, DC: AACC Press, 2001, p. 151.

49 Jones RG, Payne RB. *Clinical Investigation and Statistics in Laboratory Medicine*. London: ACB Venture, 1997, p. 196.

50 St John A, Davis TM, Goodall I, Townsend MA, Price CP. Nurse-based evaluation of point-of-care assays for glycated haemoglobin. *Clin Chim Acta* 2006; **365**: 257–63.

51 Boyd JC, Bruns DE. Quality specifications for glucose meters: assessment by simulation modeling of errors in insulin dose. *Clin Chem* 2001; **47**: 209–14.

52 Kanji S, Buffie J, Hutton B, et al. Reliability of point-of-care testing for glucose measurement in critically ill adults. *Crit Care Med* 2005; **33**: 2778–85.

CHAPTER 15
Monitoring for the adverse effects of drugs

Jamie J. Coleman, Robin E. Ferner, Jeffrey K. Aronson

There are two aspects of monitoring for the adverse effects of drugs: individual and population monitoring. Population monitoring schemes look for previously unknown adverse effects of drugs ('signals'), for example by examining spontaneous reports of suspected adverse drug reactions to discover whether a particular adverse drug reaction is more frequently reported with one drug than with another drug or series of drugs [1, 2]. To discuss these schemes here is beyond our scope. We concentrate instead on monitoring in individuals who are taking drugs in order to prevent or reduce harm from known adverse effects of those drugs.

15.1. Definitions

15.1.1. Adverse event
An adverse event is any abnormal sign, symptom, or laboratory test, or any syndromic combination of such abnormalities, any untoward or unplanned occurrence (e.g. an accident or unplanned pregnancy), or any unexpected deterioration in a concurrent illness [3]. An adverse event that occurs while a patient is taking a drug, or at some time afterwards, may or may not be attributable to it. All adverse drug effects are adverse events, but not all adverse events are adverse drug effects. In describing adverse outcomes as events rather than (drug-induced) effects, investigators acknowledge that it is often difficult, and sometimes impossible, to attribute causality.

15.1.2. Adverse reaction and adverse effect
An adverse drug reaction can be defined as an appreciably harmful or unpleasant reaction, resulting from an intervention related to the use of a medicinal product; adverse effects usually predict hazard from future administration and warrant prevention, or specific treatment, or alteration of the dosage regimen, or withdrawal of the product [3]. Adverse drug reactions can be suspected (i.e.

Evidence-based Medical Monitoring: from Principles to Practice. Edited by Paul Glasziou,
Les Irwig and Jeffrey K. Aronson. © 2008 Blackwell Publishing, ISBN: 978-1-4051-5399-7.

adverse events that are attributed to the drug) or established with varying degrees of certainty.

'Adverse reaction' and 'adverse effect' refer to the same phenomenon, but an adverse effect is seen from the point of view of the drug, while an adverse reaction is seen from the point of view of the patient—the drug causes an effect, and the patient suffers a reaction. The term 'adverse effect (or reaction)' is preferable to other terms that are commonly used in a general sense. These include 'toxic effect' and 'side effect', which have more restricted technical meanings (see below). 'Unwanted effect' is a synonym for 'adverse effect', except that the above definition of adverse drug reaction excludes very minor unwanted effects.

15.2. Monitoring the effects of drugs

Some assessment of the effects of drugs is implicit in almost all therapeutics. It may be as simple as a patient observing that her headache has improved after taking paracetamol, or it may involve complex tests, such as positron emission tomography to assess tumour regression after chemotherapy. In this chapter, we consider only planned and systematic assessment of adverse effects in our discussion of monitoring.

15.2.1. Why monitoring for adverse drug reactions is important

Drugs are very widely promoted and prescribed, but can cause adverse effects, some of which are serious. All rational therapeutic decisions implicitly or explicitly examine the likely balance between benefit and harm from treatment. Monitoring schemes that detect adverse symptoms, signs or investigational indices before more serious effects occur can make them less likely and improve the overall balance between benefit and harm. Several factors determine the extent to which monitoring schemes for adverse drug reactions in individual patients will be useful, but many monitoring schemes seem to be proposed without considering any of these factors, and are incomplete, impractical or invalidated [4].

Here we consider the ways in which various strategies for monitoring will allow clinicians to avert adverse drug reactions, or mitigate their most serious consequences, by detecting their early features [5].

Relevant factors include the nature of the adverse effect, the existence or otherwise of premonitory features or of early and reversible effects, the possibility of repeated testing for those premonitory features or early effects, the properties of the tests used, and the ability to define actions to take on the basis of the outcome of the tests [5]. When a scheme is possible, it will require the following conditions to be met:

- there is a factor that is related to the harm and that can be monitored;
- the factor can be measured with reasonable accuracy and precision;
- changes in the measurement are sensitive to potential harm;
- changes in the measurement are specific for potential harm;

- changes in the measurement are slow compared with the time between measurements;
- changes in the measurement are rapid compared with the evolution of the harm;
- actions in response to the value, or changes in the value, of the factor are defined.

While some of these factors are relevant to any monitoring scheme, some are specifically relevant to monitoring for adverse drug reactions.

15.3. The frequency of adverse drug reactions

Adverse reactions to drugs are common. Many cause little or no harm, although even medically trivial effects may be unwelcome to the patient. However, they are not infrequently serious; about 6.5% of acute general medical admissions, that is about three admissions per day in a busy district general hospital, are attributable to adverse drug effects (excluding cases of self-poisoning) [6]. Many in-patients suffer adverse drug reactions, which in half of them will prolong their stay in hospital [7].

Some adverse drug reactions are predictable and some predictable reactions can be prevented. For example, patients who receive opiates for pain relief in terminal illness often develop pruritus and become constipated; co-administration of antihistamines and laxatives will prevent this. Other adverse effects, although predictable, are not preventable. For example, headache from vasodilatation will occur when patients first take organic nitrates; this cannot be prevented, but can be eased by warning, reassurance and simple analgesic drugs. Many more serious adverse reactions are unpredictable. This is true, for example, of Stevens–Johnson syndrome, which occurs in 1:1000 or fewer patients taking carbamazepine [8].

To help clarify how and what may be monitored, we next consider a classification of the components of adverse drug reactions.

15.4. Classification of adverse drug reactions

An adverse drug reaction has the following components:
1 A drug.
2 A patient.
3 The adverse reaction, that is, the interaction between drug and patient.
The components that best define these components are as follows:
1 The *dose* of the drug, which determines its effects.
2 The *susceptibility* of the patient to the adverse effects of the drug, which determines whether the individual suffers the reaction.
3 The *time course* of the adverse reaction, which describes its pattern of occurrence.
This is illustrated in Figure 15.1.

This approach yields the system of classification of adverse drug reactions called DoTS, based on dose, time course and susceptibility [9].

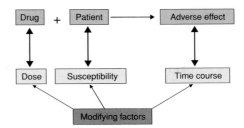

Figure 15.1 The rationale for the DoTS system of classifying adverse drug reactions.

15.4.1. Dose relatedness of adverse drug reactions

The dose–response curve (or concentration–effect curve) is a central feature of the pharmacology of a drug, some of whose principles are discussed in Chapter 1. Adverse drug reactions can be classified according to their dose relatedness by comparing the dose–response curve for harm with the dose–response curve for benefit. This yields three patterns (Figures 15.2–15.4):

- *hypersusceptibility reactions*—reactions that occur at subtherapeutic doses in susceptible patients (Figure 15.2);
- *collateral reactions* (side effects)—reactions that occur at standard therapeutic concentrations (Figure 15.3);
- *toxic reactions*—adverse reactions that occur at concentrations above those needed to produce the therapeutic effect (Figure 15.4).

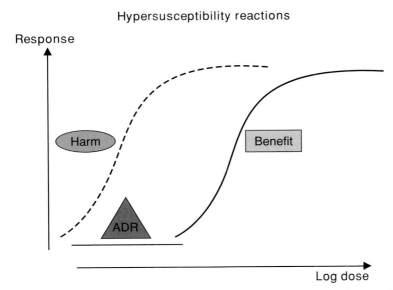

Figure 15.2 Dose relatedness of adverse drug reactions. Hypersusceptibility reactions: they occur when the dose–response curve for harm is to the left of the dose–response curve for benefit.

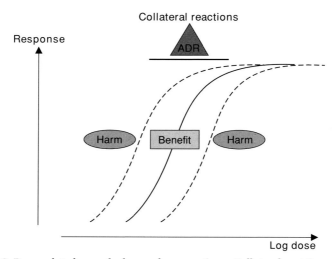

Figure 15.3 Dose relatedness of adverse drug reactions. Collateral reactions: they occur when the dose–response curve for harm is in the same range as the dose–response curve for benefit.

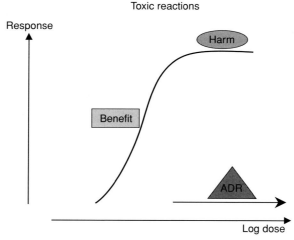

Figure 15.4 Dose relatedness of adverse drug reactions. Toxic reactions: they occur when the harm occurs at the top of the dose–response curve for benefit (or in a separate curve to the right, not illustrated).

15.4.2. Time courses of adverse drug reactions
Adverse drug reactions can be either time dependent or time independent.

15.4.2.1. Time-dependent adverse drug reactions
There are six types of time-dependent reactions. Examples of each of these types are given in Table 15.1:

Table 15.1 Time-related classification of adverse drug reactions

Type of reaction	Example(s)
Time independent	
Due to a change in dose or concentration (pharmaceutical effects)	Toxicity due to increased systemic availability
Due to a change in dose or concentration (pharmacokinetic effects)	Digitalis toxicity due to renal insufficiency
Occurs without a change in dose or concentration (pharmacodynamic effects)	Digitalis toxicity due to hypokalaemia
Time dependent	
Rapid (due to rapid administration)	Red man syndrome (vancomycin)
	Hypertension (digitalis)
	Hypotension (iodipamide)
First dose (of a course)	Hypotension (α_1 adrenoceptor antagonists and angiotensin converting enzyme inhibitors)
	Type I hypersensitivity reactions
Early (abates with repeated exposure)	Adverse reactions that involve tolerance (e.g. nitrate-induced headache)
Intermediate (risk maximum during the first few weeks or months)	Venous thromboembolism (antipsychotic drugs) Hypersensitivity reactions types II, III and IV
Late (risk increases with time)	Osteoporosis (glucocorticoids)
	Tardive dyskinesia (dopamine receptor antagonists)
	Retinopathy (chloroquine)
	Tissue phospholipid deposition (amiodarone)
	Withdrawal syndromes: opiates, benzodiazepines, hypertension (clonidine and methyldopa), myocardial infarction (beta-blockers)
Delayed	Carcinogenesis (ciclosporin, diethylstilbestrol)
	Teratogenesis (thalidomide)

- *Immediate* (rapid) reactions occur when a drug is given too quickly.
- *First-dose* reactions occur only after the first dose of a course.
- *Early* reactions occur soon after the first administration in all or most patients; some are early tolerant (they wear off with time as patients develop tolerance to them, e.g. nitrate-induced headache) and some are early persistent (e.g. corticosteroid-induced hypertension, to which tolerance does not occur).
- *Intermediate* reactions occur within the first few weeks or months of administration but not thereafter; those who are susceptible will suffer the reaction and those who are not will not (they are healthy survivors).
- *Late* reactions occur late in the course of administration, the risk increasing with time; this group includes withdrawal reactions.
- *Delayed* reactions are seen at some distant time after the initial exposure, even if the drug is withdrawn before the reaction appears.

15.4.2.2. Time-independent adverse drug reactions
Time-independent reactions are generally toxic reactions as defined above, and they occur when the effective concentration of the drug at the site of undesired action increases. This can be because the actual concentration increases; for example, as a result of pharmacokinetic changes, as when renal insufficiency reduces the excretion of digoxin. It can also be because the concentration necessary to produce the adverse effect falls as a result of pharmacodynamic changes; for example, when hypokalaemia shifts the dose–response curve for digoxin to the left (Figure 15.5).

15.4.3. Susceptibility factors in adverse drug reactions
The risk of an adverse drug reaction differs among members of an exposed population. For some reactions—for example, haemolysis due to oxidizing agents in people with glucose-6-phosphate dehydrogenase (G6PD) deficiency—some individuals are susceptible, others are not. For other reactions, susceptibility follows a continuous distribution—for example, increasing susceptibility with increasing impairment of renal function. Some susceptibility factors (such as female sex) are fixed, while others (such as co-administered medicines) change with time.

Although reasons for increased susceptibility may be unknown, several types are recognized (Table 15.2). These include
- genetic variation (including drug allergy);
- age;
- sex;
- physiological variation (e.g. pregnancy, body weight);
- exogenous factors (e.g. drugs and food);
- diseases (e.g. renal or hepatic impairment).
More than one susceptibility factor can be present in an individual.

Table 15.2 Sources of altered susceptibility to adverse drug reactions

Source of susceptibility (mnemonic GASPED)	Examples
Genetic	Porphyria
	Suxamethonium sensitivity
	Malignant hyperthermia
	CYP isoenzyme polymorphisms
Age	Neonates, e.g. chloramphenicol
	Elderly people, e.g. hypnotics
Sex	Alcohol, intoxication
	Mefloquine, neuropsychiatric effects
	Angiotensin converting enzyme inhibitors, cough
	Hydralazine, lupus-like syndrome
Physiology altered	Phenytoin in pregnancy
Exogenous factors	Drug interactions
	Interactions with food, e.g. grapefruit juice with drugs cleared by CYP3A4
Disease	Renal insufficiency, e.g. lithium
	Hepatic cirrhosis, e.g. morphine

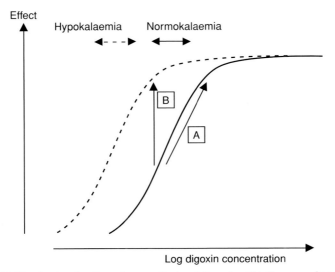

Figure 15.5 Monitoring for the adverse effects of digoxin. (A) Pharmacokinetic effects: for example, the arrow shows the effect of a reduced creatinine clearance (and therefore digoxin clearance), causing toxicity; (B) pharmacodynamic effects: for example, the effect of hypokalaemia, causing a leftward shift of the dose–response (i.e. concentration–effect) curve; the arrow shows the increased effect that would occur at the same plasma digoxin concentration. Double arrowheads represent notional target ranges.

15.5. What to monitor

Drug therapy can be monitored at any point from the issuing of the prescription for a drug to observation of the relevant outcome, which for some adverse effects may be many years after exposure to the drug.

15.5.1. Monitoring adherence to therapy

Many prescriptions issued to patients are never taken to a pharmacy to be dispensed, and drugs that are dispensed are not necessarily taken as intended, or even taken at all [10]. Adherence to therapy is relevant to monitoring for adverse drug reactions (and more often therapeutic effects), as the following examples show. If a patient has not been taking prescribed drugs and comes into hospital because of an acute illness, administration of the prescribed drugs may yield adverse effects that had otherwise been avoided by non-adherence. Methadone maintenance therapy carries a risk of opiate overdosage, both for the patient and for those to whom methadone may be diverted. Supervising methadone ingestion in pharmacies can reduce the risk of these adverse effects. Furthermore, the risks of interactions between methadone and other, illicit, opiates can be reduced by urine screening for drugs of abuse.

Experimental studies of adherence have used, for example, electronic bottle caps that record when doses have been removed from a bottle [11] or markers that can be easily detected in the blood or urine, such as riboflavin [12] or phenobarbital [13].

15.5.2. Monitoring pharmacokinetics

Drug concentration measurement is sometimes an important method for monitoring drug therapy. However, it requires certain conditions to be met if it is to be valuable. Firstly, the adverse drug effect must be toxic (in the sense defined above), so that reducing the concentration of the drug will reduce the risk of the adverse effect without vitiating the therapeutic effect. Secondly, there must be a clear understanding of the relation between concentration and effect for both the therapeutic and the toxic effect, and that must be relatively uniform in the population. Thirdly, monitoring will be worthwhile only if the drug has a narrow therapeutic range or when the dose is a very poor determinant of the concentration, since a drug with a wide therapeutic range or predictable dosing can simply be given in a dose lower than that likely to give rise to toxic concentrations. Fourthly, there must be a sufficiently long asymptomatic period to make it plausible to detect drift from the therapeutic target range before important toxicity, or loss of therapeutic effect, occurs.

There are several circumstances in which plasma drug concentration monitoring has been proposed [14]. It remains important for digoxin, lithium, aminoglycoside antibiotics and some immunosuppressant therapies. It has been widely used in the management of epilepsy with phenytoin or carbamazepine, having the perceived advantage that 'therapeutic concentrations' (i.e. concentrations in the target range) could avert seizures whose frequency was so low that it was uncertain clinically whether activity was suppressed. However, recognition of the wide variation in effective target ranges between individual patients and the ready clinical detection of signs of toxicity, such as nystagmus or ataxia, has made monitoring of phenytoin or carbamazepine concentrations to prevent adverse effects much less common.

In addition to monitoring drug concentrations, assessment of those factors that determine differences in drug concentrations between and within individuals (Table 15.3) is also important for avoiding adverse drug reactions.

15.5.3. Monitoring pharmacodynamics

The pharmacodynamic actions of a drug will depend on its concentration at its site of action. There will generally be a chain of actions leading to the clinical effect. When it is possible to measure a pharmacodynamic effect close to the clinical adverse effect, this may be helpful in monitoring. For example, warfarin inhibits the synthesis of vitamin K-dependent clotting factors. It would be possible to measure the concentration of warfarin (pharmacokinetic measurement) or a proximate pharmacodynamic effect, such as epoxide hydrolase activity, as a measure of the effect of warfarin. However, measurement of overall clotting by prothrombin time or international normalized ratio (INR) is a more helpful way of estimating the risk of bleeding (see Chapters 3 and 18). It is also a more satisfactory measure of the therapeutic effect. Other measures, such as blood pressure in patients treated with venlafaxine, are also examples of pharmacodynamic markers ('biomarkers'—see Chapter 4) that are routinely monitored.

15.5.4. Monitoring adverse effects directly

Monitoring can also simply take the form of careful observation for the early features of an important adverse effect. This can be a laboratory measure, such as the platelet count, used to detect the onset of heparin-associated thrombocytopaenia and thrombosis [15], or testing the urine for protein in patients taking penicillamine [16]. Alternatively, it may be a clinical manoeuvre, such as measuring the heart rate during digoxin therapy for atrial fibrillation, or examining for tardive dyskinesia when a patient is taking dopamine receptor antagonists. Patients can also be asked to monitor adverse effects directly, for example the occurrence of diarrhoea with colchicine.

Monitoring tests may not be specific. For example, patients taking hydralazine can develop antinuclear antibodies as an adverse effect [17], but they can also occur in idiopathic lupus erythematosus; a positive Coombs' test occurs in as many as 20% of patients taking methyldopa [18], but only a fraction of these develop significant anaemia.

15.6. Monitoring based on the DoTS classification

Monitoring should allow adverse drug reactions to be avoided or detected sufficiently early to avoid irreversible harm. Knowledge of the timing, dose

Table 15.3 Important pharmacokinetic factors that can dictate the need to monitor for adverse drug reactions

Factor	Explanation	Examples
Age—neonates	Neonates have immature renal and liver function	Chloramphenicol, which is metabolized in the liver; the 'grey baby syndrome' of cardiovascular collapse in neonates treated with chloramphenicol is a toxic adverse effect related to poor metabolism
Age—old people	Renal and hepatic function fall with age; hepatic blood flow can also be reduced in the elderly	Digoxin, lithium and aminoglycoside antibiotics, which are excreted by the kidneys; morphine and lidocaine, which are metabolized in the liver
Obesity	For drugs that are distributed into fat	Halothane, whose action is prolonged in obesity, as stores of the drug in fat are re-circulated
Polypharmacy	Because of drug interactions	
Renal and hepatic failure	As discussed above	
Heart failure	Reduced liver blood flow	Drugs with high first-pass metabolism, such as morphine and lidocaine
Thyroid disease	Reduced renal and hepatic function in hypothyroidism; increased in hyperthyroidism	Digoxin clearance is reduced in hypothyroidism and increased in hyperthyroidism
Genetic abnormalities	Altered drug metabolism	Slow metabolizers of procainamide, hydralazine and isoniazid are at greater risk of adverse effects (e.g. lupus-like syndrome with procainamide and peripheral neuropathy with isoniazid)

responsiveness and susceptibility of an effect can help to decide whether a monitoring scheme is possible. For many adverse effects, no scheme will be possible. Even if schemes are possible, they are not necessarily practicable. They are unlikely to be implemented for rare harms of rapid onset that need to be monitored by expensive, painful and inaccurate tests.

If monitoring schemes are to be efficient, tests should be most frequently done when changes are rapid or highly probable. There is no value in repeated and prolonged monitoring for adverse effects that occur early in a course of treatment; nor is there any value in starting to monitor before any effect could possibly occur.

Here we illustrate some of these points with reference to the DoTS classification of adverse drug reactions.

15.6.1. Dose relation

Hypersusceptibility effects can occur even at subtherapeutic doses. It is therefore important to avoid administering a therapeutic dose to patients who are likely to have such a reaction. The only feasible option is to screen out patients at highest risk. Possible screening criteria include a history of susceptibility to a class of drugs (e.g. penicillin allergy) and a severe reaction to a subtherapeutic test dose (e.g. iron dextran).

Important factors one should seek in avoiding hypersusceptibility reactions are as follows:

- *A history of allergic reactions.*   This is particularly important for the penicillins and sulphonamides, since the risks of allergic reactions to these groups of drugs in the general population are relatively high.
- *A history of atopic disease or hereditary angio-oedema.*   Patients with these conditions have an increased risk of allergic reactions, particularly to penicillins.
- *Recent or repeated exposure to some drugs.*   This is important for halothane, which should not be given within 3 months of a previous exposure, because of the risk of halothane hepatitis. Other drugs, for example the anthracyclines, have cumulative toxicity.

Collateral adverse effects occur at doses within the usual therapeutic range, implying that plasma concentration measurement will not be of use. In some cases, the effects can be avoided by using relatively low doses; this is the principle underlying the current use of lower doses of oestrogens in oral contraceptives than were used formerly. However, monitoring of collateral effects generally needs to be directed at the harm itself (e.g. clozapine-induced neutropenia) or some biomarker of it (e.g. the INR in patients taking warfarin).

Toxic effects of drugs occur at doses above the maximum needed for therapy in the individual patient. Consider digoxin. Its adverse effects are mostly toxic ones, and so ensuring that the digoxin concentration is less than the toxic concentration should protect against them. The plasma digoxin concentration can be monitored directly, and this can help to avoid adverse effects [19]. Kinetic factors (e.g. renal insufficiency) can increase the concentration of digoxin at the site of action, and dynamic factors (e.g. potassium depletion) can shift the dose–response (i.e. concentration–effect) curve to the left, increasing the risk of harm (Figure 15.5); monitoring those factors should be useful. Indeed, in diagnosing digoxin toxicity it is essential to measure the plasma potassium concentration, without which the plasma digoxin concentration is uninterpretable.

15.6.2. Time course

Time-dependent reactions.   The time course of an adverse effect can be an important determinant of whether a monitoring strategy is practical, and if so, the frequency of monitoring. In particular, no monitoring strategy will be possible if the onset of an effect is rapid compared with the time taken to measure it (or a related biomarker) or to institute measures to prevent or reduce its impact. In this context, it is salutary to reflect on the monitoring of warfarin treatment by measurement of the INR. A study of the changes in monitored INR before bleeding occurred suggested that with the current frequency of monitoring there is little warning of impending danger [20]. This may help to account for the high frequency of serious bleeding in patients taking warfarin—the frequency of monitoring in current schemes is too low for reliable detection of the premonitory changes that occur before haemorrhage.

The way in which the risk of an adverse effect varies with time after the start of a course of treatment can help determine how monitoring is set up. For example, harms that occur only after the first dose of a drug (such as first-dose hypotension with ACE inhibitors) need not be sought subsequently; hypotension from ACE inhibitors that is related to volume depletion in otherwise stable patients need only be sought if volume depletion is likely, for example, because of diarrhoea or diuretic therapy. On the other hand, there is no virtue in monitoring early for delayed reactions (e.g. tardive dyskinesia with neuroleptic drugs), whose risks increase with duration of therapy, and monitoring need only begin after some time.

Clozapine-induced neutropenia affords a good example of the insight that can come from the approach of observing the time course of adverse drug reactions. This is an adverse effect of intermediate time course—it occurs with maximal frequency during a window of time after initial administration, in this case the first 24 weeks [21]. During that time monitoring of the white blood cell count should be intensive (usually once a week), but thereafter vigilance can be relaxed, because almost all of those who are destined to suffer the adverse effect will have done so by 24 weeks and the almost all of unaffected survivors will not be at risk.

Time-independent reactions.   If a reaction can occur at any time during therapy, the risks will be determined by factors of dose and susceptibility and these can change with time.

15.6.3. Susceptibility

Screening procedures can define subgroups of patients at particularly high risk of harm, in whom prevention will be the best strategy. Such procedures range from simple observation (women of child-bearing age should not take thalidomide) or questioning (patients who have previously experienced facial swelling with a penicillin should not be further exposed) to laboratory testing (for G6PD deficiency, for example) or physiological measurement (patients with an ejection fraction below 55% should not receive trastuzumab). When the risks are not so high that the drug must be avoided, knowledge of those at highest risk may allow resources for monitoring to be directed at the susceptible group.

Some susceptibility factors, such as sex, can be used to predict the risk of an adverse effect, but are not monitored. The extent and importance of genetic factors in determining susceptibility to adverse drug effects is gradually emerging [22, 23]. We do not yet know what the overall contribution of assessment of genetic factors to the prevention of harms (as opposed to monitoring) will be, although it has so far been disappointing. Phenotyping may be more relevant than genotyping, but even phenotyping can be problematic: despite the fact that the association between thiopurine methyltransferase activity and the risk of adverse effects from mercaptopurine was described several years ago [24], methods for measuring the enzyme are not standardized [25] and optimal treatment is often not achieved [26].

Age, which is also an important determinant of susceptibility, is sometimes monitored, in the sense that treatment may be introduced or withdrawn when the patient's age reaches a certain value. For example, it is desirable to withdraw the oral contraceptive from women over the age of 50 years (or earlier if there are risk factors for thrombosis, such as smoking).

Acquired susceptibility factors, such as renal and hepatic impairment, can easily be monitored and can help predict which individuals are at greatest risk of adverse effects or become so during long-term therapy. This could, for example, dictate that serum concentrations of lithium should be measured, not at regular intervals, but when the patient becomes susceptible to its adverse effects, for example during a viral illness or a bout of diarrhoea [27]; however, it is still routine practice to measure the serum lithium concentration at defined intervals, and the relative benefits of the two approaches have not been compared. These types of susceptibility factors can be either pharmacokinetic (Table 15.3) or pharmacodynamic (Table 15.4) (see also Chapter 3).

15.7. Conclusions

Monitoring is most often used in drug therapy when the prescription carries a risk of adverse drug effects that are detectable by measurement. Monitoring is also beneficial if the drug can cause organ (especially liver or renal) dysfunction, which subsequently requires dosage adjustment, or when pharmacokinetic or pharmacodynamic factors change the concentration of drug in the body or its effects on target organs. A valid test is one that will measure or predict clinically significant events (see Chapter 2) so that remedial action can be taken. With adverse drug effects, withdrawal of the drug is usually sufficient, although sometimes other therapies may be required. Monitoring thereafter

Table 15.4 Important pharmacodynamic factors that can dictate the need to monitor for adverse drug reactions

Factor	Explanation	Examples
Age—old people	Old people have impaired physiological homoeostatic mechanisms	Impaired response to a fall in blood pressure (hypotensive effects of vasodilators increased); sedative effects of centrally acting drugs exaggerated
Fluid or electrolyte imbalance	Potassium depletion; volume depletion	Cardiac glycosides and antiarrhythmic drugs, whose actions are enhanced in patients with potassium depletion; volume depletion due to diuretics enhances the hypotensive action of ACE inhibitors
Liver disease	Impaired liver function in patients with liver disease and the frail elderly	Impaired synthesis of clotting factors in liver disease (increased actions of anticoagulants); increased risk of hepatic encephalopathy with potent diuretics or sedatives (unexplained)
Heart disease	Poor left ventricular function	Increased risk of cardiac arrhythmias due to antiarrhythmic drugs
Lung disease	Increased sensitivity to adverse effects on the lungs	Reversible airways obstruction increases the risk of asthma in response to beta-blockers; increased risk of amiodarone-induced lung damage in pre-existing lung disease
Peptic ulcers	Increased risk of gastrointestinal haemorrhage	Non-steroidal anti-inflammatory drugs and anticoagulants
Genetic abnormalities	Altered drug responses	Deficiency of G6PD is associated with an increased risk of haemolysis in response to some oxidant drugs; acute intermittent porphyria can be precipitated in those with a predisposition by a wide variety of drugs, including enzyme inducers

will depend on the adverse effect that has been observed; the clinician and patient will often be keen to see 'normality' restored after drug withdrawal.

The strategies used to monitor for adverse drug effects in current clinical practice are sometimes based on explicit evidence of their ability to detect warning signals of harm, and sometimes on reasonable theoretical and practical extrapolations, but many represent ingrained clinical practice that has never been judged by the rational criteria for a monitoring scheme. Guidance from the pharmaceutical industry and drug literature is often imprecise, impractical or unavailable. It often seems designed more to protect the market authorization holder than the patient, and rarely includes any evidence of effectiveness or cost-effectiveness. Clinicians and patients need feasible schemes that focus on real-life problems to enhance patient safety and reduce the burden of drug-induced harm during treatment.

References

1 Lindquist M, Stahl M, Bate A, Edwards IR, Meyboom RH. A retrospective evaluation of a data mining approach to aid finding new adverse drug reaction signals in the WHO International Database. *Drug Saf* 2000; **23**: 533–42.
2 Evans SJ, Waller PC, Davis S. Use of proportional reporting ratios (PRRs) for signal generation from spontaneous adverse drug reaction reports. *Pharmacoepidemiol Drug Saf* 2001; **10**: 483–6.
3 Aronson JK, Ferner RE. Clarification of terminology in drug safety. *Drug Saf* 2005; **28**: 851–70.
4 Ferner RE, Coleman JJ, Pirmohamed M, Constable S, Rouse AR. The quality of information on monitoring for haematological for adverse drug reactions. *Br J Clin Pharmacol* 2005; **60**: 448–51.
5 Pirmohamed M, Ferner RE. Monitoring drug treatment. *BMJ* 2003; **327**: 1179–81.
6 Pirmohamed M, James S, Meakin S, et al. Adverse drug reactions as cause of admission to hospital: prospective analysis of 18 820 patients. *BMJ* 2004; **329**: 15–19.
7 Classen DC, Pestotnik SL, Evans RS, Lloyd JF, Burke JP. Adverse drug events in hospitalized patients. Excess length of stay, extra costs, and attributable mortality. *JAMA* 1997; **277**: 301–6.
8 Mockenhaupt M, Messenheimer J, Tennis P, Schlingmann J. Risk of Stevens–Johnson syndrome and toxic epidermal necrolysis in new users of antiepileptics. *Neurology* 2005; **64**: 1134–8.
9 Aronson JK, Ferner RE. Joining the DoTS: new approach to classifying adverse drug reactions. *BMJ* 2003; **327**: 1222–5.
10 Wetzels GE, Nelemans PJ, Schouten JS, van Wijk BL, Prins MH. All that glisters is not gold: a comparison of electronic monitoring versus filled prescriptions—an observational study. *BMC Health Serv Res* 2006; **6**: 8.
11 George CF, Peveler RC, Heiliger S, Thompson C. Compliance with tricyclic antidepressants: the value of four different methods of assessment. *Br J Clin Pharmacol* 2000; **50**: 166–71.
12 Dubbert PM, King A, Rapp SR, Brief D, Martin JE, Lake M. Riboflavin as a tracer of medication compliance. *J Behav Med* 1985; **8**: 287–99.

13 Kumar S, Haigh JR, Rhodes LE, et al. Poor compliance is a major factor in unstable outpatient control of anticoagulant therapy. *Thromb Haemost* 1989; **62**: 729–32.

14 Reynolds DJ, Aronson JK. ABC of drug monitoring. Making the most of plasma drug concentration measurements. *BMJ* 1993; **306**: 48–51.

15 Warkentin TE. Platelet count monitoring and laboratory testing for heparin-induced thrombocytopenia. *Arch Pathol Lab Med* 2002; **126**: 1415–23.

16 Simon CH, Dijkmans BA, Breedveld FC. Variations in the monitoring and management of the side effects of antirheumatic drugs by means of laboratory tests. *Clin Exp Rheumatol* 1997; **15**: 633–9.

17 Russell GI, Bing RF, Jones JA, Thurston H, Swales JD. Hydralazine sensitivity: clinical features, autoantibody changes and HLA-DR phenotype. *Q J Med* 1987; **65**: 845–52.

18 Carstairs KC, Breckenridge A, Dollery CT, Worlledge SM. Incidence of a positive direct Coombs' test in patients on alpha-methyldopa. *Lancet* 1966; **2**: 133–5.

19 Campbell TJ, Williams KM. Therapeutic drug monitoring: antiarrhythmic drugs. *Br J Clin Pharmacol* 2001; **52** (Suppl 1): 21S–34S.

20 Kucher N, Connolly S, Beckman JA, et al. International normalized ratio increase before warfarin-associated hemorrhage: brief and subtle. *Arch Intern Med* 2004; **164**: 2176–9.

21 Alvir JMJ, Lieberman JA, Safferman AZ, Schwinner JL, Schaaf JA. Clozapine-induced agranulocytosis: incidence and risk factors in the United States. *N Engl J Med* 1993; **329**: 162–7.

22 Evans WE, McLeod HL. Pharmacogenomics—drug disposition, drug targets, and side effects. *N Engl J Med* 2003; **348**: 538–49.

23 Phillips KA, Veenstra DL, Oren E, Lee JK, Sadee W. Potential role of pharmacogenomics in reducing adverse drug reactions. A systematic review. *JAMA* 2001; **286**: 2270–9.

24 Lennard L, Rees CA, Lilleyman JS, Maddocks JL. Childhood leukaemia: a relationship between intracellular 6-mercaptopurine metabolites and neutropenia. *Br J Clin Pharmacol* 2004; **58**: S867–S871.

25 Armstrong VW, Shipkova M, von Ahsen N, Oellerich M. Analytic aspects of monitoring therapy with thiopurine medications. *Ther Drug Monit* 2004; **26**: 220–6.

26 Coulthard SA, Matheson EC, Hall AG, Hogarth LA. The clinical impact of thiopurine methyltransferase polymorphisms on thiopurine treatment. *Nucleosides Nucleotides Nucleic Acids* 2004; **23**: 1385–91.

27 Mitchell PB. Therapeutic drug monitoring of psychotropic medications. *Br J Clin Pharmacol* 2001; **52** (Suppl 1): 45S–54S.

PART 2
The Practice of Monitoring

CHAPTER 16

Monitoring diabetes mellitus across the lifetime of illness

Andrew J. Farmer

Diabetes mellitus is one of the leading causes of death and disability. Monitoring of the disease and its course is a major health-care activity. Early treatment of raised blood pressure can prevent cardiovascular events and monitoring for vascular and neurological changes can allow treatment to limit the progression of complications. Tight control of glycaemia is a major factor in improving disease outcomes, and the problems associated with monitoring glycaemic control are widely applicable to other areas of monitoring. The focus of this chapter is therefore on the range of variables that are used to monitor and optimize glycaemic control.

16.1. The condition

Most cases of diabetes fall into two broad categories: type 1 and type 2. Type 1 diabetes follows autoimmune destruction of the insulin-producing beta cells of the pancreas, mainly in children and young adults. Insulin is required almost immediately and therapy is life long. Type 2 diabetes is a complex metabolic disorder associated with hypertension, hyperlipidaemia and insulin resistance, with long-term loss of beta cell function; it can be initially managed with diet and exercise, and later requires oral insulin-releasing or insulin-sensitizing agents and eventually insulin.

The common feature of both types of diabetes is a high blood glucose concentration, which leads to unpleasant symptoms and eventually coma and potentially death; in the long-term, tissue damage occurs through glycation. Symptomatic control of diabetes can now be managed with relative ease, but failure to bring about near-normal blood glucose concentrations can lead to an increased risk of complications (Table 16.1). More intensive control of glycaemia brings about the risk of hypoglycaemia. The aim of glycaemic monitoring is to optimize the balance between the benefits of lower blood glucose

Evidence-based Medical Monitoring: from Principles to Practice. Edited by Paul Glasziou, Les Irwig and Jeffrey K. Aronson. © 2008 Blackwell Publishing, ISBN: 978-1-4051-5399-7.

Table 16.1 The long-term complications of glycaemia

	Complications
Microvascular disease	Retinopathy
	Maculopathy
	Renal disease
	Neuropathy
Macrovascular disease	Cerebrovascular disease
	Coronary artery disease
	Peripheral arterial disease

concentrations and the potential harms that can arise from impaired consciousness due to hypoglycaemia.

16.2. Why do we monitor?

The overall aim of blood glucose control in people with diabetes is to achieve as near normal physiological or ideal blood glucose concentrations as possible without detriment to quality of life and without causing significant hypoglycaemia.

Blood glucose concentrations vary throughout the day. People with type 1 diabetes lack the normal homoeostatic mechanism to control blood glucose concentrations, while people with type 2 diabetes have an impaired or absent response. In both types, awareness of glycaemia can lead to appropriate changes in treatment, improving glycaemic control while minimizing the risks of hypoglycaemia.

16.3. Particular challenges

Discussion of the role of monitoring in diabetes requires clarity about the disease type (type 1 or 2), the stage of the disease, particularly for type 2 diabetes (early, using oral hypoglycaemic therapy or insulin requiring) and the method used to monitor. Appropriate methods of monitoring and the characteristics of treatment vary with the course of the disease, and the different methods of monitoring can provide complementary information to help make decisions about management.

16.4. Potential measures and a causal schema

Blood glucose concentration and glycated haemoglobin (Hb_{A1c}) are the two measures of glycaemic control most often used in current practice (Table 16.2). Prospective observational and intervention studies have confirmed that both measures are related to long-term disease outcomes [1–3], and both are used in routine clinical practice to guide management. Measurement of urinary

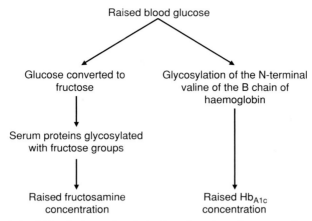

Figure 16.1 Raised blood glucose levels lead to glycation of a range of proteins in the body.

glucose concentrations remains an option for some patients who do not wish to achieve intensive glycaemic control. Raised blood glucose concentrations lead to increased rates of glycation of both Hb_{A1c} and other proteins (Figure 16.1). The more presence of larger quantities of advanced glycation products indicates poorer control.

16.5. Blood glucose concentration measurement

Blood glucose concentration measurement is a term that is frequently used without precise definition. Measurement of glucose concentration is usually carried out either on capillary or venous samples of blood. Most laboratories measure the concentration of glucose in plasma, which gives a different result from blood. Table 16.3 shows equivalent measurements in different types of blood samples from different sites. Most blood glucose concentration measurements are now made on capillary samples of whole blood using hand-held meters. However, most meters are now standardized to display results converted to a plasma-equivalent range. Thus, a 'blood glucose' measurement usually refers to either a plasma glucose concentration measurement made on a venous blood sample or a blood glucose concentration measurement made on a capillary blood sample, usually converted to a plasma glucose equivalent reading.

Fasting plasma glucose measurements are used to measure the concentrations of glucose after an overnight fast. Fasting plasma glucose concentration measurement provides information about the overnight blood glucose concentration that results either from endogenous insulin secretion or from basal amounts of injected insulin. Measurement of plasma glucose concentrations before meals indicates the adequacy of either exogenous or endogenous

Table 16.2 Measurements in monitoring glycaemic control

Underlying condition	Test	How quickly the test changes with changes in the condition or treatment	Changes in the benefit to harm balance over time detected by monitoring	Where the test is performed	Changes that result from the test	Patient	Testing frequency
Type 2 diabetes; no insulin	HbA1c	The target measurement changes only slowly (over 6–9 weeks) with changes in treatment	Important changes in the underlying medical condition occur only slowly	Laboratory	Intensify pharmacological treatment and general advice about lifestyle	Change treatment and lifestyle	6–8 weekly minimum
Type 2 diabetes	Blood glucose measured with a hand-held meter	Changes occur from minute to minute; homoeostasis should be achieved in the fasting state when not using insulin	Changes in the underlying condition occur over time; however, food intake and physical activity unpredictably affect the result	Laboratory testing is more accurate but less practical than self-testing	Intensify pharmacological treatment; the extent to which the information is useful in monitoring physical activity and diet in reducing glycaemia is not known	Change amount of insulin and lifestyle	Twice weekly; minimum three-point profile on simplest insulin regimen
Type 1 diabetes	HbA1c	Useful for assessing overall concentrations of control but not helpful in maintaining day-to-day control	Useful as a periodic check	Laboratory	Change overall insulin dose	Change treatment and lifestyle	6–8 weekly minimum
Type 1 diabetes	Blood glucose measured with hand-held meter	Hyperglycaemia and hypoglycaemia can develop rapidly	For some individuals can be an essential element in maintaining tight glycaemic control	Laboratory testing is more accurate but less practical than self-testing	Change insulin dose in relation to changes in food and physical activity	Change amount of insulin therapy and lifestyle	Twice weekly; minimum three-point profile on simplest insulin regimen

Table 16.3 Values for diagnosis of diabetes mellitus

| | Glucose concentration (mmol/l*) | | | |
| | Plasma | | Whole blood | |
Time of measurement	Venous	Capillary	Venous	Capillary
Fasting	≥7.0	≥7.0	≥6.1	≥6.1
2 h after a glucose load	≥11.1	≥12.2	≥10.0	≥11.1

Note: *1 mmol/l = 18 mg/dl.

insulin in responding to food, and post-prandial measurement (usually 2 h after food) provides information about the peak concentrations of plasma glucose after food. A single measurement of glucose after a meal may identify most patients with inadequate control [4].

In addition to measurement at defined times, additional checks on blood glucose concentrations can be made in relation to the risk of hypoglycaemia, for example before exercise or driving and in the presence of symptoms that suggest hypoglycaemia.

Although laboratory methods of blood glucose measurement are accurate (and preferred for diagnosis), the convenience of hand-held meters means that, despite their higher coefficient of variation and the possibility of user error, they are in wide use. The majority conform to international standards [5], and 95% of readings are within 0.83 mmol/l (15 mg/dl) for readings under 4 mmol/l (72 mg/dl) and within 20% for higher readings. Hand-held meters use test strips that release gluconic acid and hydrogen peroxide from a blood sample. The reaction is quantified by one of a range of methods. Problems can be minimized by careful training and consistent technique in making measurements, incorporating an allowance for the possibility of error in the reading when calculating insulin dose, and undertaking regular testing to identify results that do not fit the usual pattern, with re-testing as necessary. Nevertheless, operator error is a significant source of error, including failure to calibrate meters (some newer meters do not require external calibration), poor hand-washing technique and dirty meters [6].

16.6. Glycated haemoglobin measurement

The proportion of haemoglobin that is glycated provides an estimate of over-all glycaemic control over the preceding 6–8 weeks. Until the late 1990s the difficulties of standardization and the costs of the test made interpretation be-tween laboratories difficult and availability limited. However, many of these problems have been overcome, and the most common measured component haemoglobin A1c (Hb$_{A1c}$) is now widely accepted as a standard measure-ment of glycaemic control. However, the problem of standardization remains a matter of debate, with further developments in progress, briefly discussed at the end of this chapter [7, 8].

Human haemoglobin A is chemically altered in the presence of glucose. The increased concentrations of glucose in diabetes increase the rate of the chemical reactions involved. Hb_{A1c} results from a reaction between the β chain of haemoglobin A0 and glucose. Other compounds result from other reactions on the α and β chains of haemoglobin, and these can be measured as the total glycated haemoglobin.

Hb_{A1c} can be affected by the presence of haemoglobin variants and uraemia, but different assays can be used to obtain an accurate result. Vitamin C, haemolytic anaemia and iron deficiency anaemia can also give abnormal results. About 50% of the variance in Hb_{A1c} is determined by blood glucose concentrations over the previous month, 25% by the concentrations over 30–60 days and the remaining 25% by the concentrations over 60–120 days. For most routine purposes an interval of 3 months between tests is usually recommended, although a test after 2 months can provide additional information [9].

Because of the range of different techniques available to measure Hb_{A1c} and total glycated haemoglobin, external quality-assurance schemes are required to ensure that measurements between laboratories can be compared. The most frequently used scheme enables Hb_{A1c} measurements to be standardized to the measurements obtained in the Diabetes Control and Complications Trial [3]. Hb_{A1c} concentrations are not currently suitable for diagnosis, but current guidance for people with diabetes is to aim, if possible, for Hb_{A1c} concentrations of 6.5–7.5% [10].

Hb_{A1c} concentrations are related to blood glucose concentrations, but no method has yet been developed to relate blood glucose concentrations to Hb_{A1c} concentrations that is robust enough for use in clinical practice. For patients with type 2 diabetes who do not use insulin, a regular fasting plasma glucose concentration of 7 mmol/l would be expected to correspond to a Hb_{A1c} concentration of around 7% [11]. However, prandial elevation of blood glucose concentration makes an additional contribution to the rate of glycation, thus affecting individual results [10].

Point-of-care testing for Hb_{A1c} is now possible with analysers that can be clinic based. However, there is not yet sufficient information about benefits to justify their widespread use [12].

16.7. Symptoms, urine monitoring and fructosamine

Symptoms from hyperglycaemia are normally noticeable above a concentration of 10 mmol/l. Renal excretion of glucose is variable, but unusual below blood glucose concentrations of 8 mmol/l. At higher blood glucose concentrations, the presence of excreted glucose in the urine can be used as an indicator that the blood glucose is above 8 mmol/l. The test is semi-quantitative—higher concentrations of blood glucose are associated with higher concentrations of glucose in the urine. However, current therapy aims to lower glucose below the renal threshold, so the use of urine tests is becoming less common. Nevertheless, for an individual with good control, the presence of glucose in the urine can provide the first indication of a loss of control.

In the presence of disorders that affect the measured concentration of glycated haemoglobin (e.g. thalassaemia) or other disorders that affect erythrocyte turnover (pregnancy or anaemia), blood glucose measurement can be unreliable. Alternative blood proteins can be used to assess the rate of tissue glycation. Fructosamine is the commonest assay used for this purpose.

16.8. Choosing measures for monitoring

The choice of measure for monitoring glycaemia depends on the purpose of monitoring, which in turn depends on the type of diabetes, the time course of the disease and the treatment. For individuals who do not require intensive glycaemic control (e.g. those with a limited life expectancy) a combination of symptoms and urine monitoring may be sufficient [8].

16.8.1. Symptoms

Symptoms of hypoglycaemia closely reflect a low blood glucose concentration. However, the onset and severity of symptoms are variable, and frequent hypoglycaemia can lead to a diminished awareness of early symptoms and rapid progression to loss of consciousness. Particularly when using insulin, care should be taken to check blood glucose concentrations before tasks such as driving, operating machinery or physical activity, to check whether additional carbohydrate might be needed to prevent hypoglycaemia.

Without biochemical conformation, some symptoms of hyperglycaemia, such as faintness, thirst or polyuria, can be due to other causes and are therefore not of use in monitoring.

16.8.2. Blood glucose concentration

Fasting blood glucose concentration, measured out after an 8-h fast, can be used for people with both type 1 and type 2 diabetes. For people with type 2 diabetes not using insulin, the within-person coefficient of variation of pre-breakfast concentrations is low and measurements vary little from day to day. They are therefore useful in assessing day-to-day control and making adjustments to therapy or assessing the impact of lifestyle changes. A study of people with type 2 diabetes carried out before the routine availability of Hb_{A1c} suggested that the proportion of people with uncontrolled diabetes could be increased from 46 to 76% using fasting plasma glucose monitoring with control (fasting plasma glucose >4 to <6 mmol/l) maintained over at least 6 months [13]. For people with type 2 diabetes overnight concentrations, particularly when interpreted in the light of the previous evening's readings, indicate the effectiveness of long-acting insulin. Fasting plasma glucose concentration measurement can therefore be used to adjust medication in type 2 diabetes, including insulin.

Pre-prandial blood glucose concentrations are often equated with fasting blood glucose concentrations. However, they do not, because the fasting blood glucose concentration is measured after an 8-h fast. However, the pre-prandial concentration may be useful for evaluating the impact of a complex insulin schedule, particularly when a fast-acting analogue insulin is used [7].

Blood glucose concentrations are usually high after meals, and thus contribute to overall blood glucose control. Some studies have been interpreted to suggest that post-prandial glucose concentrations correlate better than fasting concentrations with the development of complications (or that glycaemic variability may be related to poor outcomes [14, 15]). However, attempts to titrate oral hypoglycaemic medications by taking account of post-prandial measures have not been successful [16].

The case for monitoring people with type 2 diabetes not taking oral hypoglycaemic drugs by blood glucose concentrations measurement remains unproven. It is sometime advocated for an educational benefit, for example increasing awareness of the variation in blood glucose that comes with type 2 diabetes. Fasting blood glucose concentration measurement remains, in principle, a good measure of overall glycaemic control in these patients. However, unless a laboratory measure is used, there may be an unacceptably large error when using blood glucose meters. A single measurement can also be affected by recent alcohol or exercise. Hb_{A1c} measurement is more accurate and stable than blood glucose testing, but, in areas where resources are limited, a blood glucose measurement may be the only feasible measurement.

Optimum treatment for type 1 diabetes using insulin is intended to produce a near-normal pattern of blood glucose during the day. Blood glucose measurement is therefore essential to allow the within-day variation of insulin dose that is required to allow for variations in physical activity and food. The major trial in this area included SMBG as an integral part of its intervention [17]. Glucose concentrations can change rapidly in response to lifestyle and insulin treatment, so intermittent measurement will inevitably fail to identify the full range of variation. Continuous glucose monitoring provides increasing concentrations of information about such variation, and, in combination with continuous infusion pumps, allows frequent interventions to maintain tight control.

16.8.3. Hb_{A1c}

In order to interpret blood glucose results, regular measurements are necessary. In contrast, a single Hb_{A1c} test can provide information about blood glucose control over a period of weeks rather than minutes. In addition, the within-person coefficient of variation is low. Unless people with type 2 diabetes who do not require insulin have chosen to titrate the dose of oral hypoglycaemic medication at 2 weekly intervals, Hb_{A1c} will provide sufficient information for effective clinical care, although the use of self-monitoring of blood glucose is controversial in this group of patients [18].

Hb$_{A1c}$ is therefore the measure of choice for people with type 2 diabetes who do not use insulin and for evaluating the longer term impact of treatment for people with type 1 diabetes and people with type 2 diabetes who use insulin.

16.9. Monitoring schedules

Current schedules for monitoring are based on experience with the tests over long periods. The schedules that are associated with type 1 and type 2 diabetes vary because of the different treatments used and the different physiological responses that are associated with both the presence of endogenous insulin and increased insulin resistance in type 2 diabetes. Adherence to monitoring schedules can be aided by use of educational support with recording of measurements [19].

16.9.1. Type 1 diabetes

Tight control brings with it the risk of hypoglycaemia [3]. For some people (those with a limited duration of life or who cannot make the adjustments required for tight control) intensive control is not appropriate. Accepting less tight control allows use of less complicated regimens and less frequent monitoring.

For people with type 1 diabetes who use a typical basal–bolus regimen, including three injections of short-acting insulin and one or more injections of long-acting insulin, blood glucose should be monitored on at least four occasions during the day: before breakfast, before lunch, before dinner and before bedtime. This identifies periods during the day when blood glucose concentrations are higher, and allows appropriate adjustment of the short-acting or bedtime doses. If the individual has regular routines and varies little in food intake and physical activity from day to day, monitoring can take place at a frequency of less than four tests a day; for example, a daily fasting blood glucose plus four-point sampling on one or two days a week, or testing on each day at one or more additional times, in order to build a picture over the week. However, until the dose of long-acting insulin has been established, a series of paired bedtime and fasting readings are needed.

For individuals who use conventional rather than analogue long-acting insulin, and with biphasic regimens, more frequent monitoring may be required, because of the less stable time course of the long-acting components of the insulin.

Hb$_{A1c}$ measurement complements blood glucose measurement by providing a check on the extent to which the blood glucose results provide an accurate picture of blood glucose control. A schedule of blood glucose measurements that suggests good control may need to be examined if an Hb$_{A1c}$ measurement shows that control is not so good. For example, timing of measurements and user technique may need to be re-assessed.

16.9.2. Type 2 diabetes

16.9.2.1. Diet-treated only

Recommendations about the frequency of fasting blood glucose measurements vary from once a week to once a day. However, evidence of effect of the practice is lacking, and the possible benefits in terms of motivation for any one individual have to be weighed against their facility with measurement techniques and variations in lifestyle.

16.9.2.2. Oral glucose-lowering drugs

Blood glucose monitoring may be of some help if people wish to titrate their oral medication to achieve fasting plasma glucose readings of 6 mmol/l or less. However. There is no evidence that achieving glucose targets through titration over a short period is superior to a rather slower approach using HbA1c measurements.

16.9.2.3. Insulin-treated type 2 diabetes

Most people with type 2 diabetes treated with long-acting insulin also continue to take oral hypoglycaemic drugs. The recommended schedules for monitoring are derived from trials that have sought to achieve reductions in Hb_{A1c} to within recommended concentrations [20]. However, the intensity of these schedules has not yet been evaluated in wider populations and those more representative of primary-care populations. Fasting blood glucose concentrations measured twice a week will allow weekly or 2 weekly titration of the long-acting insulin to achieve tight control. Additional four-point or seven-point profiles may be helpful every 3–4 weeks to identify patterns of blood glucose control that require further attention; for example, to address the possibility of hypoglycaemia or to identify high post-prandial glucose concentrations that require the use of a pre-meal short-acting insulin.

16.9.3. Response to treatment

16.9.3.1. Type 1 diabetes

With an active lifestyle, blood glucose concentrations vary from day to day. Changes in short-acting insulin doses can be used to achieve blood glucose concentrations of 4–6 mmol/l, but inevitably readings outside this range will be obtained. If blood glucose concentrations are higher than anticipated, a correction dose can be applied by either using a single bolus of short-acting insulin or taking extra insulin. The amount of extra insulin needed can be calculated, although it may need to be further adjusted in the light of experience. In general, one extra unit of insulin will lower the blood glucose concentration by x mmol/l where $x = 100/$total daily dose of insulin.

16.9.3.2. Type 2 diabetes

Although, in principle, the manipulation of insulin dose for people with type 2 diabetes with no remaining endogenous insulin secretion is the same for people with type 1 diabetes, the actual implementation is usually different, because people at this stage tend to be older, may often be limited by co-morbidity, are therefore less in need of intensive glycaemic control, and may also have insulin resistance, requiring much larger doses of insulin.

For people titrating basal insulin dose upwards, the initial dose can be calculated using a published formula [21] and then titrated upwards in increments of 2–4 units, depending on response, to reach the target concentration of fasting blood glucose.

16.9.3.3. Non-specific response to monitoring

Although monitoring can lead to a change of treatment by a specific response to information obtained, improvements can also be made through non-specific mechanisms. For example, regular measurement of blood glucose concentration may increase awareness of the seriousness of the disease, which may in turn affect the type of food eaten or the amount of exercise taken. Any evaluation of the impact of monitoring for an individual may need to account for the extent to which any benefit takes place through this mechanism.

16.9.3.4. Monitoring in people with hypoglycaemia

People with hypoglycaemia are vulnerable to further bouts of hypoglycaemia, so blood glucose concentrations consistently below 4 mmol/l (plasma) or even occasionally below 3.1 mmol/l should be reviewed and doses of insulin or hypoglycaemic medications reduced to avoid potential complications. Achieving a fasting plasma glucose (usually measured on a capillary blood sample) of 4–6 mmol/l in someone with type 2 diabetes will mean an 80–95% chance of achieving a Hb_{A1c} of 6.5%.

16.9.4. Maintenance schedule

16.9.4.1. What is the within-individual variation?

Blood glucose concentrations vary from day to day. There is general agreement that measurements should be repeated on at least two occasions to ensure that treatment decisions are not made on potentially inaccurate single measurements. Type 2 diabetes has a tendency to deteriorate over time, with increases in blood glucose of 0.5–1 mmol/l per year [22].

People with type 1 diabetes do not generally experience progressive changes in blood glucose concentrations once stable, unless there are lifestyle changes, such as weight gain, affecting insulin resistance.

16.9.4.2. Graphical display/control charts

Software packages are beginning to display blood glucose results and use graphical charts to help identify trends and excursions from usual concentrations of control [23]. For example, a recently developed telemedicine support system includes a display of blood glucose excursions that relate to specific insulin doses (Figure 16.2).

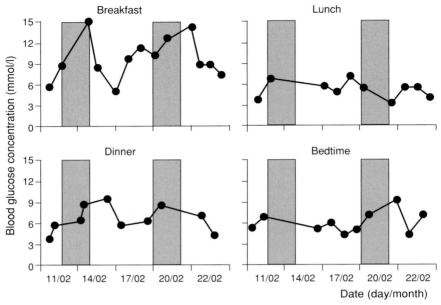

Figure 16.2 Sequential blood glucose measurements in a patient with type 1 diabetes charted by time of day to show the variation that can be addressed by changes in doses of short-acting and long-acting insulin; weekends marked in blue.

16.9.4.3. How often should we remeasure?

Remeasurement, once stable, depends on variability of lifestyle and disease type. Most current clinical practice is based on experience with individual patients. This is partly because of a recognition that individual biological variations and variability of lifestyle will limit the extent to which population data can be assembled to guide practice. However, there remains a need to characterize the wider population and subgroups of people with diabetes to shape expectations for the performance of monitoring tests in these groups and to provide estimates of the numbers of people that might benefit from different types of monitoring schedules. With type 1 diabetes, the more active person might need to continue a minimum of four readings a day, sometimes more if using additional insulin to cover snacks between meals. If lifestyle is more stable, a sample of measurements once or twice a week may be sufficient. Hb$_{A1c}$ measurements every 3–6 months are needed to detect any drifts in control that are not being revealed by the blood glucose readings (e.g. high post-prandial concentrations because of mis-timings of insulin injections).

For type 2 diabetes Hb$_{A1c}$ measurements should be taken every 3 months when not on target. Once on target, 6 monthly or even annual measurements may be sufficient, but because of the deterioration in beta-cell function, time-intervals of greater than 1 year are not desirable.

16.9.4.4. How should we alter management?

For people with type 1 diabetes, usual therapy consists of long-acting and short-acting insulin. Long-acting analogue insulin can be adjusted on the basis of the extent to which it brings about a stable plasma glucose concentration or a slight fall in concentration between bedtime and a fasting morning dose. Changes in dose at minimum intervals of 3–4 days are needed to allow the long-acting concentrations of insulin to stabilize. Prandial insulin may need changing from day to day, depending on blood glucose concentrations (higher concentrations require additional units of insulin), planned food intake and planned physical activity. Programmes such as DAFNE [24] provide detailed support and advice about the way to monitor intake of food and make appropriate adjustments in insulin dose. Insulin pumps are an alternative approach when an infusion of short-acting insulin can be used to achieve a steady state, and are particularly useful when people with active lifestyles find it difficult to achieve a balance between an adequate dose of basal insulin to maintain control between meals and avoiding hypoglycaemia after injections of short-acting insulin.

For people with type 2 diabetes, the range of available options for changing dose is limited. For people on diet only, the main purpose of blood glucose monitoring is as a supplementary check on the efficacy of losing weight in lowering blood glucose. Fasting blood glucose concentrations provide a stable indicator of progress. For people taking metformin or a sulphonylurea, fasting blood glucose is a potential mechanism for titration of dose, although the usual pattern of clinic visits every 3–4 months means that Hb_{A1c} could also be used for this purpose, coinciding titration steps with visits. The availability of short-acting insulin secretagogues has led some patients to check blood glucose before meals, then deciding on whether to take a tablet depending on blood glucose concentrations and planned food intake. However, there are no well-designed studies of this approach to therapy.

Hb_{A1c} measurements have some degree of laboratory variation and day-to-day variation, and so decisions about titration of therapy need to take this into account. Current recommended targets are for Hb_{A1c} <6.5%. However, single HbA1c readings of <7.5% should not lead to therapy changes to achieve the lower target without confirmation and monitoring for hypoglycaemia. In these circumstances, review of blood glucose measurements can be useful in reaching a decision. However, a single concentration above 7.5% is unlikely to represent a true value below the lower target, and therapy can be increased.

Individuals with type 1 diabetes need, in addition to fasting plasma glucose concentrations below 6 mmol/l, similar pre-meal readings, and to limit post-prandial excursions of glucose by use of prandial insulin.

People with type 2 diabetes who progress to insulin also require regular monitoring with blood glucose tests. Most people in the UK are now starting to use a basal insulin regimen, which can be monitored with a fasting blood glucose concentration measurement, with increments of insulin used to titrate to near a fasting plasma glucose target of <6 mmol/l. Biphasic or prandial regimens require more frequent monitoring. Individuals with type 2 diabetes tend to be older and have more stable lifestyles; therefore, day-to-day monitoring and changes in dose are less likely to be required. A fasting or pre-meal plasma glucose concentration of 4–6 mmol/l is currently the range in which control is near normal without a substantial, although slightly increased, risk of hypoglycaemia.

16.9.4.5. Evaluation of effectiveness

There is only a limited number of full trial evaluations of blood glucose monitoring. Evaluation of monitoring in people with type 1 diabetes has been incorporated into the DCCT trial, which has shown that tight control is important in preventing complications [3, 17]. Among people with type 2 diabetes some studies have attempted to review the role of monitoring. A systematic review failed to show benefit [16], but many of the included studies did not incorporate educational advice focused on blood glucose readings [25]. More recently, some studies have incorporated monitoring and educational interventions in comparisons with usual care, but again the extent to which monitoring may have added to the effectiveness of the educational element is not clear [24].

There are alternative strategies, which have not been fully evaluated. Many people simply prescribe oral hypoglycaemic medications on the basis of a raised Hb_{A1c}, with dose titration at 3 monthly intervals. Once target concentrations are reached (e.g. <6.5%) annual review is appropriate. However, if the concentration is 6.5–7.5%, 6 monthly review would be appropriate.

More intensive monitoring might be appropriate if there is uncertainty about Hb_{A1c} concentrations (e.g. 7.5% with hypoglycaemia) or concern about rapidly changing concentrations of Hb_{A1c}, for example in a younger person in whom there is uncertainty about the possibility of late-onset autoimmune diabetes.

16.10. Self-monitoring

Self-monitoring of blood glucose is an area in which adherence is poor. A small group of people are interested, but most studies confirm that unless relevant information is obtained (i.e. a rapid change with diet), the repetition of blood glucose concentrations with the same results leads to a fall-off in adherence. Conversely, taking concentrations at different times of the day can lead to concentrations that are very different, without a clear explanation of the differences, which again can demotivate, since there is no obvious course of action.

16.11. Future research

16.11.1. The future of Hb_{A1c}

Hb_{A1c} measurements vary widely, and assays are increasingly focusing on measurement of the discrete A1c component. Problems of standardization are unresolved. The main problems are the use of different assays, which are not easily standardized against current reference tests, and the potential for giving test results in units that are not consistent with current tests [6, 7]. Intensive work to resolve these issues is under way.

Hb_{A1c} monitoring is now laid down as a measure by which clinicians' performance is judged in the UK through the Quality Outcomes Framework mechanism [26]. Further work is required to evaluate this in policy terms, particularly in view of the lack of standardization of the measure and the range of uncertainty around the coefficient of variation of the measure.

References

1 DECODE Study Group on behalf of the European Diabetes Epidemiology Group. Glucose tolerance and mortality: comparison of WHO and American Diabetes Association diagnostic criteria. *Lancet* 1999; **354**: 617–21.

2 UK Prospective Diabetes Study (UKPDS) Group. Intensive blood glucose control with sulphonylureas or insulin compared with conventional treatment and risk of complications in patients with type 2 diabetes (UKPDS 33). *Lancet* 1998; **352**: 837–53.

3 The Diabetes Control and Complications Trial Research Group. The effect of intensive treatment of diabetes on the development and progression of long-term complications in insulin-dependent diabetes mellitus. *N Engl J Med* 1993; **329**: 977–86.

4 El Kebbi IM, Ziemer DC, Cook CB, Gallina DL, Barnes CS, Phillips LS. Utility of casual postprandial glucose levels in type 2 diabetes management. *Diabetes Care* 2004; **27**: 335–9.

5 International Organization for Standardization. Geneva: Switzerland. http://www.iso. org/iso/en/ISOOnline.frontpage.

6 Brunner GA, Ellmerer M, Sendlhofer G, et al. Validation of home blood glucose meters with respect to clinical and analytical approaches. *Diabetes Care* 1998; **21**: 585–90.

7 Marshall SM, Barth JH. Standardization of Hb_{A1c} measurements—a consensus statement. *Diabet Med* 2000; **17**: 5–6.

8 Home P, Chacra A, Chan J, Emslie-Smith A, Sorensen L, Crombrugge PV. Considerations on blood glucose management in type 2 diabetes mellitus. *Diabetes Metab Res Rev* 2002; **18**: 273–85.

9 Tahara Y, Shima K. The response of GHb to stepwise plasma glucose change over time in diabetic patients. *Diabetes Care* 1993; **16**: 1313–4.

10 National Institute for Clinical Excellence. *Management of Type 2 Diabetes: Management of Blood Glucose*. London: National Institute for Clinical Excellence, 2002.

11 Rohlfing CL, Wiedmeyer HM, Little RR, England JD, Tennill A, Goldstein DE. Defining the relationship between plasma glucose and Hb_{A1c}: analysis of glucose profiles and Hb_{A1c} in the Diabetes Control and Complications Trial. *Diabetes Care* 2002; **25**: 275–8.

12 Schwartz K, Monsur J, Bartoces M, West P, Neale A. Correlation of same-visit Hb_{A1c} test with laboratory-based measurements: a MetroNet study. *BMC Fam Pract* 2005; **6**: 28.

13 Howe-Davies S, Simpson RW, Turner RC. Control of maturity-onset diabetes by monitoring fasting blood glucose and body weight. *Diabetes Care* 1980; **3**: 607–10.

14 Rubin RR, Peyrot M, Saudek CD. Effect of diabetes education on self-care, metabolic control, and emotional well-being. *Diabetes Care* 1989; **12**: 673–9.

15 DECODE Study Group on behalf of the European Diabetes Epidemiology Study Group. Will new diagnostic criteria for diabetes mellitus change phenotype of patients with diabetes? Reanalysis of European epidemiological data. *BMJ* 1998; **317**: 371–5.

16 Gerstein HC, Garon J, Joyce C, Rolfe A, Walter CM. Pre-prandial vs. post-prandial capillary glucose measurements as targets for repaglinide dose titration in people with diet-treated or metformin-treated type 2 diabetes: a randomized controlled clinical trial. *Diabet Med* 2004; **21**: 1200–3.

17 The Diabetes Control and Complications Trial/Epidemiology of Diabetes Interventions and Complications (DCCT/EDIC) Study Research Group. Intensive diabetes treatment and cardiovascular disease in patients with type 1 diabetes. *N Engl J Med* 2005; **353**: 2643–53.

18 Coster S, Gulliford MC, Seed PT, Powrie JK, Swaminatham R. Self-monitoring in Type 2 diabetes mellitus: a meta-analysis. *Diabet Med* 2000; **17**: 755–61.

19 Moreland EC, Volkening LK, Lawlor MT, Chalmers KA, Anderson BJ, Laffel LMB. Use of a blood glucose monitoring manual to enhance monitoring adherence in adults with diabetes: a randomized controlled trial. *Arch Intern Med* 2006; **166**: 689–5.

20 Riddle MC, Rosenstock J, Gerich J. The Treat-to-Target Trial: randomized addition of glargine or human NPH insulin to oral therapy of type 2 diabetic patients. *Diabetes Care* 2003; **26**: 3080–6.

21 Holman RR, Turner RC. Optimizing blood glucose control in type 2 diabetes: an approach based on fasting blood glucose measurements. *Diabet Med* 1988; **5**: 582–8.

22 UK Prospective Diabetes Study (UKPDS) Group. Overview of 6 years therapy of type II diabetes: a progressive disease (UKPDS 16). *Diabetes* 1995; **44**: 1249–58.

23 Farmer AJ, Gibson OJ, Dudley C, et al. A randomized controlled trial of the effect of real-time telemedicine support on glycemic control in young adults with type 1 diabetes (ISRCTN 46889446). *Diabetes Care* 2005; **28**: 2697–702.

24 DAFNE Study Group. Training in flexible, intensive insulin management to enable dietary freedom in people with type 1 diabetes: dose adjustment for normal eating (DAFNE) randomised controlled trial. *BMJ* 2002; **325**: 746.

25 Farmer A, Wade A, French DP, Goyder E, Kinmonth AL, Neil A. The DiGEM trial protocol—a randomised controlled trial to determine the effect on glycaemic control of different strategies of blood glucose self-monitoring in people with type 2 diabetes (ISRCTN47464659). *BMC Fam Pract* 2005; **6**: 25.

26 Department of Health. *Delivering Investment in General Practice: Implementing the New GMSC Contract*. London: Department of Health, 2003.

CHAPTER 17

Oral anticoagulation therapy (OAT)

Carl Heneghan, Rafael Perera

Oral anticoagulant therapy inhibits coagulation; that is, it reduces the likelihood that blood will clot inappropriately in the blood vessels, producing thrombi or emboli. The principal mode of action of such anticoagulants is antagonism of endogenous synthesis of vitamin K-dependent clotting factors. Anticoagulants are most commonly used to treat patients with deep-vein thrombosis (DVT), pulmonary embolism, atrial fibrillation and mechanical prosthetic heart valves.

The standard measure used to monitor the adequacy of anticoagulant dose is the international normalized ratio (INR). The main anticoagulant used in the UK and the USA is warfarin. Other anticoagulants include acenocoumarol and phenprocoumon, which are used more commonly outside the USA and the UK, and phenindione. Warfarin (named after the Wisconsin Alumni Research Foundation) was patented in 1941 and has been in clinical use as an antithrombotic agent for more than 50 years [1]. It was first registered as a rodenticide in the USA in 1952 and approved for medical use in humans in 1954.

17.1. Indications for oral anticoagulation

The annual risk of thromboembolic complications is substantial in the absence of anticoagulation for selected conditions (Table 17.1) [2]. For instance, in those at moderate to high risk of stroke, oral anticoagulation therapy clearly reduces not only the frequency of such events but also their severity and the associated risk of death [3–7].

Recently there has been a marked expansion of the indications for oral anticoagulant therapy, particularly among elderly people [8]. For instance, in the UK the number of patients taking warfarin is expected to increase by about 10% per year [9]. The reasons for this include improvements in

Evidence-based Medical Monitoring: from Principles to Practice. Edited by Paul Glasziou, Les Irwig and Jeffrey K. Aronson. © 2008 Blackwell Publishing, ISBN: 978-1-4051-5399-7.

Table 17.1 Annualized risks of thrombotic complications in the absence of anticoagulant therapy

Condition	Risk of thrombosis (%)
Lone atrial fibrillation	1
Average-risk atrial fibrillation	5
High-risk atrial fibrillation	12
Dual-leaflet (St Jude) aortic valve prosthesis	10–12
Single-leaflet (Bjork–Shiley) aortic valve prosthesis	23
Dual-leaflet (St Jude) mitral valve prosthesis	22
Multiple St Jude prostheses	91

clinical outcomes with these drugs, more extensive indications for their use in common diseases [10] and improvements in anticoagulant safety [11].

17.2. Monitoring oral anticoagulation therapy

Monitoring oral anticoagulation therapy is challenging in clinical practice for a number of reasons [12]:

- oral anticoagulants have a narrow therapeutic window;
- there is considerable variability in intra-dose and inter-dose responses;
- they interact with many different drugs and dietary factors;
- they need constant laboratory monitoring, which can be difficult to standardize;
- problems in dosing occur as a result of patient non-adherence and miscommunication.

The measure used to monitor oral anticoagulation therapy is the INR. The INR was developed to eliminate problems caused by variability in the sensitivity of different commercial sources of thromboplastin to blood coagulation factor VII, which results in variability in prothrombin time (PT) measurements; the INR was developed to overcome these discrepancies [13]. The INR is calculated from the PT, as follows:

$$INR = \left(\frac{patient\ PT}{mean\ normal\ PT} \right)^{ISI}$$

or

$$Log\ INR = ISI(log\ observed\ PT\ ratio)$$

The PT is not standardized when expressed in seconds or as a ratio to the PT in plasma from a healthy subject. A calibration model [13, 14], adopted in 1982, is used to standardize reporting by converting the PT ratio measured with the local thromboplastin into an INR. The INR increases in response to depression of three of the four vitamin K-dependent coagulation proteins—factors II, VII and X. In the initial stages of warfarin administration, prolongation of the INR primarily reflects factor VII depression (since it is the vitamin K-dependent coagulation factor with the shortest half-life).

The ISI reflects the responsiveness of a given thromboplastin to reduction in the vitamin K-dependent coagulation factors compared with the primary World Health Organization (WHO) international reference preparations. Individual manufacturers give an International Sensitivity Index (ISI) for any tissue factor they make. The ISI is usually between 1.0 and 1.4; the more responsive the reagent, the lower the ISI [14].

At the onset of warfarin therapy, monitoring of the INR is usually performed after the second or third dose until the target has been achieved. The frequency of monitoring can gradually be reduced to intervals as long as every 4 weeks. If adjustments to the dose are made, more frequent monitoring should be repeated until a stable response is achieved.

17.2.1. The pharmacology of warfarin and anticoagulation control

Anticoagulation with warfarin is clinically challenging in view of its complex pharmacokinetic and pharmacodynamic profile. Warfarin is rapidly absorbed from the gastrointestinal tract and has high systemic availability [15], reaching maximal blood concentrations about 90 minutes after oral administration [13]. It has a half-life of 36–42 hours, circulates bound to plasma proteins (mainly albumin) and accumulates in the liver.

Warfarin is a racemic mixture of two enantiomers, R and S. Anticoagulant activity is mainly attributable to S-warfarin, and cytochrome P450 2C9 (CYP2C9) is the principal enzyme responsible for its metabolism. Therefore, factors that modulate the expression and activity of CYP2C9 influence plasma warfarin concentrations and determine the antithrombotic response [16].

The response to warfarin is modified by genetic and environmental factors that can influence its absorption, its clearance and its pharmacodynamics (see Figure 17.1 [16]).

Many factors, including medications, herbal products (Table 17.2), vitamins, alcohol, diet and changes in lifestyle, have been implicated in affecting anticoagulation control. However, other than the influence of dietary vitamin K intake, there is no evidence that any particular food or nutrient interacts with warfarin by altering CYP2C9 activity [17].

Fluctuations in dietary vitamin K are an important source of anticoagulant variance; however, the dose responsiveness of anticoagulation to vitamin K has yet to be established. Despite this, a constant dietary intake of vitamin K of 65–80 μg/day is the suggested practice for patients taking warfarin [18].

Despite extensive evaluation of potential causes of over- and under-anticoagulation, the isolation of a specific cause commonly cannot be determined in individual cases. The results of an evaluation of 12,897 INR values were as follows [19]:

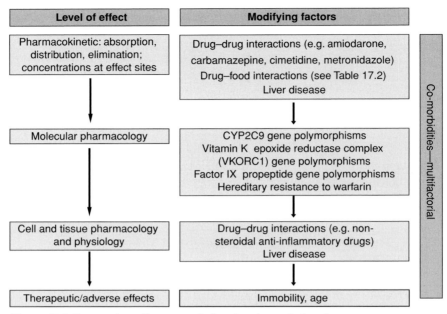

Figure 17.1 Factors that affect control of oral anticoagulation therapy.

- 6642 (52%) were within the target range,
- 8525 (66%) were within 0.2 INR units of the target range,
- 2881 (22%) were below 2.0.

The causes of under-anticoagulation were as follows:
- indeterminate in 856 (30%);
- a response to a previous change in dosage in 16%;
- non-compliance or dosing errors in 16%;
- initiation of therapy in 16%;
- changes in drugs, medical condition, dietary vitamin K intake, alcohol use and activity in 15% combined.

Table 17.2 Natural substances and foods that reportedly interact with warfarin

Potentiation (increased INR)	Antagonism (reduced INR)
Coenzyme Q	Green tea
Cranberry juice	St John's wort (*Hypericum perforatum*)
Danshen (Devil's claw; *Harpagophytum procumbens*)	
Garlic (*Allium sativum*)	
Ginkgo biloba	
Ginseng (*Panax ginseng*)	
Vitamin E	

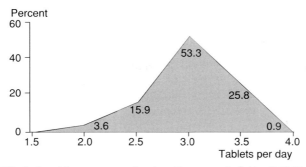

Figure 17.2 Warfarin tablet usage per day in a 5-year period (April 2000–2005). (Redrawn from www.anticoagulationeurope.com, with permission.)

The causes of over-anticoagulation (603 INR values greater than 4.0) were as follows:
- indeterminate in 43%;
- changes in medical condition in 16%;
- a response to a previous change in warfarin dosage in 11%;
- interactions with prescription drugs in 7.3%;
- poor compliance or dosing errors, initiation of therapy and change in dietary vitamin K intake in 15% combined.

Even in closely controlled individuals dosage adjustment is required, as shown in Figure 17.2.

Warfarin tablets come in strengths of 0.5, 1, 3 and 5 mg to facilitate the very variable inter-individual doses and repeated intra-individual changes in dose that are needed during INR monitoring.

17.3. Therapeutic control limits for oral anticoagulation therapy

The target range for the INR is narrow (Figure 17.3) [20]: an INR over 4.5 increases the risk of major bleeding and an INR under 2.0 increases the risk of thromboembolism [9–11]. However, the exact target varies according to the disease being treated. For example, an INR of 2.0–3.0 is adequate for the treatment and prevention of DVT. However, a higher INR is recommended for prevention of thromboembolism associated with mechanical heart valves.

Several factors impinge on the therapeutic control limits for oral anticoagulation therapy. For instance, the risk of major bleeding associated with warfarin increases with advancing age. In patients aged 65 years or older, the mean INR at the time of a major bleeding event was significantly lower than in patients under 65 years (3.1 versus 4.2). For every 1-year increase in age, mean INR at the time of a major bleeding event fell significantly by 0.03 [12, 21].

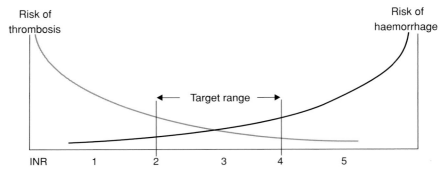

Figure 17.3 The higher the INR, the higher the risk of bleeding (black line); the lower the INR, the higher the risk of thrombosis (blue line). The target range is chosen to maximize the benefit and minimize the harm. (Redrawn from [20], with permission.)

The frequency of monitoring also affects the time spent within the control limits. When monitored monthly, about 50% of patients remain within the target range [12], compared with 85% of those who are monitored weekly [13].

Natural variation is common and expected, as long as it falls within the target range. Figure 17.4 shows the INR values over a 5-year period of an individual with 'good control' from the start of oral anticoagulation therapy. The target range for this individual was 2.5–3.5, defined by the dark blue lines

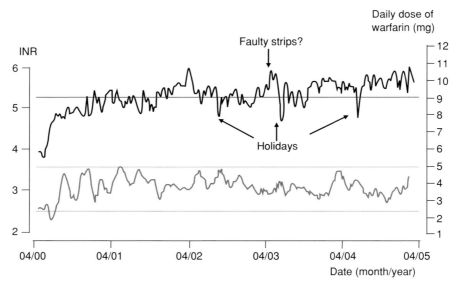

Figure 17.4 Average INRs and daily warfarin doses for one individual over 5 years. (Redrawn from www.anticoagulationeurope.org, with permission.)

Table 17.3 Differences in observed values from the same INR data sets in a randomized controlled trial of computerized decision support and near-patient testing

	Tests in range (%)	Point prevalence	Time in range (%)
Intervention	62	71	69
Control	58	64	62

in the figure. The association between INR and the initial warfarin dosage is clearly seen at the start of the 5-year period when adequate dosage was being established.

The bottom trace shows the average INR over a 6-week period (INR measured once a week). The light blue lines demarcate the control limits within which INR measures should fall. In this case the individual had close control, and the percentage of measures within the target range was 86%.

17.3.1. What should be monitored?

In terms of reporting anticoagulation data from trials of oral anticoagulation therapy, there are differences in the observed efficacy, depending on the statistic chosen, that is, the percentage of tests in range, the point prevalence or the percentage of time in range. In a randomized trial of oral anticoagulation in primary care in which computerized decision support and near-patient testing was compared with usual care (control), depending on which measure was used, the efficacy results differed by up to 10% in terms of INR control (Table 17.3) [22].

A systematic review of the reported outcome measures in trials of the effectiveness of oral anticoagulation [23] showed that there were four widely reported values:
• the proportion of time spent by individuals in the target range,
• the mean INR,
• the proportion of tests within the target range,
• the mean warfarin dose.
Other values included
• the point prevalence—the proportion of patients with therapeutic INRs at a given time,
• the proportion of tests performed.
Potential surrogate markers for the risks of thromboembolic and haemorrhagic complications in individuals are the proportion of INR values in the target range and the time spent in the target range (TTR). Of these, the proportion of tests in the target range is biased, because of the tendency for repeat testing in patients with a test outside the target range. This bias increases as the interval between tests increases. In addition, pooling of the mean percentage of tests in range between trials proves difficult, as information is often collected in two different ways—the percentage of overall tests in range and the percentage of tests of each individual in range [24].

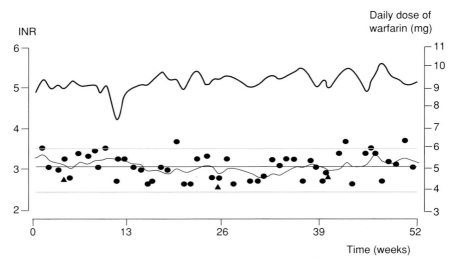

INR

Daily dose of
warfarin (mg)

Time (weeks)

Figure 17.5 Average daily warfarin, weekly INR and 6 weekly average INR values in one individual over 1 year. (Redrawn from www.anticoagulationeurope.org, with permission.)

It is important to recognize that in individuals whose anticoagulation is deemed to be controlled, natural fluctuations INR still result in isolated values that are well beyond the target limits. However, this does not necessarily mean that dosage adjustment is required (see Figure 17.5). The dots in Figure 17.5 represent the isolated weekly measures, of which 92.5% fall within the target range represented by the blue lines.

The TTR is a potentially useful surrogate marker in predicting long-term control. It is estimated by interpolating between observed test values in order to extrapolate data points daily; therefore, the TTR is the number of patient-days within the target range divided by the total number of patient days of follow-up. However, there are problems in the interpretation of the TTR; these include the following:

• it depends on the width of the target range;
• there is lack of differentiation between small and large departures from the target range;
• it is based on the linear interpolation method of Rosendaal et al. [25], which assumes that there is a linear relation between two INR values, and allocates a specific INR value to each day between tests for each patient.

However, the TTR is useful, because it is strongly related to the rate of clinical events [26–29].

In a large representative study, there was a strong relation between the TTR and major bleeds or thromboembolism for INRs above or below the target range [26]. In addition, the individual time spent in the target range (ITTR) can be used to identify patients at risk of recurrent thromboembolism or major bleeding. The 30-day ITTR is highly predictive of total treatment ITTR. In a retrospective study of 2300 consecutive patients with venous thromboembolism treated with vitamin K antagonists, an ITTR below 37% during the first 30 treatment days was highly predictive of the total treatment time ITTR below 45% (RR 24; 14–43) [30]. Since the 30-day ITTR is highly predictive of total treatment ITTR, these patients can be identified soon after the start of treatment.

17.4. Monitoring options

17.4.1. Dosing aids

Diary cards are the main dosing aid for warfarin therapy. These are often given out at the start of therapy but not always. Diaries normally include the patient's name and address, the indication for warfarin treatment, the INR reference range and whom to contact in an emergency. Patients are asked to record their INR measurements, dosage adjustments, current dosage and the date on which tests were taken. Although very few professionals check these diaries for appropriate use, they act to remind individuals of their last dose and any adjustments in therapy. However, individuals cannot obtain a sense of their overall control from these diaries, and there is usually insufficient space to record factors that may have led to deviation in INR. To counteract some of these problems, graphical representations can be helpful in understanding fluctuations in individual INR values (Figures 17.4 and 17.5). Such graphs can be used in a paper diary format, but to be more useful they should ideally be incorporated into computer software programs and decision-support technology. Such technology already exists for point-of-care testing meters (see Chapter 14).

17.4.2. Dosing adjustment

Natural fluctuations in an individual's INR can make adequate monitoring difficult. Changes in dosage that respond to isolated measurements of INR tend to produce over-adjustments (Figure 17.6) increasing the variability of the INR, therefore producing a 'ping-pong' effect (see Chapter 1) [31]: high INR → reduce warfarin dosage → low INR → increase warfarin dosage → high INR → etc. To avoid this ping-pong effect, the natural INR variation per individual should be taken into account before any dose adjustment (for rules see Chapter 7). An added complication is that target ranges for INR do not necessarily coincide with the individual limits. If this is the case, the first strategy is to reduce individual variability to within the target ranges established for the condition.

As isolated INR measures have a biological variability of 9.6% [32], warfarin dosage adjustments should be made only when extreme INR values are observed, or when there are large variations between consecutive INR values [29, 33]; this strategy should minimize over-adjustment. For instance, the biological variability of an isolated INR measurement of 3.0 would give a

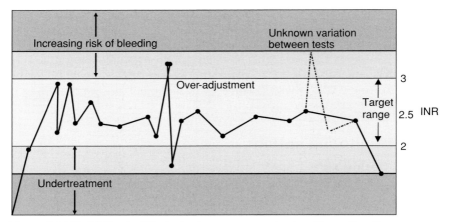

Figure 17.6 Variability in INR during long-term monitoring, illustrating the 'ping-pong' effect (see text for discussion).

range of 2.4–3.6, based on a 10% standard deviation, as in the reference range (0.8–1.2). When there are unexpected fluctuations in the INR in an individual who has previously been stable, it is worth investigating to find a possible cause. Often, one or more causes can be identified, such as an intercurrent illness, change in diet, alternating adherence, varied alcohol consumption and concomitant drug use, including over-the-counter medications.

17.4.3. Data management and computerized dosing

One of the benefits of using computers is that they remember things that we may forget (Figure 17.7). To this effect computerized dosage management is at least as effective as physician dosing for the initiation of oral anticoagulation therapy as well as long-term management [13]. A systematic review of randomized trials of computerized dosing analysed outcomes in terms of the number of tests within the target range, in addition to information on major haemorrhage or bleeding events; in seven studies with 3416 anticoagulation tests, computers generally did a little better: 65% of tests were within target compared with 59% (Figure 17.8) [34].

However, clinical benefit from the use of computer programs over conventional medical staff dosing has not yet been established. Nor can it be assumed that all computer programs will be equally successful.

17.5. Options for managing oral anticoagulation therapy

There are various options for managing anticoagulation (Figure 17.8).

Summary INR data

Target INR	3.0	
INR range	2.5–3.5	
Testing period	06/00–04/05	
Number of weeks	251	
Frequency	6.7 days	
INR tests	263	
Number of tests in range	227	86.3%
Number of tests out of range	36	13.7%
INR 3.0–3.5	131	50.8%
INR 2.5–3.0	90	34.2%
INR < 2.5	6	2.3%
INR > 3.5	30	11.4%
Average INR	3.09	
Average warfarin dose	8.98 mg/day	

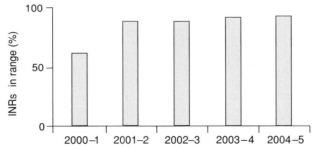

Figure 17.7 An example of a computer output of information about monitoring oral anticoagulation therapy over a 5-year period.

17.5.1. Anticoagulation management services or anticoagulation clinic

In a systematic review of published randomized or cohort studies on the effect of study setting [35]. Sixty-seven studies with 123 patient groups were identified. In all trials, patients were within the target range 64% of the time (95% CI = 62, 66%). In community practices there was significantly less control than in either anticoagulation clinics or clinical trials (−12%; 95% CI = −20, −4.8). After accounting for the clustering of groups within studies and controlling for the other group factors, study setting, drug and self-management remained significantly associated with the proportion of TTR.

Although these results suggest that the coordinated approach of an anticoagulation clinic is superior to usual care, some of the studies were not randomized. Only two studies were truly population-based and only two studies included all INR measurements and not just those performed for monitoring at a particular laboratory. Moreover, there are worldwide difficulties in determining the exact features that comprise management by a family physician.

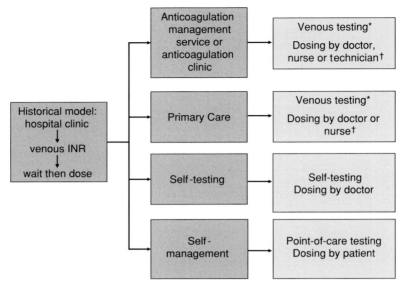

Figure 17.8 Anticoagulation management: different settings and techniques. (*Point-of-care testing can be used as an alternative to venous testing in these settings; †computer decision systems can be used to support dosing decisions.)

17.5.2. Point-of-care testing

Point-of-care testing devices allow the patient to measure the INR with a drop of whole blood [14]; the hand-held devices that are used have proved sufficiently reliable [15, 16]. Many studies [12] have reported on the accuracy and precision of point-of-care testing instruments. However, potential problems include differences compared with standard plasma-based methods as the INR increases above the target range, incorrect calibration of the ISI of the point-of-care instruments and problems in calculating a mean normal PT.

17.5.3. Patient self-testing and patient self-management

Self-testing provides a convenient opportunity for increased frequency of testing when necessary. The use of the same instrument provides a degree of consistency.

Patients can either
- self-test and self-adjust therapy according to a predetermined dose/INR schedule or self-management schedule,
- self-test and call a clinic to tell them the appropriate dosage adjustment.

The potential advantages of self-monitoring include improved convenience for patients, better adherence to treatment, more frequent monitoring and fewer thromboembolic and haemorrhagic complications [23]. Although no single trial of self-monitoring alone has been statistically significant, a meta-analysis has shown a significant one-third reduction in death from all causes

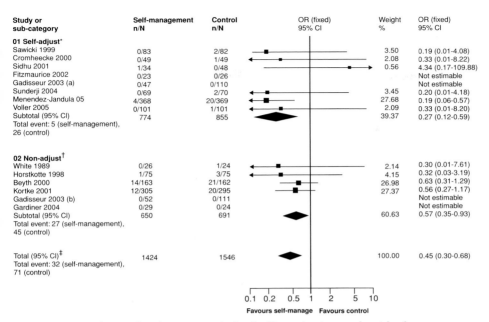

Study or sub-category	Self-management n/N	Control n/N	OR (fixed) 95% CI	Weight %	OR (fixed) 95% CI
01 Self-adjust*					
Sawicki 1999	0/83	2/82		3.50	0.19 (0.01-4.08)
Cromheecke 2000	0/49	1/49		2.08	0.33 (0.01-8.22)
Sidhu 2001	1/34	0/48		0.56	4.34 (0.17-109.88)
Fitzmaurice 2002	0/23	0/26			Not estimable
Gadisseur 2003 (a)	0/47	0/110			Not estimable
Sunderji 2004	0/69	2/70		3.45	0.20 (0.01-4.18)
Menendez-Jandula 05	4/368	20/369		27.68	0.19 (0.06-0.57)
Voller 2005	0/101	1/101		2.09	0.33 (0.01-8.20)
Subtotal (95% CI)	774	855		39.37	0.27 (0.12-0.59)
Total event: 5 (self-management), 26 (control)					
02 Non-adjust[†]					
White 1989	0/26	1/24		2.14	0.30 (0.01-7.61)
Horstkotte 1998	1/75	3/75		4.15	0.32 (0.03-3.19)
Beyth 2000	14/163	21/162		26.98	0.63 (0.31-1.29)
Kortke 2001	12/305	20/295		27.37	0.56 (0.27-1.17)
Gadisseur 2003 (b)	0/52	0/111			Not estimable
Gardiner 2004	0/29	0/24			Not estimable
Subtotal (95% CI)	650	691		60.63	0.57 (0.35-0.93)
Total event: 27 (self-management), 45 (control)					
Total (95% CI)[‡]	1424	1546		100.00	0.45 (0.30-0.68)
Total event: 32 (self-management), 71 (control)					

0.1 0.2   0.5   1   2   5   10
Favours self-manage   Favours control

Figure 17.9 The results of a meta-analysis of self-monitoring on the risk of thromboembolic events. (Adapted from [23].)

and a reduction in thromboembolism by 55% (Figure 17.9). Moreover, there is a tendency for self-adjustment to be better than self-testing only. However, not all patients can self-monitor. In randomized trials of self-monitoring, the average number of people that could not (or would not) take part was 62% (range 31–88%). In trials that included older populations [23], the exclusion rates were much higher. Of the patients who were assigned to the intervention, 22% (range 9–43%) were unable to complete self-monitoring. The main reasons were problems with the device, physical limitations preventing self-monitoring, problems with attending the training assessments or failing the assessment.

Individuals who self-monitor undertake more tests than individuals in usual care or managed services [23]. On average, individuals perform tests once a week after the start of therapy, and the expected maximum test frequency occurs in studies with the shortest durations. The ratio of tests in self-monitoring groups compared with control groups in randomized trials ranged from 1.69 to 4.98; that is, self-monitoring patients test 2–5 times more often than control patients. In addition, self-monitoring improves the percentage of tests in range compared with usual care. The possible reasons for these benefits include the increased frequency of testing, improved educational input and the subsequent enhancement of learned behaviour that comes with self-monitoring. A potential pitfall is the variability in the quality of care in comparison groups, which can affect the rate of testing and hence the benefit and safety of standard anticoagulation monitoring. Specialist programmes may improve outcomes by the same mechanism as self-monitoring, improving the TTR and reducing the frequency of adverse outcomes.

17.6. Conclusions

Potential areas that need addressing include pre-treatment problems, such as the lack of training of health-care professionals and failure to initiate therapy when indicated. In addition, poor communication needs to be addressed between secondary and primary care and the suitability of actions' plan for many individuals taking oral anticoagulants.

Other problems include inadequate patient-held information, problems with translation of information into other languages and problems with loading dose errors. The appropriate use of computer dosing algorithms has yet to be determined. There is insufficient support for individuals and inadequate safety checks at repeat prescribing and repeat dispensing in the community. There is still confusion over management during dentistry, surgery and other procedures. Moreover, ill-considered co-morbidity, co-prescribing, prescribing errors and dosage adjustment errors still occur. There is much to be learnt about improving the monitoring of oral anticoagulation therapy, from the use of computer dosing aids to increasing the numbers of individuals who self-test and self-manage. The main goal should be to increase the proportion of tests in range and the TTR, so that morbidity and mortality are effectively reduced. Patients who take oral anticoagulants spend much of their time outside of the target range. The translation of changes in anticoagulation control to differences in true outcome rates requires further study. Furthermore, there is a lack of true population-based studies [34] of anticoagulation control that give an unbiased assessment of anticoagulation control.

References

1 Pirmohamed M. Warfarin: almost 60 years old and still causing problems. *Br J Clin Pharmacol* 2006; **62**: 509–11.
2 Stein PD, Alpert JS, Bussey HI, Dalen JE, Turpie AG. Antithrombotic therapy in patients with mechanical and biological prosthetic heart valves. *Chest* 2001; **119** (1 Suppl): 220S–7S.
3 The Boston Area Anticoagulation Trial for Atrial Fibrillation Investigators. The effect of low-dose warfarin on the risk of stroke in patients with nonrheumatic atrial fibrillation. *N Engl J Med* 1990; **323**: 1505–11.
4 Hylek EM, Go AS, Chang Y, et al. Effect of intensity of oral anticoagulation on stroke severity and mortality in atrial fibrillation. *N Engl J Med* 2003; **349**: 1019–26.
5 Go AS, Hylek EM, Chang Y, et al. Anticoagulation therapy for stroke prevention in atrial fibrillation: how well do randomized trials translate into clinical practice? *JAMA* 2003; **290**: 2685–92.

6 Stroke Prevention in Atrial Fibrillation Investigators. Adjusted-dose warfarin versus low-intensity, fixed-dose warfarin plus aspirin for high-risk patients with atrial fibrillation. Stroke Prevention in Atrial Fibrillation III randomised clinical trial. *Lancet* 1996; **348**: 633–8.

7 Caro JJ, Flegel KM, Orejuela ME, Kelley HE, Speckman JL, Migliaccio-Walle K. Anticoagulant prophylaxis against stroke in atrial fibrillation: effectiveness in actual practice. *CMAJ* 1999; **161**: 493–7.

8 Majeed A, Moser K, Carroll K. Trends in the prevalence and management of atrial fibrillation in general practice in England and Wales, 1994–1998: analysis of data from the general practice research database. *Heart* 2001; **86**: 284–8.

9 Sudlow M, Rodgers H, Kenny RA, Thomson R. Population based study of use of anticoagulants among patients with atrial fibrillation in the community. *BMJ* 1997; **314**: 1529–30.

10 Manotti C, Moia M, Palareti G, Pengo V, Ria L, Dettori AG. Effect of computer-aided management on the quality of treatment in anticoagulated patients: a prospective, randomized, multicenter trial of APROAT (Automated PRogram for Oral Anticoagulant Treatment). *Haematologica* 2001; **86**: 1060–70.

11 Ansell J, Hirsh J, Dalen J, et al. Managing oral anticoagulant therapy. *Chest* 2001; **119**: 22S–38S.

12 Ansell J, Jacobson A, Levy J, Voller H, Hasenkam JM. Guidelines for implementation of patient self-testing and patient self-management of oral anticoagulation. International consensus guidelines prepared by International Self-Monitoring Association for Oral Anticoagulation. *Int J Cardiol* 2005; **99**: 37–45.

13 Ansell J, Hirsh J, Poller L, Bussey H, Jacobson A, Hylek E. The pharmacology and management of the vitamin K antagonists. The Seventh ACCP Conference on Antithrombotic and Thrombolytic Therapy. *Chest* 2004; **126**: 204S–33S.

14 Kirkwood TB. Calibration of reference thromboplastins and standardisation of the prothrombin time ratio. *Thromb Haemost* 1983; **49**: 238–44.

15 Breckenridge A. Oral anticoagulant drugs: pharmacokinetic aspects. *Semin Hematol* 1978; **15**: 19–26.

16 Greenblatt DJ, von Moltke LL. Interaction of warfarin with drugs, natural substances, and foods. *J Clin Pharmacol* 2005; **45**: 127–32.

17 Ioannides C. Effect of diet and nutrition on the expression of cytochromes P450. *Xenobiotica* 1999; **29**: 109–54.

18 Booth SL, Centurelli MA. Vitamin K: a practical guide to the dietary management of patients on warfarin. *Nutr Rev* 1999; **57**: 288–96.

19 Wittkowsky AK, Devine EB. Frequency and causes of overanticoagulation and underanticoagulation in patients treated with warfarin. *Pharmacotherapy* 2004; **24**: 1311–6.

20 Fitzmaurice DA, Kesteven P. How to evaluate the performance of oral anticoagulation clinics. *Br J Cardiol* 2003; **10**: 370–2.

21 Wittkowsky AK, Whitely KS, Devine EB, Nutescu E. Effect of age on international normalized ratio at the time of major bleeding in patients treated with warfarin. *Pharmacotherapy* 2004; **24**: 600–5.

22 Fitzmaurice DA, Hobbs FD, Murray ET, Holder RL, Allan TF, Rose PE. Oral anticoagulation management in primary care with the use of computerized decision support and near-patient testing: a randomized, controlled trial. *Arch Intern Med* 2000; **160**: 2343–8.

23 Fitzmaurice DA, Kesteven P, Gee KM, Murray ET, McManus R. A systematic review of outcome measures reported for the therapeutic effectiveness of oral anticoagulation. *J Clin Pathol* 2003; **56**: 48–51.

24 Heneghan C, Alonso-Coello P, Garcia-Alamino JM, Perera R, Meats E, Glasziou P. Self-monitoring of oral anticoagulation: a systematic review and meta-analysis. *Lancet* 2006; **367**: 404–11.

25 Rosendaal FR, Cannegieter SC, van der Meer FJ, Briet E. A method to determine the optimal intensity of oral anticoagulant therapy. *Thromb Haemost* 1993; **69**: 236–9.

26 Stroke Prevention in Atrial Fibrillation Investigators. Warfarin versus aspirin for prevention of thromboembolism in atrial fibrillation. Stroke Prevention in Atrial Fibrillation II Study. *Lancet* 1994; **343**: 687–91.

27 Cannegieter SC, Rosendaal FR, Wintzen AR, van der Meer FJ, Vandenbroucke JP, Briet E. Optimal oral anticoagulant therapy in patients with mechanical heart valves. *N Engl J Med* 1995; **333**: 11–17.

28 Connolly SJ, Laupacis A, Gent M, Roberts RS, Cairns JA, Joyner C. Canadian Atrial Fibrillation Anticoagulation (CAFA) Study. *J Am Coll Cardiol* 1991; **18**: 349–55.

29 Palareti G, Leali N, Coccheri S, et al. Bleeding complications of oral anticoagulant treatment: an inception-cohort, prospective collaborative study (ISCOAT). Italian Study on Complications of Oral Anticoagulant Therapy. *Lancet* 1996; **348**: 423–8.

30 Veeger NJ, Piersma-Wichers M, Tijssen JG, Hillege HL, van der Meer J. Individual time within target range in patients treated with vitamin K antagonists: main determinant of quality of anticoagulation and predictor of clinical outcome. A retrospective study of 2300 consecutive patients with venous thromboembolism. *Br J Haematol* 2005; **128**: 513–9.

31 Lassen JF, Kjeldsen J, Antonsen S, Hyltoft PP, Brandslund I. Interpretation of serial measurements of international normalized ratio for prothrombin times in monitoring oral anticoagulant therapy. *Clin Chem* 1995; **41**: 1171–6.

32 Introcaso G, Cuboni A, Ratto A, Foieni F. Mathematical derivative applied to international normalised ratio and analytical variations in oral anticoagulant therapy control. *Haemostasis* 2000; **30**: 281–9.

33 Introcaso G, Gesu G. Significance of consecutive international normalized ratio (INR) outcomes using statistical control rules in long-term anticoagulated patients. Optimization of laboratory monitoring and interpretation of borderline measurements. *Clin Chem Lab Med* 2004; **42**: 294–9.

34 Chatellier G, Colombet I, Degoulet P. Computer-adjusted dosage of anticoagulant therapy improves the quality of anticoagulation. *Medinfo* 1998; (9 Pt 2): 819–23.

35 Van Walraven C, Jennings A, Oake N, Fergusson D, Forster AJ. Effect of study setting on anticoagulation control: a systematic review and metaregression. *Chest* 2006; **129**: 1155–66.

CHAPTER 18

Monitoring cholesterol-modifying interventions

Paul P. Glasziou, Les Irwig, Stephane Heritier

Cholesterol is one of several modifiable risk factors for cardiovascular disease. Others include high blood pressure and smoking, which will need monitoring to manage overall cardiovascular risk. However, in this chapter we shall confine ourselves to considering how and when to monitor lipid profiles in patients with hyperlipidaemias taking an HMG-CoA reductase inhibitor (a 'statin'). We shall not discuss the question of how or even whether to monitor the use of statins in preventing cardiovascular disease in apparently healthy individuals. The mechanism of action of statins is illustrated in Figure 18.1.

Cholesterol monitoring is now a common clinical activity. With widening indications for treatment over the past decade, cholesterol-lowering medications gave become the highest cost pharmaceutical items in the National Health Service in the UK. Correspondingly, cholesterol screening, treatment and lipid monitoring have increased. For example, in Oxfordshire there was a 2.5-fold increase in the total number of cholesterol tests performed between 1996 and 2004, making serum cholesterol the most common single test ordered (J Kay, T James, personal communication).

18.1. Why should we monitor lipids in patients with hyperlipidaemias?

To achieve adequate risk reduction, most guidelines suggest 5.0 mmol/l as an upper limit to the target range. However, while most guidelines on lipid management provide clear statements about the number and interpretation of initial measurements, they do not specify a subsequent monitoring schedule. Among those that do, there is some variation. For example, the PRODIGY guidelines in the UK suggest rechecking annually [1], whereas the NCEP

Evidence-based Medical Monitoring: from Principles to Practice. Edited by Paul Glasziou, Les Irwig and Jeffrey K. Aronson. © 2008 Blackwell Publishing, ISBN: 978-1-4051-5399-7.

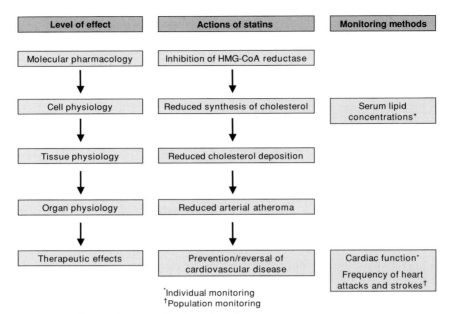

Figure 18.1 The mechanism of action of statins.

guidance in the USA suggests that 'patients can be monitored for response to therapy every 4–6 months, or more often if considered necessary' [2]. The Australian National Heart Foundation guidelines suggest measurement of the lipid profile every 6–12 months [3]. However, the basis for these intervals is unclear, and the guidelines do not explicitly mention the within-person variability or the likely rates of change over time on a fixed dosage regimen. Furthermore, simulation studies have suggested that frequent monitoring is more likely to mislead than to help [4].

In the following sections, we shall use data obtained from the LIPID trial, a randomized trial of patients with known ischaemic heart disease randomized to pravastatin 40 mg/day or matching placebo and followed for an average of 6.1 years [5]. The trial included 12 monthly cholesterol measurement, as well as information on compliance and 'drop-in' to other medications. In all, 9014 patients were recruited at 87 centres (67 in Australia and 20 in New Zealand). They had either an acute myocardial infarction or a hospital discharge diagnosis of unstable angina at 3–36 months before study entry. The patients entered an 8-week, single-blind, placebo run-in phase, during which they received dietary advice aimed at reducing their fat intake to less than 30% of total energy intake. For patients to qualify for the study, the plasma total cholesterol concentration measured 4 weeks before randomization was required to be 4.0–6.9 mmol/l and the fasting triglyceride concentration less than 5.0 mmol/l.

Table 18.1 Criteria for lipid measurements*

Lipid	CV(a+b)* (%)	Change with statin (%)	Signal-to-noise ratio	Cost
Total cholesterol	8.8	18	2.0	£3.77
LDL	12	25	2.1	£11.82
HDL	10	5	0.5	£3.94

Note: * Data from [6].

18.2. Choosing the main lipid measurement for monitoring

Combinations of lipid measures, such as LDL/HDL or total cholesterol/HDL, are generally found to be the best measures of risk. Initial assessment is based on a full lipid profile, including LDL, HDL and triglycerides, for a full assessment of risk. However, multiple tests generate high within-person variability, and so subsequent monitoring can rely on a single measurement. Since therapy is usually aimed at lowering LDL or total cholesterol, these have generally been used for monitoring, and other measured lipid elements are obtained only if needed.

Table 18.1 shows the coefficients of variation, responses to statin treatment and the ratios of these [7]. For monitoring overall risk a full profile would still be best, but to monitor response and continuing statin treatment, either total cholesterol or LDL is equivalent, and the former is clearly cheaper. We shall therefore focus on total cholesterol. However, similar principles apply to LDL.

18.3. Initial response to treatment

In the LIPID trial 9012 patients were randomized to placebo or pravastatin, with an average pre-treatment cholesterol concentration of 5.65 mmol/l (SD 0.82; range 3.0–9.2). At the start of the study, the median age of the patients was 62 years; 83% were men, 64% had had a myocardial infarction, and 36% had unstable angina. Details of the changes in cholesterol concentrations at 6 and 72 months are shown in Table 18.2.

Treatment with pravastatin 40 mg/day led to an average initial drop in cholesterol of 1.16 mmol/l (SD 0.75). Figure 18.2 shows the changes in cholesterol concentrations in the pravastatin and placebo groups over the 6 years of the study (the last value being carried forward for drop-outs or drop-ins). The difference between the groups was largely maintained, but in both groups there was a small increase in cholesterol over the 6 years. In those who took pravastatin the average increase was around 0.14 mmol/l by 5 years (from 6 to 60 months), or about 0.5% per year on average.

Table 18.2 Average cholesterol concentrations in LIPID in the placebo and pravastatin groups at 0, 6 and 72 months*

Group	Time	n	Mean (mmol/l)	Standard deviation	Interquartile range
Placebo	Baseline	4502	5.65	0.81	5.1–6.2
	6 mo	4307	5.67	0.84	5.1–5.6
	6 yr	2709	5.66	0.93	5.0–6.2
Pravastatin	Baseline	4512	5.65	0.82	5.1–6.2
	6 mo	4318	4.49	0.81	3.9–5.0
	6 yr	2837	4.60	0.87	4.0–5.1

Note: * Data from [5].

18.4. Maintenance schedule

18.4.1. Within-person variation

To estimate the short-term variability, we used two methods. Firstly, we used the cholesterol concentrations during the run-in period (excluding the first measurement), which were taken only a few weeks apart, to provide an estimate of very short-term variability. Secondly, we used a linear backward extrapolation from the longer term measures, asking what the apparent variance at time 0 would have been (this method is known as a 'variogram'). We also looked at the variability between pairs of serial measurements to judge the stability of the estimates with time.

To estimate long-term variability, we take the average squared difference of the cholesterol concentrations compared with baseline (i.e. cholesterol at time *t* minus cholesterol at time 0), where time *t* is 6, 12, 18 months, etc (see

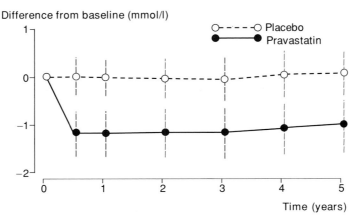

Figure 18.2 Changes in total cholesterol concentrations from baseline to year 5 for pravastatin and placebo groups in the LIPID study. (Adapted from [5].)

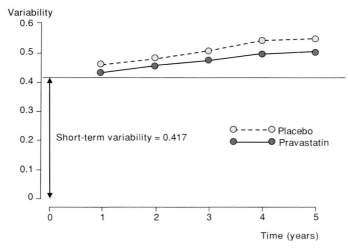

Figure 18.3 Changes in within-person variability over 5 years in the LIPID study. (Adapted from [5].)

Figure 18.3). The within-person variability for each of the different periods is half the variance of the difference. By comparing the short-term variability with the long-term variability, we estimated the degree of 'random drift' with time, and hence the likelihood that a patient's true cholesterol concentration had drifted beyond the control limits around the target.

Because we want to estimate change in those taking stable treatment, a key problem is how to cope with patients who drop in or drop out of treatment. Hence, when patients dropped in to cholesterol-lowering medication, we 'censored' the data and replaced values thereafter with the last value carried forward for each of the subsequent measurements.

To estimate any systematic changes, we examined the group mean cholesterol concentration at each time point (using the imputed values for those who had dropped in to cholesterol-lowering medication) and the mean individual changes. Both methods have small (and opposing) biases, so we looked for discrepancies between the methods.

Based on estimates from a subsample, the within-person variability was about 0.63 mmol/l (corresponding to a coefficient of variation of under 10%). With the 4507 patients in LIPID on a fixed dose of pravastatin, we calculated that we had adequate (over 80%) power to detect changes in cholesterol between periods of as little as 0.03 mmol/l.

Table 18.3 shows the standard deviations of the differences between (a) the baseline (i.e. time 0) and (b) cholesterol measurements at 6 months and subsequently. The initial 0–6-month variability was 0.46 in the placebo group and 0.53 in the pravastatin group. The latter is likely to be higher, because it includes not only short-term biological variability but also a component of variation in response to statin treatment.

Table 18.3 Within-person standard deviations (calculated from half the variance of the differences) comparing (a) baseline concentrations and (b) 6-month cholesterol concentrations at times from 6 months to 6 years

Time	n	Placebo		Pravastatin	
		(a) From baseline	(b) From 6 mo	(a) From baseline	(b) From 6 mo
6 mo	4307	0.46		0.53	
Year 1	4252	0.46	0.46	0.54	0.43
Year 3	3881	0.52	0.51	0.58	0.48
Year 5	3602	0.54	0.55	0.60	0.51

We cannot directly measure the variation in response to treatment, because of the intrinsic variability between measurements. However, Table 18.3 shows that there is a slightly greater variation in the changes with pravastatin than with placebo. This excess variation represents the variation in response to treatment with pravastatin, and is a standard deviation of 0.26 (calculated as the square root of the difference in squared standard deviations). This average change is thus more than four standard deviations from no change, and virtually all treated patients will have some change. The range of responses to pravastatin treatment can be estimated as 1.16 ± 0.51, or a 95% range of true response from 0.65 to 1.66 mmol/l.

18.4.2. Establishing the baseline before treatment

If we want to detect whether a person has responded adequately to treatment, we need to have a clear idea where they started. The high intra-individual variation suggests that we need to make several measurements in order to establish a firm baseline. This is important for two reasons. Firstly, it establishes that the cholesterol is 'abnormal' and that treatment is truly indicated. Secondly, repeated measurements give a clearer baseline from which to estimate changes in an individual patient.

18.4.3. Longer term monitoring

18.4.3.1. Change in within-person variability over time

The placebo group shows the small increase over time in this within-person variability from a standard deviation of 0.46 mmol/l (coefficient of variation 8%) between the 0 and 6 month measurements to 0.57 mmol/l (coefficient of variation 10%) for the 0–72-month measurements, that is, a 23% relative increase in the standard deviation over 6 years. This small relative increase of around 4% per year suggests that most of the variation over the period of the study is due to short-term biological variability and analytical variability.

Table 18.4 Estimated numbers of true-positive and false-positive cholesterol measurements over a threshold of 5 mmol/l at initial true concentrations of 4.5 or 4.0 mmol/l

Initial true concentration	Year	True-positive (TP) rate	False-positive (FP) rate	Ratio FP/TP
4.5 mmol/l	1	0.0002	0.12	6600
	3	0.06	0.15	2.3
	5	0.17	0.16	0.94
4.0 mmol/l	1	0.0000	0.01	—
	3	0.00012	0.019	157
	5	0.0031	0.025	8.0

18.4.4. Determining the target range

18.4.4.1. When should measurements be repeated?

What are the implications of these results for different monitoring intervals? After the serum cholesterol concentration has stabilized during treatment there are two elements that can lead to a rise in cholesterol: the average drift of the whole group over time and random variation. Based on the LIPID trial figures, we have calculated the likelihood of different degrees of drift over time. If we are interested in whether a patient has truly exceeded a target of 5.0 mmol/l, the rate of true positives and false positives is as shown in Table 18.4. We can also interpret the figures in Table 18.4 as the likelihood of a 0.5 or 1.0 mmol/l true drift at different time points.

The data from the LIPID study suggest that true long-term changes in cholesterol concentration occur relatively slowly and that most of the variation seen is due to either analytical variation or short-term biological variation.

The changes found in LIPID, such as the within-person coefficient of variation of 8% (0.46/5.65), are comparable to those found in other similar studies. For example, cholesterol concentration measurements made 1 year apart in the 14,600 patients in the MRC trial of mild hypertension showed a within-person coefficient of variation of 7% [8]. However, the estimates vary with the time between measurements. For example, in a study of 41 healthy volunteers there was a coefficient of variation of 2–3% for measurements 24 hours apart, rising to 4–5% at 4 weeks apart. Similarly, in a study of 458 patients there was a coefficient of variation of 3% at a median of 4 days between blood samples, and the geometric mean of the within-person standard deviation was 0.13 mmol/l [6]. The rise in cholesterol of 0.5% per year is a little less than the 1% seen in cohort studies [9], but this may be due to either dietary adherence or to monitoring and the addition of further cholesterol-lowering therapy in some patients in LIPID.

There is generally a weak signal-to-noise ratio in cholesterol monitoring. The signal of a small rise in cholesterol (around 1% per year) will be difficult to detect against the background of short-term variability of 8%.

18.5. Conclusions

The main implication of our findings is that cholesterol monitoring should be less frequent than current practice. Much current testing will detect only false positives, that is, changes that are due to either short-term biological variation or analytical error. Based on the results in Table 18.4, re-testing every 3–5 years would be more appropriate. Clinicians may be concerned about such a long delay, because of concerns about adherence to therapy. However, other means of assessing adherence may be preferable, such as prescription refill records or non-threatening ways of inquiring about it [10].

Acknowledgements

We should like to thank the LIPID investigators for making available the data from the LIPID trial.

References

1 Prodigy guidance. Lipids management. Available from www.prodigy.nhs.uk/ProdigyKnowledge/Guidance/WholeGuidanceView.aspx?GuidanceId=3738 (last accessed 7 October 2006).

2 Grundy SM, Cleeman JI, Merz CN, et al. Implications of recent clinical trials for the National Cholesterol Education Program Adult Treatment Panel III guidelines. *Circulation* 2004; **110**: 227–39.

3 Cardiac Society of Australia and New Zealand National Heart Foundation. Position statement on lipid management—2005. Available from www.heartfoundation.com.au.

4 Shepard DS. Reliability of blood pressure measurements: implications for designing and evaluating programs to control hypertension. *J Chronic Dis* 1981; **34**: 191–209.

5 The Long-Term Intervention with Pravastatin in Ischaemic Disease (LIPID) Study Group. Prevention of cardiovascular events and death with pravastatin in patients with coronary heart disease and a broad range of initial cholesterol levels. *N Engl J Med* 1998; **339**: 1349–57.

6 Rotterdam EP, Katan MB, Knuiman JT. Importance of time interval between repeated measurements of total or high-density lipoprotein cholesterol when estimating an individual's baseline concentrations. *Clin Chem* 1987; **33**: 1913–5.

7 Tsalamandris C, Panagiotopoulos S, Allen TJ, et al. Long-term intraindividual variability of serum lipids in patients with type I and type II diabetes. *J Diabetes Complications* 1998; **12**: 208–14.

8 Thompson SG, Pocock SJ. The variability of serum cholesterol measurements: implications for screening and monitoring. *J Clin Epidemiol* 1990; **43**: 783–9.

9 Pereira MA, Weggemans RM, Jacobs DR Jr, et al. Within-person variation in serum lipids: implications for clinical trials. *Int J Epidemiol* 2004; **33**: 534–41.

10 Bakx JC, van den Hoogen HJ, Deurenberg P, van Doremalen J, van den Bosch WJ. Changes in serum total cholesterol levels over 18 years in a cohort of men and women: The Nijmegen Cohort Study. *Prev Med* 2000; **30**: 138–45.

CHAPTER 19

Monitoring levothyroxine replacement in primary hypothyroidism

Andrea Rita Horvath

19.1. Primary hypothyroidism

Adult primary hypothyroidism is a common and insidious condition with a prevalence in the UK of 7.5–9.3% in women and 1.3–2.8% in men [1–3]. In elderly people, the prevalence of mild to overt hypothyroidism is even higher: 12–21% in women and 5–16% in men [4–7]. The ratio of overt to mild hypothyroidism is about 1:6 to 1:8 [4, 7].

Hypothyroidism often presents with subtle non-specific symptoms (such as weight gain, cold intolerance, fatigue), which may be attributed to many other illnesses. In iodine-replete areas the commonest cause is chronic autoimmune disease, most commonly Hashimoto's thyroiditis, or destructive treatment for hyperthyroidism, which may account for up to one-third of cases. In primary hypothyroidism of autoimmune origin, the earliest biochemical abnormality is the development of antibodies to thyroid peroxidase (TPO) and a subsequent increase in serum thyroid stimulating hormone (TSH), associated with normal serum concentrations of total thyroxine (T4), free thyroxine (fT4), total tri-iodothyronine (T3) and free tri-iodothyronine (fT3), an intermediate state that is called mild thyroid failure or subclinical hypothyroidism (Figure 19.1). Well-conducted longitudinal studies provide good evidence that subclinical hypothyroidism can progress to overt hypothyroidism, particularly in elderly women and if there are antithyroid antibodies [3]. This intermediate phase is followed by a reduction in serum fT4 concentration and a further increase in TSH. At this point, most patients have multiple symptoms of overt hypothyroidism and benefit from treatment with levothyroxine (Figure 19.1).

Evidence-based Medical Monitoring: from Principles to Practice. Edited by Paul Glasziou, Les Irwig and Jeffrey K. Aronson. © 2008 Blackwell Publishing, ISBN: 978-1-4051-5399-7.

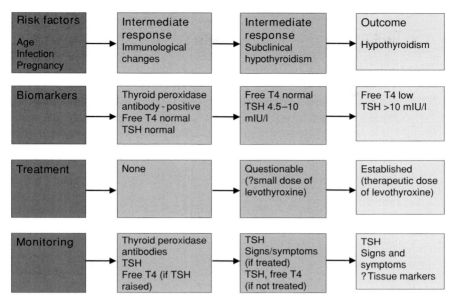

Figure 19.1 Causal relation between the pathophysiology, diagnosis, treatment and monitoring of primary autoimmune hypothyroidism.

19.2. Treatment of hypothyroidism

In the early immunological phase of the condition, no treatment is needed. However, there is a debate about whether patients benefit from replacement in the subclinical phase of thyroid disease and whether early treatment improves morbidity, mortality and patient-related outcomes [8–12].

The treatment of choice in *overt* primary hypothyroidism is levothyroxine, with the aim of restoring clinical euthyroidism. Replacement with levothyroxine is usually life long, although about one-fifth of patients with Hashimoto's thyroiditis revert to normal spontaneously [13]. After ingestion of levothyroxine, serum T4 concentrations peak at 2–4 hours and remain high for up to 6–9 hours [13, 14]. Levothyroxine has a relatively long half-life (6–7 days), and is converted to T3; thus, once-daily administration provides a stable and physiological concentration of T3 in most patients. T3 as liothyronine (the laevorotatory isomer) can also be used, and after oral administration produces a peak concentration of T3 at the same time as T4, but its half-life is much shorter (1 day) [15]. Thus, once-daily dosing does not maintain a narrow band of therapeutic concentrations.

Animal research has generated increasing interest in combination treatment with levothyroxine and liothyronine [16]. However, data on combination therapy are controversial in humans, and a recent systematic review of 9 trials [17] and a meta-analysis of 11 randomized controlled trials [15] showed no difference in the effectiveness of combination therapy versus monotherapy.

Therefore, in the rest of this chapter, I shall limit discussion to thyroid monitoring in patients taking levothyroxine monotherapy. The mechanism of action of levothyroxine at different pharmacological levels is shown in Table 19.1.

19.3. Rationale for monitoring treatment in primary hypothyroidism

Levothyroxine has a narrow toxic-to-therapeutic ratio, making regular monitoring necessary. The different phases of a thyroid monitoring strategy (pre-treatment, initial titration, maintenance and re-establishment of control) are discussed in detail below. The key objectives of thyroid monitoring are to regain euthyroidism and to avoid the adverse effects of under-treatment or over-treatment and thus the consequences of clinical or subclinical hypothyroidism and hyperthyroidism, which can affect cardiac function, bone metabolism, psychological and neurological functions, quality of life, fertility and reproductive function, and overall morbidity and mortality. Biochemical investigations of thyroid function are used to monitor thyroid status during replacement therapy. Current guidelines universally recommend using serum TSH measurements to assess thyroid status and adherence to treatment, with the goal of normalizing TSH [12, 18–21].

Although guideline recommendations are available, several studies have reported that many patients receive either excessive or insufficient thyroid replacement. For example, in one study only 56% of the patients taking levothyroxine replacement received the minimal recommended monitoring, and many errors were identified at all stages of follow-up in tertiary care [22]. This study also showed that patients who received the recommended monitoring had significantly fewer levothyroxine-related adverse effects than those who did not (1% versus 6%). In studies from the UK, USA, Finland and Spain about 60% of patients had normal serum TSH concentrations, about one-fifth of patients were under-treated or over-treated, and in 12% even the ultrasensitive TSH was undetectable [5, 23–27]. Therapy was changed by testing in only a small proportion of patients and the outcome of treatment was unknown in most cases [5, 23, 24, 28–30].

In a comparison of actual and recommended practices in primary care in Scotland, stable patients taking levothyroxine were monitored with measurement of both TSH and fT4 more often than with TSH alone [27]. In spite of the questionable quality and outcome of care provided to these patients, one TSH test was performed for every six of the population in 1999 [31]. The costs of reagents for all thyroid investigations (not including labour, equipment or overheads) were £20 million in the UK and £19 million per annum in British Columbia, Canada; one-third of the costs were for the purposes of monitoring levothyroxine replacement therapy [20, 31]. These data suggest that thyroid monitoring is wrongly or insufficiently carried out in many countries and that current practices are not effective either clinically or economically.

Table 19.1 Relation between the pharmacological effects and potential methods of monitoring of levothyroxine replacement

Level of effect	Actions of and events induced by levothyroxine replacement	Potential monitoring methods
Pharmacokinetics	Conversion of T4 to T3 by • type I deiodinase in peripheral tissues • type II deiodinase in pituitary and central nervous system	T3/fT3 Ratio of T4: T3 or ratio of fT4: fT3
Molecular pharmacology	Binding of fT3 to nuclear thyroid hormone receptors of peripheral tissues	Nuclear thyroid hormone receptor activity
Cellular biochemistry	• Regulation of gene transcription by thyroid hormone receptor stimulation • Altered thyroid–pituitary feedback	• Transcripts of thyroid hormone-responsive genes (e.g. SREBP2-mediated hepatic LDL receptor gene) • TSH/TRH
Tissue physiology	Change in metabolic rate	Metabolic markers: • Enzymes: creatine kinase, cardiac and liver enzymes • Lipids: cholesterol, HDL-C, LDL-C, lipoprotein(a) • Homocysteine • Bone markers • Urine sodium
Organ physiology	Effect of levothyroxine replacement on • Myocardium • Metabolism • Bone • Nervous system • Gastrointestinal system • Coagulation • Reproductive organs	Changes in • Systolic time interval, pulse rate • Weight • Mood, ankle reflex time • Factor VII, VIII, IX, XI activity • Menstrual cycle, LH response to LHRH
Clinical outcome	Short-term effects of levothyroxine treatment on target condition: • Adequate replacement: euthyroidism • Under-replacement: clinical or subclinical hypothyroidism • Over-replacement: clinical or subclinical hyperthyroidism	Clinical markers: • Signs, symptoms • Systolic time intervals, pulse rate • Weight • Ankle reflex time • Mood Surrogate markers: • TSH or TSH + fT4 or TSH + fT3

(Continued)

Table 19.1 (*Continued.*)

Level of effect	Actions of and events induced by levothyroxine replacement	Potential monitoring methods
	Long-term effects of inadequate treatment on • Morbidity and mortality • Cardiovascular disease • Bone metabolism • Psychiatry, psychology, quality of life • Reproductive function, fertility	Clinical markers: • Morbidity • Systolic time intervals, pulse rate • Bone markers • Psychometric measures, scores on quality-of-life questionnaire • Number of regular cycles, markers of ovulation

HDL-C, high-density lipoprotein cholesterol; LDL-C, low-density lipoprotein cholesterol; LH, luteinizing hormone; LHRH, luteinizing hormone-releasing hormone.

Several controversial questions remain unsolved in thyroid monitoring:
- What is the best testing strategy and test(s) for thyroid monitoring during levothyroxine replacement?
- Do the commonly used monitoring strategies apply appropriately timed assessments?
- How can we assess the tissue or organ effects of levothyroxine treatment?
- How frequently should we monitor patients?
- What is the therapeutic target and what is considered 'adequate' thyroxine replacement?
- Has net benefit of the monitoring strategy been demonstrated in practice?

Therefore, in the rest of this chapter I shall review the currently available evidence relating to the monitoring of adult patients with overt hypothyroidism taking levothyroxine, with special emphasis on these questions. I shall not explore monitoring strategies for patients with subclinical or secondary (i.e. pituitary) hypothyroidism, patients taking liothyronine or combination levothyroxine and liothyronine therapy, patients with congenital hypothyroidism, treatment in pregnancy or patients taking suppressive doses of levothyroxine as part of the 'block-replacement' strategy in thyroid cancer or nodular goitre.

I shall illustrate how some of the basic principles of monitoring, as described in Part I, can be applied in practice, focusing on the application of the following items of the monitoring framework:
- The relation between the pathophysiology of hypothyroidism, the mechanism of action of levothyroxine replacement and the development of a monitoring schedule (see Chapters 3 and 4).
- Test selection for monitoring levothyroxine replacement therapy (see Chapters 4 and 5).

- Setting treatment targets for levothyroxine replacement (see Chapter 7).
- Developing a thyroid monitoring schedule (see Chapter 8).
- Evaluating the effectiveness of thyroid monitoring (see Chapter 12).

19.4. Relation between the pathophysiology of hypothyroidism, the mechanism of action of levothyroxine replacement and the development of a monitoring schedule

A brief description of normal thyroid hormone physiology and regulation helps in understanding the pathophysiology of hypothyroidism and the responses to exogenous levothyroxine during replacement therapy. In physiological circumstances, T4 is only produced by the thyroid gland. In euthyroid individuals, 20% of T3 is deiodinated from T4 in the thyroid gland and 80% is produced in peripheral tissues [13]. Serum fT3 the biologically active hormone at the peripheral tissues level binds to nuclear receptors in the liver, kidney, heart, brain, skeletal muscle, bone, and skin and regulates transcription of cell-specific thyroid hormone-responsive genes [32–34]. The multiple cellular effects of thyroid hormones on these end organs explain the various signs and symptoms of hypothyroidism. Free T4 is primarily responsible for negative feedback on pituitary TSH secretion. In other words, fT3 is active at the peripheral tissue level, while fT4 is the key regulator at the pituitary level.

A key principle in thyroid regulation is that each individual has a genetically determined set-point for fT4 at the level of the pituitary, and any deviation from this set point will cause an amplified (log/linear) inverse response in TSH secretion. This explains why a small fall in fT4 concentration, even within the population reference range, results in a noticeable increase in TSH in the subclinical phase of thyroid failure. Therefore, measurement of serum TSH is currently considered the most sensitive indicator of thyroid status. When using TSH as a marker of thyroid function, it has to be borne in mind that TSH secretion by the pituitary responds to any changes in peripheral thyroid hormone status with a delay of 6–12 weeks.

During levothyroxine replacement, the lack of thyroid hormone production and reduced peripheral conversion of T4 to T3 significantly alter a patient's thyroid status. Free T4 concentrations may exceed euthyroid reference ranges when the TSH and fT3 remain closer to normal, resulting in an increased ratio of T4 to T3 [14, 35–41]. Furthermore, the serum TSH concentration only reflects the feedback effect of thyroid hormones at the level of the hypothalamic–pituitary axis, but not necessarily at the tissue or end-organ levels. Potential markers of tissue and end-organ responses to levothyroxine replacement are shown in Table 19.1 and discussed in detail below.

Table 19.2 Correlations (Spearman's rank correlation) between thyroid hormone concentrations and markers of tissue hypothyroidism in 49 patients with overt untreated hypothyroidism*

Marker	Reference range	Median (range)	Correlation with TSH		Correlation with fT4		Correlation with T3	
			r value	P value	r value	P value	r value	P value
Ankle reflex time (ms)	290–410	440 (310–815)	0.32	0.02	−0.71	<0.0001	−0.73	<0.0001
Clinical score (points)		5 (0–11)	0.17	0.28	−0.62	<0.0001	−0.53	<0.001
Total cholesterol (mmol/l)	3.0–5.2	7.0 (3.4–14.2)	0.04	0.81	−0.58	<0.0001	−0.39	<0.01
Creatine kinase (U/l)	40–160	151 (28–2170)	0.20	0.19	−0.61	<0.0001	−0.55	<0.001

Note: *Adapted from [42], with permission.

19.5. Test selection for monitoring thyroxine replacement therapy

Selection of the most appropriate tests for monitoring should be driven by the causal relation between the natural history of primary hypothyroidism and the pharmacological effects of treatment (Figure 19.1 and Table 19.1) (see also Chapters 3 and 4). During monitoring, the patient's thyroid status can be assessed by investigating

1 the function of the hypothalamo–pituitary–thyroid axis,
2 the responses of peripheral tissues and end organs to replacement,
3 signs and symptoms.

In this section I shall discuss the advantages, disadvantages and diagnostic usefulness of these potential biomarkers of thyroid monitoring.

19.5.1. Tests for assessing the function of the hypothalamo–pituitary–thyroid axis

As the definition of hypothyroidism relies on assessment of the function of the hypothalamo–pituitary–thyroid axis, monitoring conventionally also targets its investigation. Two thyroid function tests are available for this purpose: dynamic function testing of the release of TSH by thyrotrophin-releasing hormone (TRH) stimulation, and single measurement of concentrations of TSH and the peripheral thyroid hormones.

19.5.1.1. TRH function testing

Serial measurement of TSH after TRH stimulation indirectly assesses the activity of the thyroid gland. TSH response to TRH stimulation is blunted or accentuated, depending on whether the thyroid gland is currently underactive or overactive. Dynamic measurements after TRH stimulation are still considered by some authors as the reference standard in thyroid function testing. In practice, however, they are invasive, time-consuming, expensive and not easily reproducible, and are therefore not routinely used in the assessment of thyroid function. With the development of highly sensitive (third- and fourth-generation) automated assays, TSH and measurements of T4 and fT4 have become the accepted reference standards and even part of the definition of thyroid conditions. In studies that have explored the response of TSH to TRH stimulation in thyroid replacement or have compared the performance of sensitive TSH assays and dynamic TRH tests, highly sensitive basal TSH measurements provided the same information as a TRH test [43, 44]. Several authors have evaluated the optimal dose of levothyroxine with the TRH test and have titrated the dose of levothyroxine until the TSH response to TRH was normal [45–48]. Indirect evidence is provided by a study in which the diagnostic value of TRH testing was re-evaluated using second- and third-generation TSH assays of differing functional sensitivities. This study showed that basal TSH values correlated with the TRH-induced TSH peak only if measured with a third-generation assay. Therefore, only at least the third-generation TSH assays (with a functional sensitivity of $\leq 0.01–0.02$ mIU/l) seem to be able to replace TRH testing [49].

19.5.1.2. TSH and peripheral thyroid hormone assays

Because there is a logarithmic relation between *endogenous* peripheral hormone concentrations and the feedback response of the pituitary, TSH is believed to reflect the tissue effects of thyroid hormones much earlier than peripheral hormones do. Evidence supports this view strongly, and therefore all guidelines recommend the use of a single, preferably third- or fourth-generation, TSH assay for both diagnosis and monitoring. The diagnostic accuracy of third-generation TSH assays has been evaluated in a systematic review of the results in hospitalized patients, which reported a positive likelihood ratio of 11.1 at a TSH cut-off point of >20 mIU/l [50, 51]. However, there have been no studies of the accuracy of TSH tests in monitoring.

When using TSH for monitoring, it is worth knowing that it has a diurnal rhythm, with a peak concentration at midnight and a trough concentration at around 1400–1500 h. The difference between the concentrations at peak and nadir is about twofold, which can affect the interpretation of test results, particularly in special cases, for example, shift workers, patients with sleep disturbance or patients with other forms of dyssynchronization [19, 52, 53]. The nocturnal TSH surge, absent in overt hypothyroidism, can be restored by replacement with levothyroxine [53]. Further studies are needed to establish whether restoration of the TSH surge could be used as a marker of efficacy of treatment in patients taking levothyroxine.

In the absence of a true and reliable reference standard for the assessment of thyroid status at the tissue or organ levels, it has become challenging to prove whether TSH is an equally good marker of exogenous as well as of endogenous T4 metabolism. When considering this point, it has to be remembered that *exogenous* T4 has a different effect on thyroid status, and patients taking levothyroxine commonly have supranormal fT4 (the key regulator of TSH feedback), while fT3 (the key regulator of tissue effects) is normal [26, 35, 37, 41]. Therefore, logic may dictate that T3 or fT3 would be a better marker of thyroid status at the tissue and end-organ levels. In practice, many clinicians use a combination of peripheral hormone and TSH assays, particularly when poor patient adherence to therapy is suspected [23, 26, 38, 54, 55]. In one study, however, about 42% of fT4 tests were performed unnecessarily in patients with normal TSH concentrations taking levothyroxine replacement [27].

It is commonly also believed that the magnitude of the increase in TSH reflects the severity of tissue hypothyroidism. A recent, but widely criticized, publication therefore correlated tissue markers and clinical scores of hypothyroidism with thyroid hormone concentrations in untreated, overtly hypothyroid patients [26, 30, 42]. Table 19.2 summarizes these results, and the authors concluded that there is no correlation between the different parameters of tissue hypothyroidism and serum TSH, and that free hormone concentrations better reflect the degree of tissue function in severe cases [29, 42 56–58]. These findings suggest that initiation of T4 treatment should be guided by the clinical and metabolic presentation and thyroid hormone concentrations, particularly fT4, and not simply by serum TSH results [42]. However, most of these studies have had drawbacks: they have had small sample sizes, they have investigated the relation between thyroid hormones and tissue markers in untreated patients, and interpretation of the results is hampered by the fact that they have used non-specific clinical and biochemical markers, shown to be rather insensitive tools for assessing tissue hypothyroidism (for a detailed explanation, see the text and Table 19.3).

Several pre-analytical, biological and analytical problems need to be considered when using fT4 or fT3 measurements during levothyroxine replacement. Free T4 concentrations remain raised by about 13% for up to 6–9 hours after administration of a dose of levothyroxine and thus fluctuate more, owing to variations in sampling times during clinic visits [13, 14]. Therefore, if fT4 values are to be measured, the daily dose should be withheld before phlebotomy. Free hormone measurements are also available on many automated analysers, but they are less robust than TSH measurements and may cost more. Even though free hormones have lower intra-individual biological variation than TSH (Table 19.3), interpretation of values is hampered by the fact that each patient has an individual set-point for maintaining euthyroidism and a normal TSH feedback response. Therefore, the wide population reference ranges cannot be used when individuals are monitored and free hormone concentrations are not informative without another marker of thyroid status (e.g. TSH).

19.5.2. Measures of thyroid status at peripheral tissue and end-organ levels

Thyroid hormone deficiency causes numerous changes in different tissues and end-organs (Table 19.1). Related laboratory findings often provide the diagnosis before symptoms occur. Hypothyroidism is discovered in 4–14% of patients presenting with hypercholesterolaemia, because of reduced LDL clearance [3, 60], and there is evidence of a beneficial effect of levothyroxine replacement in lowering LDL cholesterol in mild hypothyroidism [61, 62]. Myopathy with raised creatine kinase activity, hyponatraemia, hyperhomocysteinaemia, hyperprolactinaemia, hypoglycaemia, anaemia, increased lipoprotein(a), altered liver enzymes and altered coagulation are also common findings in hypothyroidism [34, 63]. There have been no studies of the diagnostic accuracy of these laboratory tests in hypothyroidism but, as many of these parameters can change for a number of other reasons, it is expected that these tests would have low sensitivity and specificity. Currently, therefore, they can be used more as additional tests of diagnosis and risk assessment, rather than as definite markers of thyroid hormone function at the tissue level. Organ-specific changes in hypothyroidism have also been reviewed widely [33, 34, 64]. However,

Table 19.3 Characteristics of potential measures for monitoring thyroid status during thyroxine replacement

Test	Analytical imprecision goal CV$_a$ (%)	Signal-to-noise ratio Intra-individual biological variation CV$_i$ (%)	Total variation* (noise) CV (%)	CD value‡ (signal) (%)	Validity (diagnostic accuracy)	Responsiveness	Practicality	Comments
TSH	10	6 wk: 21 1 yr: 22	23 25	64 68	+LR = 11 (at TSH >20 mIU/l)	6–8 wks	++	Third- or fourth-generation tests recommended
fT4	4.8	6 wk: 5.3 1 yr: 9.2	7.0 10	20 29	ND	6–7 days	++	Miss one daily dose before measurement
fT3	4.0	6 wk: 5.6 1 yr: 12	7.0 13	19 35	ND	1 day	+	Assay is less robust than fT4 and TSH
TRH stimulation test	ND	ND	–	–	ND	ND	–	Obsolete, time-consuming, costly
Cholesterol	3	6	7.0	16	ND	ND	++	Non-specific
Signs/symptoms	ND	ND	–	–	+LR = 2 (in-patients) [50] +LR = 1.0–3.88 –LR = 0.42–1.0 (out-patients) [59]	Slow	+	LRs are shown for individual signs. Combination of more signs gave slightly higher LRs (see text) Non-specific
Pulse rate	ND	ND	–	–	+LR = 3.88 [59]	Quick	++	Liable to many interferences, non-specific
Systolic time intervals	ND	ND	–	–	ND	ND	–	Requires special skills and instruments; non-specific; costly
Ankle reflex time	High	ND	–	–	+LR = 3.41 [59]	Slow	–	Subjective
Mood	High	High	–	–	ND	Slow	–	High variability, subjective
Bone density	ND	ND	–	–	ND	Slow	–	Requires special skills and instruments Non-specific, costly

Note: *(CV$_a^2$ + CV$_i^2$)$^{1/2}$.

‡Critical difference (CD%) between two consecutive test results at 95% probability: $2^{1/2} \times Z \times (CV_a^2 + CV_i^2)^{1/2}$ Z = 1.96 (95% probability).

ND, no data; CV$_a$, analytical coefficient of variation; CV$_i$, intra-individual biological variation (data obtained from the NACB guideline, 2002 [19]); +LR, positive likelihood ratio; –LR, negative likelihood ratio.

many of the available assays for monitoring end-organ function lack specificity, sensitivity and reproducibility; are difficult to carry out routinely and are costly. Here I list a few better-studied markers, but most are still restricted to research use only.

The cardiovascular changes in hypothyroidism are characterized by bradycardia, systemic hypertension, cardiac dilatation and pericardial effusion, decreased contractility with impaired ventricular systolic and diastolic function and increased peripheral vascular resistance [34, 64]. In addition to pulse rate measurement and electrocardiography, several tests of left ventricular performance have been used to detect the effect of levothyroxine on cardiac function; they include measurement of systolic time intervals (prolongation of the pre-ejection period, PEP, and reduction of the left ventricular ejection period, LVEP, and their ratio), the isovolumetric relaxation time (IRT) of the left ventricle and the increased velocity of circumferential fibre shortening (VCF). Two recent systematic reviews of endogenous and exogenous subclinical thyroid disease have provided insights into the usefulness of these tests in measuring the effects of thyroid dysfunction on the heart [65, 66].

Because of reduced cardiac output, hypothyroid patients have impaired renal function and reduced free water clearance, contributing to hyponatraemia. Detrimental effects of over-replacement with levothyroxine on skeletal integrity have been shown in many studies, particularly in patients taking suppressive doses of levothyroxine for thyroid cancer. As monitoring tools, measurements of bone density and urinary and serum bone markers have been used in these studies, and the results have been summarized in recent systematic reviews and meta-analyses [67–71]. In none of these reviews, however, has the diagnostic or monitoring usefulness of these tests been investigated; instead, their use as surrogate markers of clinical outcomes has been studied (for more details, see Section 19.8).

19.5.3. Clinical investigation of signs and symptoms

With the availability of automated thyroid hormone assays, clinical evaluation of the classical signs and symptoms of hypothyroidism (fatigue, cold intolerance, coarse skin, constipation, impaired memory, depression, carpal tunnel syndrome, muscle weakness, bradycardia, menstrual disturbance, hoarseness, goitre, periorbital and pretibial oedema, weight gain, galactorrhoea, prolonged ankle reflex time) is less popular [31]. In a case-control study only 30% of patients with newly diagnosed hypothyroidism had typical signs and symptoms, compared with 17% of euthyroid controls, and the positive predictive value was only 8–12% [57]. The literature on the signs and symptoms of thyroid disease in hospitalized patients has been systematically reviewed and the diagnostic accuracy of these clinical tests quantified [50, 51]. In 2210 individuals using patient self-reports for clinical symptoms of hypothyroidism the positive likelihood ratio was 2.0 for reduced appetite, 2.0 for hoarse voice, 2.2 for a fuller face, 2.2 for dry skin and 2.3 for a personal history of thyroid disease. In one small blinded study ($n = 135$, 7% thyroid dysfunction), the positive likelihood ratios for thyroid disease were 6.75, 1.14 and 0.20 respectively for 5, 2–4 and 0–1 symptoms. This analysis shows that clinical signs are often unhelpful in hospitalized patients with many non-thyroid co-morbidities and in whom the prevalence of overt thyroid disease is low. The accuracy of physical examination in the diagnosis of hypothyroidism has been investigated in a cross-sectional double-blind study in 130 out-patients in a rural tertiary hospital in India [59]. No single sign discriminated euthyroidism from hypothyroidism; the range of positive likelihood ratios was 1.0–3.9 and of negative likelihood ratios only 0.42–1.0. Combining signs with the highest likelihood ratios (coarse skin, bradycardia and delayed ankle reflex time) still produced very modest accuracy, with a positive likelihood ratio of 3.75 and a negative likelihood ratio of only 0.48. The authors therefore concluded that signs and symptoms cannot be used in isolation to guide treatment in hypothyroidism.

A retrospective study in patients taking levothyroxine showed that clinical assessment was correct in only 67% of cases. In particular, over-replacement was more difficult to recognize, as only 10% of patients with a suppressed TSH were correctly identified [72]. In a large community-based controlled study of 597 patients taking adequate levothyroxine replacement and with normal TSH concentrations, the frequency of psychological dysfunction and self-reported scores for well-being using a 'General Health' and a 'Thyroid Symptoms' questionnaire were investigated. The authors concluded that patients taking levothyroxine, even with a normal TSH, had significantly worse scores than age- and sex-matched healthy controls [73]. In a small randomized, controlled, crossover trial in 19 controls and 22 patients, with normal thyroid function tests but at least three signs and symptoms of hypothyroidism, T4 100 μg/day was no better than placebo in improving cognitive function and psychological well-being in both patients and controls [74].

Assessment of clinical signs and symptoms needs special skills and experience, and many studies in this field therefore suffer from observer bias and poor reproducibility. Furthermore, many studies have been poorly controlled for confounding factors. The above-mentioned studies highlight the non-specificity of signs and symptoms in thyroid disease and the difficulty in assessing them. The potential methodological shortcomings of various instruments used in measuring symptoms, health status and quality of life in hypothyroidism make it difficult to compare and synthesize trial data in this area. The validity of instruments used for measuring quality of life in hypothyroidism has been studied in two systematic reviews [75, 76]. Both highlighted numerous pitfalls in using these questionnaires and emphasized the need for thoroughly validated, sensitive and reproducible toolboxes that are also responsive and able to detect relevant changes in health-related quality of life over time as a result of therapeutic intervention with levothyroxine. Consequently, a psychometric questionnaire (ThyTSQ) has been published and validated for specifically measuring patient satisfaction with levothyroxine treatment. It is expected that this tool will be suitable for standardizing assessments in both clinical trials and routine monitoring of treated patients with hypothyroidism [77].

19.5.4. Diagnostic usefulness of tests for monitoring thyroid function

As described in Chapters 2 and 5, selection of the best monitoring test depends on:

- *validity* (how well the test predicts clinically significant events),
- *responsiveness* (how quickly the test responds to changes in the condition or treatment),
- *practicality* (whether the test is simple, non-invasive and affordable),
- *a high signal-to-noise ratio* (whether a single test result is likely to detect a clinically significant change and differentiate it from background variation).

The first three of these items have been discussed in detail above. Table 19.3 summarizes these test characteristics and presents data on 'noise' in the laboratory tests used for thyroid testing. It also provides estimates for critical difference (CD) values, that is, the minimum clinically significant difference between two consecutive test results, to enable clinicians to interpret thyroid test results accurately when monitoring patients taking levothyroxine replacement (for details, see the section on Maintenance schedule below).

Summarizing the data on test selection, it can be concluded that signs and symptoms are non-specific, that their assessment is subjective and that they have very low diagnostic accuracy in both the detection and the monitoring of hypothyroidism. However, their role in the initial investigation and subsequent follow-up of patients should not be ignored, and they should be used as baseline estimates, keeping in mind their limitations when the results are interpreted. Most organ-specific investigations lack specificity, have poor reproducibility and slow responsiveness, and their performance needs special skills or instruments. These tests are time-consuming and less practical for routine monitoring.

Other laboratory measurements, such as cholesterol, creatine kinase and liver enzymes, lack specificity and can be influenced by a number of unrelated conditions. Their use is limited to monitoring risks, rather than for judging the tissue effects of levothyroxine.

The TRH test has become obsolete. However, its role as an independent reference standard could be re-evaluated in well-designed studies of its diagnostic accuracy. The TRH test is clearly more expensive and time-consuming than single thyroid hormone concentration measurements, and reproducibility could also be a problem. Therefore, until more evidence emerges to the contrary, it cannot be routinely recommended for monitoring purposes, for reasons of practicality.

Peripheral thyroid hormone measurements in isolation are unhelpful, as the individual set-point of patients for maintaining the euthyroid state is unknown. Furthermore, these tests are susceptible to pre-analytical variations, which could grossly mislead therapeutic decisions.

The TSH assay in isolation is not the most ideal test for monitoring, as it has large biological variation and thus a relatively small signal-to-noise ratio. In addition, it reflects the effect of exogenous T4 on the pituitary secretion of TSH rather than its effects on tissues and end-organ function. In the absence of appropriate evidence, further studies are needed on the diagnostic usefulness of TSH alone or in combination with fT4 or T3/fT3 measurements in monitoring patients taking levothyroxine replacement and in predicting treatment outcomes.

19.6. Setting treatment targets for levothyroxine replacement

Recommendations on thyroid monitoring, published in the last 15 years, vary greatly regarding the target range of TSH for optimal replacement (Table 19.4) [12, 13, 18–22, 34, 78–85]. This lack of consensus is also due to a heated debate about what is considered 'normal' thyroid function. Most laboratories still use TSH reference ranges around 0.4–4.5 mIU/l, based on reference range estimates coming from populations that were later shown to be contaminated by 'healthy', symptom-free individuals with positive TPO antibodies and occult autoimmune thyroid dysfunction. Guidelines and expert consensus, based on evidence emerging from follow-up of the Wickham cohort, set an empiric range of 0.3–3.0 mIU/l [3, 21]. Recent reports on properly selected controls have proposed that the 'true' TSH reference range should be even lower, at <2.5 mIU/l [19, 83, 86], a view that is not currently shared by all [12, 87].

The comparison of 16 guidelines and expert recommendations shown in Table 19.4 suggests that in 11 a more cautious approach of maintaining TSH values in the reference range was applied, while four more recent recommendations set the target closer to the lower end of the reference range [18, 19, 34, 84]. It is common knowledge among endocrinologists that many patients report a sense of well-being only if their fT4 concentration is slightly raised and TSH is low-normal or low [29]. In contrast, many patients with a normal TSH still report symptoms of hypothyroidism [73, 74]; this could be explained by the differing effects of exogenous T4 at the pituitary and peripheral tissue levels. However, some hyperthyroxinaemic patients, despite having normal fT3 concentrations and feeling clinically euthyroid, have cardiac dysfunction and altered TSH responses to TRH, and reducing the dose of levothyroxine normalized both cardiac function and the TSH response to TRH stimulation [54, 55]. Therefore, some authors have suggested that monitoring should be done by a combination of peripheral hormone and TSH assays, particularly when the TSH is abnormal. This group of experts, along with the widely held consensus in most guidelines (Table 19.4), has also recommended that both peripheral hormones and TSH should be normalized for optimal dosing and in order to avoid adverse drug effects at the tissue and end-organ levels [23, 26, 30, 38, 54, 55]. In summary, the currently available evidence does not support a recommendation that titration of the serum TSH to the lower half of the reference range improves clinical outcomes.

19.7. Developing a thyroid monitoring schedule

19.7.1. Assessment of the initial response to levothyroxine replacement

The TSH threshold for initiating therapy and the starting dose should be patient-specific and dependent on age, aetiology, the severity and duration of the condition, the presence of co-morbidities or susceptibility factors (e.g. diabetes, hypertension, smoking), a family history of cardiac disease and concurrent use of other medications [13]. The standard initial dose of levothyroxine required to restore euthyroidism and to normalize TSH is about 1.6 µg/kg/day in uncomplicated cases. After the initial load, the optimal dose can be further titrated by using increments of 25–50 µg and repeat measurements of TSH 2–3 months after a change in dosage [12]. In a prospective, randomized, double-blind study in patients with primary hypothyroidism and no cardiac symptoms or risk, a full starting dose of 1.6 µg/kg/day was compared with a low initial dose of 25 µg/day, increased stepwise monthly; a full starting dose was safe and probably more convenient and cost-effective than the low initial dose and gradual build-up [88, 89].

Lower doses (25–50 µg/day) are used in patients over 65 years of age, as thyroid hormone metabolism diminishes with age [13]. The recommended initial dose in patients with known heart disease is 12.5–25 µg/day [12, 13, 90], with increments of 25 µg at intervals of 2–3 months until the TSH normalizes. The NACB guideline even sets a somewhat higher therapeutic target range for high-risk elderly patients than for young uncomplicated cases [19]. Higher doses are needed in infants (10–15 µg/kg) and children (>2 µg/kg). However, in a systematic review the evidence was found to be too weak for a beneficial effect on cognitive development, growth or behaviour to justify initial regimens that use high or standard doses in congenital hypothyroidism [91].

The cause of the condition influences dosing. For example, higher doses of levothyroxine are needed in patients with spontaneous hypothyroidism than in those whose hypothyroidism was caused by radiotherapy for Graves' disease, probably because of the action of circulating thyroid-stimulating antibodies on the remaining thyroid tissues. Empirical data have also suggested that higher doses of levothyroxine are required in patients with severe hypothyroidism and higher TSH concentrations, that is, the baseline TSH and the dose of levothyroxine are positively correlated [13].

Several medications and circumstances can increase dosage requirements of levothyroxine, including drugs that inhibit levothyroxine absorption (e.g. colestyramine, ferrous sulphate), increase T4 clearance (e.g. rifampicin, carbamazepine), block T4 to T3 conversion (e.g. amiodarone) or enhance the binding of T4 to proteins and thus reduce the fT4 fraction (e.g. pregnancy and

Table 19.4 Recommendations for monitoring levothyroxine treatment in primary hypothyroidism

Guideline/ recommendation	During start of treatment and when changing the dose		Monitoring stable patients—surveillance phase		Therapeutic target	Comments
	Test	Frequency	Test	Frequency		
Mandel et al. 1993 [13] (expert advice based on systematic review)	TSH	6–8 wk	TSH*	Annually	TSH: 0.5–3.0 mIU/l	*Monitor TSH and fT4 if poor adherence to therapy
Toft 1994 [78] (personal expert review)	TSH + fT4	12–16 wk	TSH*	Annually	TSH: 0.5–3.5 mIU/l**	*Monitor TSH and fT4 if poor adherence to therapy **TSH functional sensitivity: 0.05–0.1 mIU/l
Oppenheimer et al. 1995 [79] (personal expert review)	TSH + fT4	8 wk	TSH	Annually*	TSH: 0.25–5.0 mIU/l**	*Recommend more frequent monitoring in pregnancy and if interfering drugs given **Use third-generation TSH assay
Singer et al. 1995 [80] American Thyroid Association (consensus guideline for primary care)	TSH	6–8 wk	TSH and physical examination	6–12 monthly	TSH in reference range	
Vanderpump et al. 1996 [18] Royal College of Physicians and Society of Endocrinology, UK (consensus statement)	TSH	6 wk	TSH	Annually	Normal or below normal TSH*	*With normal or slightly raised T4 and normal T3; measure fT4 if TSH is abnormal Highlights the need for adequate patient information and the use of thyroid registers

HAS–ANAES Guideline 1999 [81] Haute Autorité de la Santé–Agence Nationale d'Accréditation et d'Evaluation en Santé, France (consensus statement)	TSH (+ fT4 if necessary)	6–8 wk/8–12 wk*	TSH**	6 monthly or annually	No detail	*First monitoring 6–8 wk after beginning therapy; 8–12 wk in the case of a change in dose **Monitor TSH and fT4 if poor adherence to therapy, or if unexplained instability, or taking amiodarone
Woeber 2000 [82] (personal expert review)	TSH	4–8 wk	TSH + fT4	Initially 6 monthly, then annually	TSH in reference range	
AACE Guideline 2002 [21] American Association of Clinical Endocrinologists (guideline, updated in 2006)	TSH + fT4	6 wk	TSH, patient's history and physical examination	Initially 6 monthly, then annually	TSH in reference range*	*TSH functional sensitivity: ≤0.02 mIU/l Recommends patient information and education to improve adherence to treatment
NACB Guideline 2002 [19] National Academy of Clinical Biochemistry, USA (expert consensus guideline)	TSH	6–8 wk	TSH*	Annually	TSH: 0.5–2.0 mIU/l** TSH: 0.5–3.0 mIU/l in elderly	*Monitor TSH and fT4 if poor adherence to therapy, but in this case omit the daily dose of levothyroxine **TSH functional sensitivity: ≤0.02 mIU/l Provides information on future likelihood of lowering reference range to 0.4–2.5 mIU/l

(*Continued*)

Table 19.4 (*Continued.*)

Guideline/ recommendation	During start of treatment and when changing the dose		Monitoring stable patients—surveillance phase		Therapeutic target	Comments
	Test	Frequency	Test	Frequency		
Zimmerman 2003 [83] (personal expert review)	TSH	6–12 wk	TSH	Annually	TSH: 0.4–3.0 mIU/l	Points to the likelihood of lowering the upper limit of the reference range to ~2.0 mIU/l
Roberts and Ladenson 2004 [34] (expert advice based on systematic review)	TSH	4–6 wk	TSH*	Annually**	TSH in the lower half of the reference range: ~1.0 mIU/l	*Monitor TSH and fT4 if non-compliant **Monitor more frequently if symptomatic
Stelfox et al. 2004 [22] (expert opinion based on literature review and consensus)	TSH + fT4	6–12 wk	TSH*	Annually	TSH: 0.5–5.0 mIU/l	*Monitor TSH + fT4 if TSH is out of target range
British Columbia Medical Association Guideline 2004 [20] (evidence-based guideline)	TSH	6–8 wk	TSH*	Annually	TSH in reference range**	*Monitor TSH + fT4 if TSH is subnormal **If TSH is reduced but measurable and patient is asymptomatic, do not change the dose

EBM Guidelines 2004 [84] (evidence-based guideline)	TSH	–	TSH	TSH near lower limit of reference range*	*If fT4 is normal and patient asymptomatic Daily dose of levothyroxine must not be taken if fT4 and TSH are to be measured
PRODIGY Guidance 2005 [85]	TSH	6 wk	TSH	TSH in reference range	Provides discussion points for patients
UK Guidelines 2006 [12] Association of Clinical Biochemists—British Thyroid Association—British Thyroid Foundation (evidence-based guideline)	TSH + fT4 and clinical signs	8–12 wk	TSH*	TSH in reference range**	*Monitor TSH and fT4 if poor adherence to therapy; in that case, standardize the timing of testing in relation to the daily dose of levothyroxine **With normal or slightly raised fT4 **TSH functional sensitivity: ≤0.02 mIU/l **Finds the evidence for lowering the TSH reference range to 2.5 mIU/l unconvincing Computerized thyroid registers may support successful follow-up

oestrogen replacement) [92]. It is beyond the scope of this chapter to list all potential interferences, and the interested reader is referred to the published literature [13, 93, 94].

Most recommendations ($n = 10$) have advocated the use of a single TSH measurement and six guidelines have also proposed fT4 measurements in the initial titration phase of replacement (Table 19.4). Only one UK guideline mentions monitoring signs and symptoms in the initial phase of monitoring. The recommended testing frequency, both at initiation and after any dosage adjustments later in the monitoring schedule, shows some variation, but overall it is 6–8 weeks, until euthyroidism is achieved (Table 19.4). The adequacy of out-patient monitoring in a US hospital in the different phases of the follow-up schedule has been investigated [22]. At the start of treatment, 76% of patients satisfied the monitoring criteria, with an average of six errors per 100 criteria. All patients had their baseline TSH measured and levothyroxine prescribed, but most monitoring errors (24 per 100 criteria) occurred with baseline evaluations of fT4.

19.7.2. Maintenance schedule: surveillance, re-adjustment and long-term follow-up

Once patients achieve biochemical and clinical euthyroidism while taking a maintenance dose, clinic visits can be reduced. Some guidelines initially recommend a testing frequency of 6 months, and annual follow-up is sufficient if patients remain stable. Most guidelines recommend the use of a single TSH assay annually. For avoidance of adverse drug reactions and subclinical hyperthyroidism, some guidelines recommend the use of at least third-generation TSH assays with a functional sensitivity of less than 0.02 mIU/l [12, 19, 21, 79].

Free T4 measurements are particularly helpful if poor adherence to therapy is suspected. TSH concentrations, if tested at appropriate intervals, act as long-term markers of thyroid status. In patients who have a raised TSH and a high normal or high fT4, it is most likely that adherence to treatment is random and that the clinic visit prompted the patient to take the medication. Some guidelines also highlight the importance of pre-analytical factors when fT4 is used for monitoring, and recommend avoidance of the daily dose of levothyroxine before clinic visits. No guidelines recommend the use of T3 or fT3 assays in any phases of thyroid monitoring. One guideline from Canada explicitly prohibits the performance of T3 hormone assays in hypothyroidism and, for economical considerations, also strictly regulates when fT4 tests can be carried out [20]. One study showed that most monitoring errors occurred at surveillance and follow-up visits (25 and 10 monitoring errors per 100 criteria) [22]. Even though the population studied was relatively small ($n = 99$) and the monitoring criteria were not validated to draw far-reaching conclusions, the results were similar to the findings of others: that is, 25% of patients did not satisfy baseline evaluation criteria, 28% did not comply with surveillance and 39% with surveillance response criteria, and 10% failed to fulfil follow-up visit criteria [5, 23, 25–27].

Two British recommendations have highlighted the finding that access to a computerized thyroid disease register improves surveillance [12, 28], and three sets of guidelines have emphasized the need to provide information for patient education [18, 21, 85]. However, a randomized controlled trial in three UK general practices over 3 months showed no improvements in health, TSH concentrations or adherence to medication after an educational booklet and reminder card were given to hypothyroid patients [95]. It is possible that the results of this study were confounded by the fact that patients and controls involved in a trial are more likely to adhere to treatment instructions anyway, and so the difference between the control and intervention groups was less significant.

Only two American sets of guidelines mention the use of clinical history and physical investigations during follow-up, pointing to an over-reliance on laboratory testing and less attention to patients' signs and symptoms. As discussed above, clinical signs have poor specificity and low diagnostic accuracy. However, it should not be forgotten that clinical queries and investigations may have positive psychological effects on patients, and the individual who notices that his physician cares about him and does not simply treat a laboratory result is more likely to follow instructions and advice [96]. Clinical assessment is also mandatory, as laboratory errors can sometimes misguide management [97].

During long-term follow-up, the most difficult question that clinicians face is when to consider that a monitoring test result is clinically significantly different from previous test results, and whether the observed change warrants adjustment of treatment. A few studies have shown that most primary-care physicians do not capture the concept of 'critical difference' (CD) between consecutive test results, and this can lead to errors in monitoring and treatment decisions [98, 99]. The CD is defined as the minimum difference needed between two consecutive test results to be certain (with a given degree of confidence) that the two results are truly different and not simply a result of analytical imprecision (CV_a) or intra-individual biological variation (CV_i). Table 19.3 shows the analytical and biological variation inherent in thyroid measurements, which will be responsible for baseline 'noise', from which a true change ('signal') should be differentiated when monitoring replacement [19]. Using a published formula, the CD for optimal analytical circumstances of low imprecision (i.e. good reproducibility of test results) and zero bias (i.e. no calibration change of and no bias between instruments if different instruments have been used) has been calculated; an example is shown in Table 19.3. From these data it follows that TSH has the biggest CD value, owing to its relatively high intra-individual biological variation and imprecision of the assay, particularly at lower values of TSH. This means that if the laboratory repeats the TSH test after 6–8 weeks with an analytical imprecision of 10%, a normal TSH concentration of 3 mIU/l can be anything between 1.1 and 4.9 mIU/l (with 95% probability), simply due to analytical and biological variation. A clinically significant change after treatment must therefore be greater than the

CD value, that is, TSH has to change by more than 65% to call that change clinically relevant.

Awareness of these CD values clearly has an impact on interpreting therapeutic target ranges and excursions from those ranges during monitoring. Setting the therapeutic target at the lower end of the TSH reference range, as some recommendations in Table 19.4 have suggested (i.e. at around 0.5–1.0 mIU/l), carries the risk that patients are over-replaced, if the CD values are not taken into consideration before dosage adjustment. Therefore, if the TSH concentration is only slightly raised or lowered, it is advisable to repeat the TSH tests after 6–8 weeks; analysis of the trends on control charts can aid decisions about dosage adjustment [79].

It is important to emphasize that the CD values shown in Table 19.3 and the above example are for guidance only, as intra-individual variation also has some uncertainty. Calculations can also vary from laboratory to laboratory, depending on local analytical performance and thus variations in the CV_a values of thyroid hormone assays. However, as long as the CV_a of the laboratory is less than half of the CV_i (the analytical precision goal), it will not influence the CD values much. It is more important to remember that, as thyroid hormone measurements are not well standardized, TSH values may also show variations because of methodological bias between laboratories, making comparison of test results difficult. Physicians are therefore advised to use the same laboratory, or at least laboratories with the same type of method, when monitoring individual patients. It is the responsibility of laboratory professionals to inform their clinicians about assay performance or changes in assay methods and their effect on test interpretation. In one study there was a modest reduction (4.7%) over 3 years in the proportion of under-replaced patients as a result of interpretative comments on laboratory reports to general physicians [100]. However, the proportion of over-treated patients also increased by 2.3%, and the study was poorly controlled. Therefore, more carefully designed, well-controlled and preferably randomized studies are needed to investigate whether additional information or comments by laboratory personnel have an educational impact on doctors' practices and improve treatment-related outcomes in patients.

19.8. Evaluating the effectiveness of thyroid monitoring

Monitoring any condition is only valuable if the treatment is associated with short-term or long-term adverse effects that can be prevented by tight control and appropriate follow-up. The short-term effects of levothyroxine treatment are as follows:
- euthyroidism, if replacement is adequate;
- clinical or subclinical hypothyroidism when patients are under-replaced;
- clinical or subclinical hyperthyroidism caused by over-replacement.

There is debate about the long-term effects of inadequate treatment on overall morbidity and mortality, cardiovascular risk, bone metabolism, reproductive function, psychiatric and psychological functions and quality of life. In a retrospective study, there was no increase in morbidity or mortality among patients taking levothyroxine whose TSH was <0.05 mIU/l compared with those with a normal TSH [101]. It is beyond the scope of this chapter to evaluate critically the vast amount of literature behind all the above-listed treatment outcomes, and I shall therefore limit discussion to the two best-studied and systematically reviewed areas only, the potential skeletal and cardiovascular adverse effects of levothyroxine replacement.

19.8.1. Adverse effects of levothyroxine on bone metabolism

The effects of thyroid hormone on skeletal integrity have been studied widely, particularly in patients taking *suppressive* doses of levothyroxine. Hyperthyroxinaemia increases bone turnover and affects the cortical bones (hip and forearm) more than the trabecular ones (e.g. the spine). Research evidence has been summarized in three systematic reviews and two meta-analyses, but the conclusions are greatly limited by small sample sizes and incomplete follow-up, inappropriately defined and heterogeneous patient populations, poor methodological quality, different study designs poorly controlled for confounders and differing techniques for measuring both TSH suppression and bone density [67–71]. The two earlier meta-analyses of cross-sectional studies showed reduced bone mass in postmenopausal but not premenopausal women taking suppressive doses of levothyroxine, but both suffered from heterogeneity in the primary data [67, 68]. Because of continuing debate and confusion, the authors of three subsequent qualitative reviews critically re-evaluated and synthesized the most recent literature, re-analysed data according to subgroups and made recommendations for current practice and future research [69–71]. Although in all the reviews the results were equivocal on the deleterious effects of TSH suppression on bone, the authors concluded that exogenous hyperthyroidism may adversely affect bone and increases the risk of hip fracture, particularly in postmenopausal women. Therefore, until better evidence is available from large high-quality studies, they recommended careful titration of the dose of levothyroxine during suppressive therapy, together with periodic assessment of bone mass at cortical sites, and the consideration of preventive interventions in higher risk postmenopausal patients (e.g. exercise, replacement of oestrogen, vitamin D and calcium, and the use of bisphosphonates).

In three of the above-mentioned reviews, the effect on bone of levothyroxine *replacement* was also investigated [68, 69, 71]. One showed reduced bone density at the spine and hip in premenopausal but not postmenopausal women [68], and in spite of heterogeneous and conflicting data, no overall clinically significant skeletal effects were found in premenopausal or postmenopausal women taking replacement doses. Another group did not find an increased risk of overall fractures or fractured neck of femur in patients whose TSH was suppressed during levothyroxine replacement therapy [101].

19.8.2. Adverse effects of levothyroxine on cardiac function

Thyroxine excess, either endogenously or due to treatment with levothyroxine, can cause atrial fibrillation, tachyarrhythmias, bouts of palpitation and exacerbation of angina pectoris. In patients over the age of 60 years, a low TSH (≤ 0.1 mIU/l) was associated with a three-fold relative risk of atrial fibrillation in the next decade [102]. Cardiac complications can arise in patients with underlying ischaemic heart disease, even during restoration of euthyroidism, and about 40% of these patients cannot tolerate a full replacement dose, hence the use of a lower starting dose and a somewhat higher treatment target in such high-risk patients [19, 64]. Patients under 65 years taking levothyroxine had an increased prevalence of ischaemic heart disease than the general population, but surprisingly the risk was no different between those with suppressed TSH (<0.05 mIU/l) and normal TSH [101]. However, more insight into the evidence base that has accumulated since that study has come from a systematic review of 12 primary studies of the effects of subclinical thyroid dysfunction on the heart [65]. Heart rate was increased in only six studies and in two studies it was unchanged. The prevalence and incidence of atrial fibrillation were higher in elderly patients with subclinical hyperthyroidism, and atrial extra beats were also increased in younger adults. In five studies systolic function was increased, but in three it was unchanged. In all studies left ventricular mass was increased, but the prognostic significance of this is unknown. Research data are mainly concerned with investigation of the effects of suppressive doses of levothyroxine on the heart, and little is known about cardiac function in cases of levothyroxine replacement. However, based on the currently available best evidence, it is strongly recommended that subnormal TSH values should be avoided in elderly patients and those with cardiac risks, and that beta-blockade be considered in those with adrenergic hyperresponsiveness to levothyroxine to prevent irreversible or fatal cardiac adverse effects [65].

Another area of interest is investigation of the relation between thyroid status and risk factors for coronary heart disease (CHD), such as increased cholesterol, LDL cholesterol, C reactive protein (CRP) and homocysteine. The Rotterdam Study provided strong evidence that subclinical hypothyroidism is associated with a greater prevalence of atherosclerosis and CHD-related death [6]. A recent systematic review also showed that subclinical hypothyroidism is associated with an increased risk of CHD (summary OR for CHD after adjustment for demographic characteristics = 1.81; 95% CI = 1.38, 2.39) [68]. There is still more controversy about the effect of levothyroxine treatment on lipid concentrations. Two meta-analyses have shown modest mean falls in cholesterol of –0.4 mmol/l (CI = –0.2, –0.6) and –0.2 mmol/l (CI = –0.09, –0.34), and LDL cholesterol was also reduced (–0.26 mmol/l, CI = –0.12, –0.41) [61, 103]. HDL and triglyceride concentrations, as well as apolipoprotein AI, lipoprotein(a), total homocysteine, and CRP were unchanged [11, 61, 62]. There were similar results in the placebo-controlled, double-blind Basel Thyroid Study, which estimated a 9–31% potential reduction in cardiovascular mortality from the observed improvements in lipid parameters [62]. However, some authors have argued that levothyroxine-induced changes in lipid concentrations are subtle, and that patients at increased risk are better treated with lipid-lowering medications than levothyroxine. Recent guidelines also do not recommend levothyroxine treatment in these cases unless TSH is higher than 10 mIU/l [12].

The above studies, however, focused on the association of *subclinical* hypothyroidism with an increased risk of atherosclerosis and whether screening for the condition and treating these cases with levothyroxine is beneficial. This evidence can only therefore be applied indirectly to cases of *overt* hypothyroidism. In a meta-analysis of the effect of thyroid replacement in a subset of cases of overt hypothyroidism, the reduction in cholesterol concentrations was highly dependent on pre-treatment values: -1.2 mmol/l (CI = -0.9, -1.5) at cholesterol concentrations up to 8 mmol/l and -3.4 mmol/l (CI = -3.0, -3.7) if baseline concentrations were higher than 8 mmol/l [103]. Again, these changes caused by levothyroxine replacement are insufficient to reduce the risk of CHD, and supplementation of treatment with lipid-lowering medication is therefore warranted.

In summary, evidence on the long-term effects of thyroid replacement on clinical outcomes related to cardiac function and bone metabolism is controversial. More research is needed to define the best strategy and the optimal therapeutic targets for monitoring these patients to avoid potential long-term adverse effects of levothyroxine replacement.

Acknowledgements

The author thanks Joseph Watine (Rodez, France), Eva Nagy (Szeged, Hungary), Sverre Sandberg (Bergen, Norway), and Paul Glasziou and Jeffrey Aronson (Oxford, UK) for their valuable comments and contributions to the writing of this chapter. Part of this work was initiated by the Aspley Guise Task Force on evidence-based laboratory medicine in 1997–1999. This work has been supported by the Committee on Evidence-Based Laboratory Medicine of the International Federation of Clinical Chemistry and Laboratory Medicine.

References

1 Tunbridge WM, Evered DC, Hall R, et al. The spectrum of thyroid disease in the community: the Wickham survey. *Endocrinology* 1977; **7**: 481–93.
2 Sawin CT, Castelli WP, Hershman JM, McNamara P, Bacharach P. The aging thyroid. Thyroid deficiency in the Framingham Study. *Arch Intern Med* 1985; **145**: 1386–8.
3 Vanderpump MP, Tunbridge WM, French JM, et al. The incidence of thyroid disorders in the community: a twenty-year follow up of the Wickham Survey. *Clin Endocrinol* 1995; **43**: 55–68.

4 Parle JV, Franklyn JA, Cross KW, Jones SC, Sheppard MC. Prevalence and follow-up of abnormal thyrotrophin (TSH) concentrations in the elderly in the United Kingdom. *Clin Endocrinol* 1991; **34**: 77–83.

5 Canaris G, Manowitiz N, Mayor G, Ridgway C. The Colorado thyroid disease prevalence study. *Arch Intern Med* 2000; **160**: 526–34.

6 Hak AE, Pols HA, Visser TJ, Drexhage HA, Hofman A, Witteman JC. Subclinical hypothyroidism is an independent risk factor for atherosclerosis and myocardial infarction in elderly women: the Rotterdam Study. *Ann Intern Med* 2000; **132**: 270–8.

7 Hollowell JG, Staehling NW, Flanders WD, et al. Serum TSH, T(4), and thyroid antibodies in the United States population (1988 to 1994): National Health and Nutrition Examination Survey (NHANES III). *J Clin Endocrinol Metab* 2002; **87**: 489–99.

8 Helfand M. Screening for subclinical thyroid dysfunction in nonpregnant adults: a summary of the evidence for the US Preventive Services Task Force. *Ann Intern Med* 2004; **140**: 128–41.

9 Surks MI, Ortiz E, Daniels GH, et al. Subclinical thyroid disease: scientific review and guidelines for diagnosis and management. *JAMA* 2004; **291** (2): 228–38.

10 Wilson GR, Curry RW. Subclinical thyroid disease. *Am Fam Phys* 2005; **72**: 1517–24.

11 Beyhan Z, Erturk K, Uckaya G, Bolu E, Yaman H, Kutlu M. Restoration of euthyroidism does not improve cardiovascular risk factors in patients with subclinical hypothyroidism in the short term. *J Endocrinol Invest* 2006; **29** (6): 505–10.

12 Association for Clinical Biochemistry (ACB), the British Thyroid Association (BTA) and the British Thyroid Foundation (BTF). UK guidelines for the use of thyroid function tests. July 2006. Available from www.acb.org.uk.

13 Mandel SJ, Brent GA, Larsen PR. Levothyroxine therapy in patients with thyroid disease. *Ann Intern Med* 1993; **119** (6): 492–502.

14 Ain KB, Pucino F, Shiver TM, Banks SM. Thyroid hormone levels affected by time of blood sampling in thyroxine-treated patients. *Thyroid* 1993; **3**: 81–5.

15 Grozinsky-Glasberg S, Fraser A, Nahshoni E, Weizman A, Leibovici L. Thyroxine–triiodothyronine combination therapy versus thyroxine monotherapy for clinical hypothyroidism: meta-analysis of randomized controlled trials. *J Clin Endocrinol Metab* 2006; **91**: 2592–9.

16 Escobar-Morreale HF, Escobar del Rey F, Obregón MJ, de Escobar G. Review: only the combined treatment with thyroxine and triiodothyronine ensures euthyroidism in all tissues of the thyroidectomized rat. *Endocrinology* 1996; **137**: 2490–502.

17 Escobar-Morreale HF, Botella-Carretero JI, Escobar del Rey F, Morreale de Escobar G. Review: treatment of hypothyroidism with combinations of levothyroxine plus liothyronine. *J Clin Endocrinol Metab* 2005; **90**: 4946–54.

18 Vanderpump MPJ, Ahlquist JAO, Franklyn JA, Clayton RN. Consensus statement for good practice and audit measures in the management of hypothyroidism and hyperthyroidism. *BMJ* 1996; **313**: 539–44.

19 Demers LM, Spencer CA (eds). NACB (National Academy of Clinical Biochemistry): laboratory support for the diagnosis and monitoring of thyroid disease. NACB, 2002, p. 125. Available from
www.nacb.org/lmpg/thyroid_LMPG_Word.stm.

20 British Columbia Medical Association Guideline. Thyroid function tests in the diagnosis and monitoring of adults with thyroid disease. 2004. Available from www.healthservices.gov.bc.ca/msp/protoguides.

21 AACE Thyroid Task Force. American Association of Clinical Endocrinologists medical guidelines for clinical practice for the evaluation and treatment of hyperthyroidism and hypothyroidism. *Endocr Pract* 2002; **8** (6): 457–69. The amended version, produced in 2006, is downloadable from the AACE website: http://www.aace.com/pub/pdf/guidelines/hypo_hyper.pdf.

22 Stelfox HT, Ahmed SB, Fiskio J, Bates DW. An evaluation of the adequacy of outpatient monitoring of thyroid replacement therapy. *J Eval Clin Pract* 2004; **10**: 525–30.

23 Ross DS, Daniels GH, Gouveia D. The use and limitations of a chemiluminescent thyrotropin assay as a single thyroid function test in an outpatient endocrine clinic. *J Clin Endocrinol Metab* 1990; **71**: 764–9.

24 Parle JV, Franklyn JA, Cross KW, Jones SR, Sheppard MC. Thyroxine prescription in the community: serum thyroid stimulating hormone level assays as an indicator of undertreatment or overtreatment. *Br J Gen Pract* 1993; **43**: 107–9.

25 Diez J. Hypothyroidism in patients older than 55 years: an analysis of the etiology and assessment of the effectiveness of therapy. *J Gerontol* 2002; **57**: M315–M320.

26 Crilly M. Thyroid function tests and hypothyroidism: reducing concentrations further would be harmful. *BMJ* 2003; **326**: 1086.

27 Eskelinen SI, Isoaho RE, Kivela SL, Irjala KM. Actual practice vs guidelines in laboratory monitoring of older patients with primary hypothyroidism in primary care. *Aging Clin Exp Res* 2006; **18** (1): 34–9.

28 De Whalley P. Do abnormal thyroid stimulating hormone level values result in treatment changes? A study of patients on thyroxine in one general practice. *Br J Gen Pract* 1995; **45**: 93–5.

29 Toft AD, Beckett GJ. Thyroid function tests and hypothyroidism: measurement of serum TSH alone may not always reflect thyroid status. *BMJ* 2003; **326**: 295–6.

30 Vanderpump MP, Franklyn JA. Thyroid function tests and hypothyroidism: restoring TSH to reference range should be the goal of replacement. *BMJ* 2003; **326**: 1086–7.

31 O'Reilly D StJ. Thyroid function tests—time for a reassessment. *BMJ* 2000; **320**: 1332–4.

32 Brent GA, Moore DD, Larsen PR. Thyroid hormone regulation of gene expression. *Annu Rev Physiol* 1991; **53**: 17–35.

33 Ridgway EC. Modern concepts of primary thyroid gland failure. *Clin Chem* 1996; **42** (1): 179–82.

34 Roberts CGP, Ladenson PW. Hypothyroidism. *Lancet* 2004; **363**: 793–803.

35 Pearce CJ, Himsworth RL. Total and free thyroid hormone concentrations in patients receiving maintenance replacement treatment with thyroxine. *BMJ* 1984; **288**: 693–5.

36 Pearce CJ, Himsworth RL. Serum iodothyronine concentrations during introduction of thyroxine replacement therapy in hypothyroidism. *Clin Endocrinol (Oxf)* 1986; **25**: 301–11.

37 Wennlund A. Variation in serum levels of T3, T4, FT4 and TSH during thyroxine replacement therapy. *Acta Endocrinol (Copenh)* 1986; **113**: 47–9.

38 Liewendahl K, Helenius T, Lamberg BA, Nahonen H, Wagar G. Free thyroxine, free triiodothyronine, and thyrotropin concentrations in hypothyroid and thyroid carcinoma patients receiving thyroxine therapy. *Acta Endocrinol (Copenh)* 1987; **116** (3): 418–24.

39 Fish LH, Schwartz HL, Cavanaugh J, Steffes MW, Bantle JP, Oppenheimer JH. Replacement dose, metabolism, and bioavailability of levothyroxine in the treatment of hypothyroidism. Role of triiodothyronine in pituitary feedback in humans. *N Engl J Med* 1987; **316**: 764–70.

40 Browning MC, Bennet WM, Kirkaldy AJ, Jung RT. Intra-individual variation of thyroxin, triiodothyronine, and thyrotropin in treated hypothyroid patients: implications for monitoring replacement therapy. *Clin Chem* 1988; **34**: 696–9.

41 Woeber KA. Levothyroxine therapy and serum free thyroxine and free triiodothyronine concentrations. *J Endocrinol Invest* 2002; **25**: 106–9.

42 Meier C, Trittibach P, Guglielmetti M, Staub JJ, Müller B. Serum thyroid stimulating hormone in assessment of severity of tissue hypothyroidism in patients with overt primary thyroid failure: cross sectional survey. *BMJ* 2003; **326**: 311–2.

43 Wheatley T, Clark PM, Clark JD, Raggatt PR, Edwards OM. Thyroid stimulating hormone measurement by an ultrasensitive assay during thyroxine replacement: comparison with other tests of thyroid function. *Ann Clin Biochem* 1987; **24** (6): 614–9.

44 De Rosa G, Testa A, Giacomini D, et al. Comparison between TRH-stimulated TSH and basal TSH measurement by a commercial immunoradiometric assay in the management of thyroid disease. *Q J Nucl Med* 1996; **40** (2): 182–7.

45 Evered D, Young ET, Ormston BJ, Menzies R, Smith PA, Hall R. Treatment of hypothyroidism: a reappraisal of thyroxine therapy. *Br Med J* 1973; **3**: 131–4.

46 Stock JM, Surks MI, Oppenheimer JH. Replacement dosage of L-thyroxine in hypothyroidism: a re-evaluation. *N Engl J Med* 1974; **290**: 529–33.

47 Erne P, Staub JJ, Althaus B, Fleig Y, Girard J. Evaluation of the optimal thyroxine dose with the TRH test for replacement and suppression therapy. *Schweiz Med Wochenschr* 1983; **113** (50): 1922–3.

48 Carr D, McLeod DT, Parry G, Thornes HM. Fine adjustment of thyroxine replacement dosage: comparison of the thyrotrophin releasing hormone test using a sensitive thyrotrophin assay with measurement of free thyroid hormones and clinical assessment. *Clin Endocrinol (Oxf)* 1988; **28**: 325–33.

49 Christ-Crain M, Meier C, Roth CB, Huber P, Staub JJ, Muller B. Basal TSH levels compared with TRH-stimulated TSH levels to diagnose different degrees of TSH suppression: diagnostic and therapeutic impact of assay performance. *Eur J Clin Invest* 2002; **32** (12): 931–7.

50 Attia J, Margetts P, Guyatt G. Diagnosis of thyroid disease in hospitalized patients: a systematic review. *Arch Intern Med* 1999; **159**: 658–65.

51 Bauer DC. Review: sensitive thyrotropin testing in unselected inpatients has low diagnostic accuracy. *Evid Based Med* 2000; **5**: 29.

52 Bartalena L, Martino E, Falcone M, et al. Evaluation of the nocturnal serum thyrotropin (TSH) surge, as assessed by TSH ultrasensitive assay, in patients receiving long term L-thyroxine suppression therapy and in patients with various thyroid disorders. *J Clin Endocrinol Metab* 1987; **65** (6): 1265–71.

53 Sturgess I, Thomas SH, Pennel DJ, Mitchell D, Croft DN. Diurnal variation in TSH and free thyroid hormones in patients on thyroxine replacement. *Acta Endocrinol (Copenh)* 1989; **121** (5): 674–6.

54 Jennings PE, O'Malley BP, Griffin KE, Northover B, Rosenthal FD. Relevance of increased serum thyroxine concentrations associated with normal serum triiodothyronine values in hypothyroid patients receiving thyroxine: a case for 'tissue thyrotoxicosis'. *Br Med J (Clin Res Ed)* 1984; **289**: 1645–7.

55 Grund FM, Niewoehner CB. Hyperthyroxinaemia in patients receiving thyroid replacement therapy. *Arch Intern Med* 1989; **149** (4): 921–4.

56 Ridgway EC, Cooper DS, Walker H, et al. Therapy of primary hypothyroidism with L-triiodothyronine: discordant cardiac and pituitary responses. *Clin Endocrinol (Oxf)* 1980; **13**: 479-88.

57 Canaris GJ, Steiner JF, Ridgway EC. Do traditional symptoms of hypothyroidism correlate with biochemical disease? *J Gen Intern Med* 1997; **12**: 544–50.

58 Zulewski H, Muller B, Exer P, Miserez AR, Staub JJ. Estimation of tissue hypothyroidism by a new clinical score: evaluation of patients with various grades of hypothyroidism and controls. *J Clin Endocrinol Metab* 1997; **82**: 771–6.

59 Indra R, Patil SS, Joshi R, Pai M, Kalantri SP. Accuracy of physical examination in the diagnosis of hypothyroidism: a cross-sectional, double-blind study. *J Postgrad Med* 2004; **50**: 7–10.

60 Diekman T, Lansberg PJ, Kastelstein JJ, Wiersinga WM. Prevalence and correction of hypothyroidism in a large cohort of patients referred for dyslipidaemia. *Arch Intern Med* 1995; **155**: 1490–5.

61 Danese MD, Ladenson PW, Meinert CL, Powe NR. Effect of thyroxine therapy on serum lipoproteins in patients with mild thyroid failure: a quantitative review of the literature. *J Clin Endocrinol Metab* 2000; **85**: 2993–3001.

62 Meier C, Staub J-J, Roth C-B, et al. TSH-controlled L-thyroxine therapy reduces cholesterol levels and clinical symptoms in subclinical hypothyroidism: a double blind placebo-controlled trial (Basel Thyroid Study). *J Clin Endocrinol Metab* 2001; **86** (10): 4860–6.

63 Gullu S, Sav H, Kamel N. Effects of levothyroxine treatment on biochemical and hemostasis parameters in patients with hypothyroidism. *Eur J Clin Endocrinol* 2005; **152** (3): 355–61.

64 Toft AD, Boon NA. General cardiology: thyroid disease and the heart. *Heart* 2000; **84**: 455–60.

65 Biondi B, Palmieri EA, Lombardi G, Fazio S. Effects of subclinical thyroid dysfunction on the heart. *Ann Intern Med* 2002; **137**: 904–14.

66 Rodondi N, Aujesky D, Vittinghof E, Cornuz J, Bauer DC. Subclinical hypothyroidism and the risk of coronary heart disease: a meta-analysis. *Am J Med* 2006; **119**: 541–51.

67 Faber J, Galloe AM. Changes in bone mass during prolonged subclinical hyperthyroidism due to L-thyroxine treatment: a meta-analysis. *Eur J Clin Endocrinol* 1994; **130** (4): 350–6.

68 Uzzan B, Campos J, Cucherat M, Nony P, Boissel JP. Effects on bone mass of long-term treatment with thyroid hormones: a meta-analysis. *J Clin Endocrinol Metab* 1996; **81**: 4278–89.

69 Greenspan SL, Greenspan FS. The effect of thyroid hormone on skeletal integrity. *Ann Intern Med* 1999; **130**: 750–8.

70 Quan ML, Pasieka JL, Rorstad O. Bone mineral density in well-differentiated thyroid cancer patients treated with suppressive thyroxine: a systematic overview of the literature. *J Surg Oncol* 2002; **79**: 62–70.

71 Schneider R, Reiners C. The effect of levothyroxine therapy on bone mineral density: a systematic review of the literature. *Exp Clin Endocrinol Diabetes* 2003; **111**: 455–70.

72 Thomas SH, Sturgess I, Wedderburn A, Wylie J, Croft DN. Clinical versus biochemical assessment in thyroxine replacement therapy: a retrospective study. *J R Coll Phys Lond* 1990; **24** (4): 289–91.

73 Saravanan P, Chau WF, Roberts N, Vedhara K, Greenwood R, Dayan CM. Psychological well-being in patients on 'adequate' doses of l-thyroxine: results of a large, controlled, community-based questionnaire study. *Clin Endocrinol (Oxf)* 2002; **57** (5): 577–8.

74 Pollock MA, Sturrock A, Marshall K, et al. Thyroxine treatment in patients with symptoms of hypothyroidism but thyroid function tests within the reference range: randomised double blind placebo controlled cross-over trial. *BMJ* 2001; **323**: 891–5.

75 Razvi S, McMillan CV, Weaver JU. Instruments used in measuring symptoms, health status and quality of life in hypothyroidism: a systematic qualitative review. *Clin Endocrinol* 2005; **63**: 617–24.

76 Watt T, Groenvold M, Rasmussen AK, et al. Quality of life in patients with benign thyroid disorders: a review. *Eur J Endocrinol* 2006; **154**: 501–10.

77 McMillan C, Bradley C, Razvi S, Weaver J. Psychometric evaluation of a new questionnaire measuring treatment satisfaction in hypothyroidism: the ThyTSQ. *Value Health* 2006; **9** (2): 132–9.

78 Toft AD. Thyroxine therapy. *N Engl J Med* 1994; **331** (3): 174–80.

79 Oppenheimer JH, Braverman LE, Toft A, Jackson IM, Ladenson PW. A therapeutic controversy: thyroid hormone treatment: when and what? *J Clin Endocrinol Metab* 1995; **80** (10): 2873–6.

80 Singer PA, Cooper DS, Levy EG, et al. Treatment guidelines for patients with hyperthyroidism and hypothyroidism. *JAMA* 1995; **273**: 808–12.

81 HAS–ANAES (Haute Autorité de la Santé–Agence Nationale d'Accréditation et d'Evaluation en Santé). Recommendations: diagnostic et surveillance biologique de l'hypothyroïdie de l'adulte, Janvier 1998. Available from www.has-sante.fr/portail/upload/docs/application/pdf/Hypothyr.pdf

82 Woeber KA. Update on the management of hyperthyroidism and hypothyroidism. *Arch Fam Med* 2000; **9**: 743–7.

83 Zimmerman RS. What is the target TSH level in thyroid hormone replacement for primary hypothyroidism. *Cleve Clin J Med* 2003; **70** (4): 329–30.

84 EBM Guidelines: laboratory testing of thyroid function. 5 April 2004. Available from www.terveysportti.fi/pls/ebmg/.

85 PRODIGY Guidance. Hypothyroidism. Available from www.prodigy.nhs.uk/hypothyroidism (last revised in February 2005).

86 Wartofsky L, Dickey RA. The evidence of a narrower thyrotropin reference range is compelling. *J Clin Endocrinol Metab* 2005; **90**: 5483–8.

87 Surks MI, Goswami G, Daniels GH. The thyrotropin reference range should remain unchanged. *J Clin Endocrinol Metab* 2005; **90**: 5489–96.

88 Roos A, Linn-Rasker SP, van Domburg RT, Tijssen JP, Berghout A. The starting dose of levothyroxine in primary hypothyroidism treatment. *Arch Int Med* 2005; **165** (15): 1714–20.

89 Wartofsky L. Levothyroxine therapy for hypothyroidism: should we abandon conservative dosage titration? *Arch Intern Med* 2005; **165**: 1683–4.

90 Landis SE, Collins LJ. How should thyroid replacement be initiated? *J Fam Pract* 2004; **53** (11): 4.

91 Hrytsiuk I, Gilbert R, Logan S, Pindoria S, Brook CG. Starting dose of levothyroxine for the treatment of congenital hypothyroidism: a systematic review. *Arch Pediatr Adolesc Med* 2002; **156** (5): 485–91.

92 Alexander EK, Marqusee E, Lawrence J, Jarolim P, Fischer GA, Larsen PR. Timing and magnitude of increases in levothyroxine requirements during pregnancy in women with hypothyroidism. *N Engl J Med* 2004; **351**: 241–9.

93 Arafah BM. Increased need for thyroxine in women with hypothyroidism during estrogen therapy. *N Engl J Med* 2001; **344**: 1743–9.

94 Meier CA, Burger AG. Effects of drugs and other substances on thyroid hormone synthesis and metabolism. In: Braverman LE, Utiger RD (eds), *Werner and Ingbar's The Thyroid: A Fundamental and Clinical Text*, 8th edn. Philadelphia: JB Lippincott-Raven, 2000, pp. 265–80.

95 Crilly M, Esmail A. randomised controlled trial of a hypothyroid educational booklet to improve thyroxine adherence. *Br J Gen Pract* 2005; **55**: 362–8.

96 Weetman AP. Whose thyroid hormone replacement is it anyway? *Clin Endocrinol* 2006; **64** (3): 231–3.

97 Ismail AA, Walker PL, Barth JH, Lewandowski KC, Jones R, Burr WA. Wrong biochemistry results: two case reports and observational study in 5310 patients on potentially misleading thyroid-stimulating hormone and gonadotropin immunoassay results. *Clin Chem* 2002; **48**: 2023–9.

98 Skeie S, Thue G, Sandberg S. Use and interpretation of Hb_{A1c} testing in general practice. Implications for quality of care. *Scand J Clin Lab Invest* 2000; **60**: 349–56.

99 Skeie S, Nordin G, Oosterhuis WP, et al. Post-analytical external quality assurance of blood glucose and Hb_{A1c}: an international survey. *Clin Chem* 2005; **51** (7): 1145–53.

100 Kilpatrick ES. Can addition of interpretative comments to laboratory reports influence outcome? An example involving patients taking thyroxine. *Ann Clin Biochem* 2004; **41**: 227–9.

101 Leese GP, Jung RT, Guthrie C, Waugh N, Browning MC. Morbidity in patients on L-thyroxine: a comparison of those with a normal TSH to those with a suppressed TSH. *Clin Endocrinol* 1992; **37** (8): 500–3.

102 Sawin CT, Geller A, Wolf PA, et al. Low serum thyrotropin concentrations as a risk factor for atrial fibrillation in older persons. *N Engl J Med* 1994; **331** (10): 1249–52.

103 Tanis BC, Westendorp GJ, Smelt HM. Effect of thyroid substitution on hypercholesterolaemia in patients with subclinical hypothyroidism: a reanalysis of intervention studies. *Clin Endocrinol (Oxf)* 1996; **44** (6): 643–9.

CHAPTER 20

Monitoring in renal transplantation

Nicholas B. Cross, Jonathan Craig

Renal transplantation is the best treatment for patients whose kidneys have failed and who would otherwise face a lifetime of dialysis treatment or death from end-stage kidney disease. Compared with dialysis, renal transplantation confers improved survival [1] and quality of life [2] and is less costly [3]. The demand for kidneys suitable for transplantation exceeds supply by about three times, and so long-term graft survival for patients who have been transplanted is a major goal of post-transplant care.

Graft survival depends on non-immunological and immunological factors. Because the recipient's immune system recognizes a transplanted kidney as foreign (unless the donor is genetically identical to the recipient), immunosuppressant drugs are used to prevent immune-mediated recognition and damage (rejection). These drugs are very effective. A kidney transplant recipient has about a 90% chance of having a functioning transplant 1 year after operation. The corresponding figure at 5 years is about 80% [4, 5].

Patients are typically well enough to be discharged home within 7 days of transplantation and are then monitored closely as out-patients. The monitoring interval during this immediate post-transplant phase is very short, and patients return for clinical examination and laboratory testing as often as daily. They may also be asked to self-monitor certain variables at home, such as temperature, weight, blood pressure and urine output. Other tests (radiology, histopathology) are also used. As time passes, the frequency of observations reduces, depending on clinical progress, including the perceived risk of adverse events, graft function and co-morbidities. Monitoring of the patient and graft function continues until the graft is lost or the patient dies, typically over decades of follow-up.

Evidence-based Medical Monitoring: from Principles to Practice. Edited by Paul Glasziou, Les Irwig and Jeffrey K. Aronson. © 2008 Blackwell Publishing, ISBN: 978-1-4051-5399-7.

20.1. Why might we monitor?

The primary aim of monitoring renal transplant recipients is the detection of renal dysfunction or the development of other complications in the recipient, such as infection, allowing timely interventions to improve outcomes [6].

Additional reasons for monitoring include the opportunity for patient education, adjustment of drug doses based on blood concentration or kidney function and reinforcement of the need to take the immunosuppressive drugs as prescribed to minimize the risk of rejection and infection.

Kidney transplant recipients are monitored extensively. In an 85-page guideline on kidney transplant surveillance published in 2000, monitoring of 36 separate conditions and targets was recommended in all transplant recipients [6]. However, there are few data to support these recommendations, and most conditions do not fulfil the criteria for monitoring described in other chapters. Instead, the implicit basis for most monitoring is the high value placed on a functioning kidney transplant, by the recipient, the clinicians and society at large, together with a high risk of complications, such as catastrophic infection and rejection.

In these guidelines and in routine clinical practice, disease consequences are given the most weight when considering what and when to monitor. The decision to monitor transplant recipients is usually made because a condition is common, iatrogenic or devastating. Less consideration is given to other important criteria for monitoring, such as the ability of the tests to detect real changes against the background of measurement variability, and the availability of interventions to treat adverse changes detected by monitoring. For example, renal transplant recipients develop osteoporosis through exposure to steroids on a background of altered bone metabolism due to previous chronic renal insufficiency; this leads to an increased risk of fracture. Monitoring for bone disease is recommended in guidelines from the USA [6] and Europe [7], including specific recommendations about which test and testing interval in the US guidelines (bone densitometry is recommended at the time of transplantation, 6 months later, and every 12 months if abnormal), even though there is no evidence that any intervention can prevent fractures in renal transplant recipients [8]. Recommendations for monitoring are based on extrapolation from the effects of treatments on a surrogate outcome (i.e. bone densitometry), a test whose performance in predicting the clinical outcome (i.e. fractures) in transplant patients is uncertain, and from the use of treatments that are of proven benefit in other patients (postmenopausal osteoporosis) but may be ineffective in transplant recipients because of different pathophysiology [9].

There are many conditions for which monitoring is undertaken, but here we shall restrict ourselves to the monitoring of kidney graft function. The maintenance of a well-functioning graft is the primary aim of transplantation, because it is the major determinant of patient survival and quality of life. Monitoring of transplant function also serves as a good example of the way

Table 20.1 Important causes of reduction in renal graft function, with respect to monitoring

Cause	Time to graft loss after transplantation	Proportion of all transplants affected	Natural history from inception to graft loss	Treatment available	Probability of graft loss with treatment
Vascular thrombosis [10, 11]	Hours to less than 30 days	1.9%	Minutes to hours	Yes	~100%
Acute rejection	Days to months	15–30% [12–14]	Days to weeks	Yes	~15%[4]
Systemic infections	Days to years	3.5% per annum [15]	Hours to days	Yes	~35%[16]
BK virus nephropathy	Weeks to months	5–10%	Weeks to months	Experimental	Up to 70% [17]
Chronic allograft nephropathy	Months to years	Ubiquitous eventually [18]	Months to years	No	Accounts for 50% of all grafts lost per annum

in which the interaction of disease, test and patient factors determines the appropriate monitoring test and schedule.

20.2. Causes of reduced transplant function

Baseline transplant function varies between individuals. This is partly predictable, based on donor and pre-transplantation factors, such as donor age and pre-existing diseases such as hypertension. For each individual an approximate baseline level of function is established over a series of sequential measurements. Monitoring is then undertaken to detect changes in test results that reflect changes in renal function. When a change greater than the range of the normal within-patient variability is detected, a cause is sought. Any cause of renal insufficiency may reduce function in the transplanted kidney, but in the post-transplant patient specific causes need to be considered (Table 20.1) [4, 10–18].

For monitoring of renal function to be useful in detecting the occurrence of a complication after transplantation, the complication must
- be detectable by changes in renal function,
- be treatable once detected,
- have better outcomes when detected and treated earlier than would be possible without monitoring,
- have a natural history such that detection is possible with a feasible monitoring interval,
- be sufficiently common and/or severe to warrant the expense and inconvenience to the patient of monitoring.

There are many causes of graft dysfunction, including vascular thrombosis (which typically occurs very early—at hours to days), acute rejection (early—days to months) and chronic allograft nephropathy (late—months to years). The relation between likely causes of graft dysfunction, effectiveness of treatment and time frame from transplant is explored in Figure 20.1.

20.2.1. Acute rejection
Monitoring for acute rejection using measures of renal function fulfils these criteria. Acute rejection occurs in 20–40% of transplant recipients, particularly in the early phase (days to months) after transplantation, and if untreated leads to graft loss. It leads to a reduction in renal function that occurs over days, is detectable with frequent (daily) blood tests and presents with clinical signs and symptoms only very late when treatment is relatively ineffective, but if detected by routine monitoring is generally treatable [4].

20.2.2. Calcineurin inhibitor toxicity
Monitoring renal function is also useful for the detection of acute drug toxicity, particularly from calcineurin inhibitors. The calcineurin inhibitors include ciclosporin and tacrolimus and are used as part of immunosuppressive regimens for most renal transplant recipients. They have dose-related adverse effects, including renal dysfunction. While the concentration of each drug is

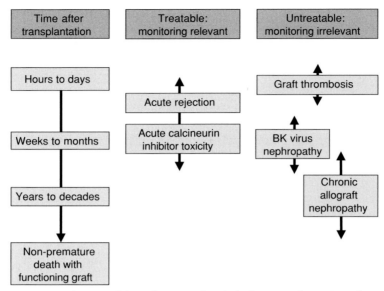

Figure 20.1 How the treatability of causes of graft dysfunction determines the monitoring strategy.

also commonly monitored, reversible renal dysfunction due to toxicity can develop despite drug concentrations in the usual target range. This can occur in the absence of any other symptoms or signs of overdose and can then only be diagnosed after exclusion of rejection.

20.2.3. Vascular thrombosis

Vascular thrombosis is not amenable to monitoring using measures of renal function. It is an uncommon cause of graft damage, but is catastrophic if it occurs. There are case reports of retrieval of thrombosed grafts by urgent surgical or percutaneous intervention [19], but most are rapidly and irreversible damaged [20]. The extreme rapidity of the natural history makes monitoring by any intermittent observation impractical, and surgery to remove the clot ineffective because secondary ischaemic damage to the kidney is untreatable.

20.2.4. Serious bacterial infections

Serious bacterial infections are common in renal transplant recipients and often lead to reversible reduction in renal function. However, infection usually leads to symptoms before the occurrence of reduced renal function. Therefore, monitoring or self-monitoring of symptoms is likely to be more effective at detecting this complication than monitoring renal function per se.

20.2.5. Chronic allograft nephropathy

Monitoring measures of renal function for detecting chronic allograft nephropathy is feasible but only useful for prognostic information because of a lack of effective treatments.

In summary, when considering the merits of monitoring renal function after transplantation with respect to disease characteristics, it is predominantly the detection of dysfunction due to acute rejection (and calcineurin inhibitor drugs in conjunction with drug concentration monitoring) that should guide decisions about the choice of test and monitoring strategy.

20.3. Tests of kidney function

Renal excretory function can be expressed in terms of the glomerular filtration rate (GFR), measured as volume per unit time (ml/min). The filtrate is the fluid component of plasma that appears in the bladder as urine, after processing by the kidney. GFR is proportional to the size of an individual, and is therefore often corrected for body surface area in order to improve comparability between individuals. This is not necessary for intra-individual comparisons (monitoring), when surface area is more or less constant. Several tests are used to estimate GFR. GFR is reduced in acute and chronic kidney diseases, and the degree to which it is reduced is a measure of the severity of the kidney disease.

20.3.1. Measured GFR

The gold standard for measuring GFR had been inulin clearance, although for practical reasons this has been supplanted by the use of radioisotope-labelled compounds (e.g. ^{51}Cr-EDTA, ^{99m}Tc-DTPA or ^{125}I-iothalamate) or x-ray contrast media (iothalamate, iohexal). Such compounds pass from the kidneys at a rate proportional to GFR. After administration of a standard dose, GFR can be calculated by measuring the change in concentration or radioactivity from timed samples of plasma and/or urine.

20.3.2. Serum creatinine concentration and estimated GFR

While measurements of exogenously administered substances (such as inulin or radioisotopes) are both accurate and precise (see below), they are expensive and time-consuming. Therefore, concentrations of endogenously produced molecules that are excreted by the kidney are more commonly used to estimate renal function, but obviously rely on the assumption of a fixed rate of production, which is only approximately true. The serum creatinine concentration is the most commonly used measurement. It is available in all biochemistry laboratories and can be measured rapidly using automated techniques.

Skeletal muscle liberates creatinine continuously and at a constant rate in health. A small proportion of circulating creatinine is derived from dietary sources (animal protein). It is freely filtered at the glomerulus, but a small proportion of total excretion occurs by tubular secretion; thus, any measure of creatinine excretion systematically overestimates GFR slightly. This is proportionally more important as GFR falls. The concentration of creatinine in the peripheral blood is therefore inversely related to kidney function.

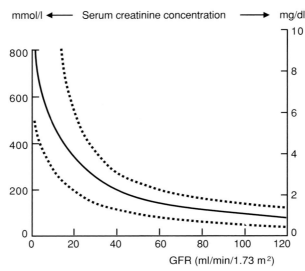

Figure 20.2 Relation of serum creatinine concentration to measured GFR; the solid line represents the mean data and the dotted lines the extremes. GFR was measured as the renal clearance of ^{125}I-iothalamate and serum creatinine concentration by a kinetic alkaline picrate assay. (Adapted from [22], with the permission of the American College of Physicians, which is not responsible for the accuracy of the representation.)

Production of creatinine from muscle is proportional to muscle bulk, which varies greatly between individuals. Age, sex, ethnicity and body mass predict muscle bulk and can be used to estimate GFR (eGFR) after measurement of serum creatinine. Several equations use such anthropomorphic data to provide an estimate of GFR. The most commonly used ones were developed in healthy normal individuals (Cockcroft and Gault equation [21], initially developed to estimate creatinine clearance) and in American patients with renal insufficiency (Modification of Diet in Renal Disease (MDRD) equations [22]).

The rate of removal of serum creatinine for a given degree of renal function depends on its concentration in plasma, so the relation between serum creatinine and underlying renal function (GFR) is not linear (Figure 20.2). This has important implications for its use as a monitoring test. In patients with lower (more normal) creatinine concentrations, a small fall in renal function can lead to a change in serum creatinine that is imperceptible from background sources of variability. The signal produced (the change in creatinine concentration) from any given change in renal function is smaller at more normal creatinine concentrations. This phenomenon also leads to poorer precision of equations for estimating GFR from serum creatinine at more normal degrees of renal function, with more variability and less agreement with measured GFR

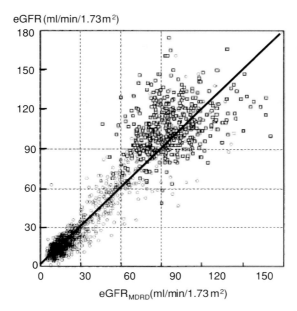

eGFR (ml/min/1.73m²)

eGFR$_{MDRD}$(ml/min/1.73 m²)

Figure 20.3 Association of eGFR using the MDRD equation with inulin-measured GFR (iGFR) in out-patients with chronic kidney disease (circles) and potential kidney donors (squares); dotted lines subclassify GFR on the basis of Kidney Disease Outcomes Quality Initiative stages. eGFR is plotted on the horizontal axis and iGFR is plotted on the vertical axis. (Reproduced with permission from [23].)

(Figure 20.3) [23]. As a result, any laboratories that report eGFR are encouraged not to report an absolute value when the eGFR is greater than 60 ml/min (about half normal) [24]. For short-interval monitoring, when the relevant comparison is not with the healthy population but to a prior measurement in an individual, anthropometric variables are unlikely to be helpful. The use of estimating equations can therefore only introduce a source of error and cannot provide any advantage over the use of serum creatinine alone.

To avoid introducing bias when monitoring using serum creatinine, or eGFR based on creatinine, the same method of laboratory analysis (and the same equation) should be used each time. The ability of eGFR to estimate measured GFR is not as good when the method for measuring creatinine differs from that used in the original studies from which the equation was derived [25]. The practical implication of this is that when monitoring patients, it is important whenever possible to use the same laboratory for every measurement. When comparing results from two different laboratories, any observed difference may be due at least in part to variability in sample handling, processing and reporting. Laboratories should also communicate clearly with clinicians when they change their methods, and report the likely effect of such changes.

Table 20.2 Tests of renal function and factors affecting their use in monitoring renal transplant function

Method of measuring renal function	Serum creatinine	eGFR (four-variable MDRD estimate)	Measured GFR (using exogenous compounds such as iohexol)
Validity (effectiveness of treatment after change in test due to acute rejection)	High	High	High
Coefficient of variation (intra-individual over days to weeks)	4.3%	4.3%	5.6%
Responsiveness to change in function	Low to moderate; better at higher serum creatinine concentrations (lower creatinine clearances)	Low to moderate; better at higher creatinine concentrations (lower values of eGFR)	High
Patient acceptability	High	High	Low
Special resource use	Nil	Nil	High
Cost	Minimal	Minimal	High (about US$136) [22]

20.4. Application of tests for monitoring renal transplant function

20.4.1. Serum creatinine concentration monitoring

In the immediate post-transplant period, testing must occur several times per week, because of the rapid natural history of the target condition (acute rejection). The serum creatinine concentration is the most appropriate measure—it is easy to perform, inexpensive, reliable for short-interval observations, acceptable to patients and not resource intense. It also has low intra-individual and analytical variability (Table 20.2), making it desirable as a monitoring test [26, 27].

Serum creatinine concentration measurement is not a perfect monitoring test. There is a poor signal-to-noise ratio at normal concentrations for detecting small degrees of change in GFR. Low-grade rejection can lead to a small reduction in function that is not translated into a rise in serum creatinine. However, if acute rejection occurs soon after transplantation, the change in renal function is usually dramatic and sudden, yielding detectable changes in serum creatinine from baseline.

20.4.2. Monitoring by renal biopsy

The reference standard test for acute rejection is renal biopsy. This is usually only performed once rejection is suspected on the basis of a change in renal function, because there are important differential diagnoses and treatment varies depending on the type and severity of rejection. In other words, a diagnosis of acute rejection is generally made in the presence of reduced renal function and typical biopsy appearances. However, histological changes associated with acute rejection can occur in the absence of changes in renal function. The presence of histological features of rejection without a rise in baseline serum creatinine is termed subclinical rejection. Whether this represents undiagnosed disease with consequences for long-term outcomes or overdiagnosis of clinically unimportant mild disease is unclear. There is uncertainty whether subclinical rejection leads to poorer graft outcomes; some studies suggest that there is a correlation [28], while others have shown no association [29].

There is some evidence that monitoring for and treatment of subclinical rejection improves outcomes, although this has been limited to only one randomized controlled trial in 72 patients [30]. The patients were randomized to receive biopsies at 1, 2, 3, 6 and 12 months, and were treated for histological changes of rejection irrespective of serum creatinine if seen on biopsies taken after 1–3 months (intervention arm) or to receive biopsies at 6 and 12 months only without any additional treatment (control arm). The primary outcome was the degree of chronic scarring seen on the 6 and 12 month biopsy specimens, which correlates positively with the risk of impaired graft function later [28]. More severe degrees of chronic scarring (a surrogate that predicts early graft loss) were seen in 24% of the control group compared with 6% of the treatment group ($P = 0.04$). The mean serum creatinine concentration at 24 months after transplantation was 133 µmol/l in the treatment arm and 183 µmol/l in the control arm ($P < 0.05$). However, while this was a randomized study, it had several flaws, including: important baseline differences in the groups, favouring the protocol biopsy group; unclear allocation concealment; and non-intention-to-treat analysis. Such design and conduct faults may have led to an overestimate of the real intervention effect.

Rejection is a condition with a wide spectrum of severity, varying from subclinical to hyperacute (leading to almost immediate graft loss). An appropriate monitoring test should detect a spectrum of disease that confers a prognostic disadvantage, but be treatable. Subclinical rejection, detectable by biopsy, is reversible, but mild rejection, which does not progress or damage the kidney significantly, may be overdetected.

While there are uncertain benefits for detecting subclinical rejection, there are also potential harms. In the randomized trial of protocol biopsies and treatment of subclinical rejection [30], there was a trend to an increased incidence

Table 20.3 Non-analytical causes of variability in serum creatinine concentration in transplant recipients

	Cause	Example
Inter-individual		
Renal function	GFR	Lower in older donors
	Tubular excretion	Increased in African Americans
Creatinine production	Muscle mass	Lower in women, with age
	Race	Higher in African Americans
	Chronic illness	Lower in patients with cirrhosis, heart failure, cancer
Intra-individual		
Renal function	GFR	Acute rejection
	Tubular excretion	Trimethoprim
Creatinine production	Muscle mass	Steroid-induced muscle wasting
	Diet	Animal protein → creatinine↑

of pneumonia in the treatment arm, with eight episodes compared with three in the control arm ($P = 0.11$), which may have been caused by increased exposure to immunosuppressive drugs in the treatment arm. There are also risks associated with the biopsy procedure. In addition, the frequency of testing required to detect a significant number of episodes of acute rejection early in their course, given the time course of days to weeks, is such that routine histological examination is not feasible [31].

20.4.3. Monitoring measured GFR

While measurement of GFR is too cumbersome and expensive for the very frequent monitoring required in the early post-transplant period, it may be preferable to serum creatinine concentration in the longer term. The test performance characteristics depend on the compound used and the analysis technique. The combined intra-individual and analytical variability of serum creatinine concentration is low, with a combined coefficient of variation of around 4–7% [32, 33]. Because of the non-renal determinants of the serum creatinine concentration (Table 20.3), intra-individual variability in serum creatinine increases with increasing intervals between observations, leading to increasingly poor sensitivity to changes in underlying GFR. An individual may have a serum creatinine concentration that remains relatively stable over years, while measured GFR changes substantially [34]. Over years of long-term follow-up rather than weeks in the early monitoring phase, non-renal determinants of serum creatinine concentration, such as age and weight, can be expected to change. The tempo of the target conditions is slow, and less frequent monitoring (1–2 times per year) is sufficient, overcoming some of the problems of inconvenience and resource intensity associated with measuring GFR.

However, the lack of effective treatments for the major diseases that cause changes in GFR over the months to years after renal transplantation, such as chronic allograft nephropathy (Figure 20.1), make detection of changes in renal function less important at this late stage.

20.4.4. Monitoring estimated GFR

How eGFR, based on transformations of serum creatinine, fits into monitoring is unclear. In the short term, the other determinants of eGFR (e.g. weight and age using the Cockcroft and Gault formula [21], and age alone with the MDRD formula [22]) are constant. Thus, any imprecision or bias in serum creatinine concentration measurement will be reflected to the same degree in the eGFR. Changes in eGFR cannot more accurately reflect changes in renal function than the measure on which any change is based (the serum creatinine concentration).

Over the longer term, eGFR might be expected to have some advantage over serum creatinine concentration alone, because changes in non-renal determinants of serum creatinine, such as age and weight, are adjusted for. However, changes in a number of other non-GFR determinants of serum creatinine that are not taken into account in eGFR equations will also affect the relation (e.g. drug changes, efficacy of tubular secretion of creatinine). Data on the performance of estimation equations in long-term monitoring of renal transplant recipients is sparse. In one study of 81 patients in whom 45 had iohexol and serum creatinine data to 21 months post-transplant, the slope of the reduction in GFR described by eGFR was greater than that of the reference method. By the iohexol GFR measure, the mean rate of reduction was 3 ml/min/yr, and various equations estimated a 5.0–7.4 ml/min/yr reduction in eGFR. This was due to more significant overestimation of eGFR in the early post-transplant period, leading to a more pronounced slope when later estimates were less biased. It may be that this was due to a change in muscle bulk in these patients with time, as they were all taking part in a trial of corticosteroid withdrawal [35]. The monitoring performance of serum creatinine alone was not reported.

The relative uses of each of three methods of monitoring renal function following transplantation are summarized in Table 20.2.

In conclusion, the best schedule at any given stage for monitoring graft function after transplantation depends on a number of factors and may be different between individuals and in different settings. Monitoring in the early transplant period needs to be frequent, and therefore simple and rapid, with less stress on detecting subtle change in function; in this case the serum creatinine concentration is the appropriate measure. However, with time, the test performance of the serum creatinine concentration is likely to decline because of increasing intra-individual variability and therefore a worsening signal-to-noise ratio. In addition, subtle changes in function over a longer time frame are the pattern for diseases that affect the graft. Thus, infrequent measures with better performance, albeit resource intense and inconvenient, such as measurement of GFR by iohexol, might be more appropriate if treatments for such conditions are developed. The role of eGFR based on serum creatinine concentration measurement for monitoring of renal transplant function is ill defined.

20.5. Future research

Given that acute rejection occurs in up to one-third of patients, research is needed to change the way that monitoring of renal transplantation occurs.

20.5.1. Graphical display/control charts

Control charts (see Chapter 7) have not previously been used in the monitoring of renal transplant recipients, although the frequency of serum creatinine concentration measurement and low intra-individual variability would make this technique appropriate. Whether this would lead to improvements in clinical outcomes is unclear, although this should be explored.

20.5.2. Randomized controlled trial data of the efficacy of treatment (including treatment of subclinical rejection)

A major weakness of monitoring strategies that are promoted for renal transplant recipients is the lack of evidence of improved outcomes with treatment of abnormalities detected with the tests, and more trials are required in many areas. For example, BK virus nephropathy can occur after transplantation, leading to a high risk of progressive graft dysfunction and early graft loss. Viral replication is detectable in the blood. Almost all patients with BK nephropathy have detectable viral replication, but not all patients with viral replication have BK nephropathy. There are drugs with in vitro activity against BK virus, and treatment might be contemplated for patients with histological evidence of BK nephropathy or for all patients with BK viraemia. Treatment can consist of antiviral drugs and/or a reduction in immunosuppressive drugs. Both treatments are potentially hazardous. Reduced immunosuppression can lead to rejection, and available treatments have important adverse effects, including renal toxicity. Randomized controlled trials with clinically important outcomes (graft and patient survival) are lacking for both strategies [36].

20.5.3. Improved renal function monitoring tests or strategies to detect the risk of rejection at an even earlier phase

When there is evidence that an intervention is beneficial, the methods used to define the disease need to be specified, and equivalent tests should be used in clinical practice. Using a different test will potentially cause misclassification and reduce the overall benefit of the intervention [37]. This is especially important when treatments are toxic. If a new test is more sensitive without improvement in specificity, more patients will be falsely classified as having the disease and will be exposed to the adverse effects of the intervention. This could lead to overall reduced net benefit, in which case the harms may even outweigh the benefits.

A potential change in disease definition is important when deciding to select a different test for monitoring changes in renal function as a method of detecting acute rejection. For example, consider the treatment of subclinical rejection (histological evidence of rejection without a change in renal function) with increased immunosuppression. These patients may either represent earlier detected cases of acute rejection (if we waited long enough, their renal function would have deteriorated), mild self-limiting cases that would resolve without intervention or a distinct 'slow grumbling' rejection that may or may not lead to insidious long-term consequences (such as chronic allograft nephropathy) without causing acute changes in renal function that may or may not be amenable to treatments available. Applying an established but toxic treatment for acute rejection may or may not lead to benefits for this group. Further randomized trials of the strategy of performing protocol biopsies and of the treatments in patients identified are required before this approach can be recommended. Using a more sensitive test for change in renal function than monitoring with serum creatinine, without any improvement in specificity would lead to more false positives (patients with lesser degrees of dysfunction previously ignored and patients without dysfunction) being selected for treatment. We would then require evidence, preferably from randomized controlled trials, that patients selected using this test benefit from treatment of their rejection, taking potential harms into account. For example, for eGFR to displace serum creatinine for monitoring for acute rejection in renal transplant recipients, we need evidence that classification as diseased (rejection) by eGFR improves outcomes with established treatment.

20.5.4. Development of specific new tests for individual diseases

Another important approach is to develop new tests for the specific diseases (acute rejection, chronic allograft nephropathy), rather than relying on monitoring the organ dysfunction and then applying secondary diagnostic tests to define the cause. This approach could allow earlier recognition of causes of perturbation (even before they caused graft dysfunction) and allow earlier treatment. For example, chronic allograft nephropathy can currently only be diagnosed once it has caused irreversible pathological changes. Ideally, for early treatments to be developed and tested, a test needs to be developed to allow detection of this disease before it reaches the advanced stage at which it can be detected using renal function monitoring. With respect to acute rejection, being able to detect this condition before renal dysfunction develops in patients who were going to develop dysfunction (i.e. the same spectrum of disease currently treated with benefit) might allow less intense treatment to be used to prevent rejection. This could reduce many of the adverse effects that transplant recipients experience from chronic immunosuppression.

20.6. Conclusions

There is extensive use of monitoring after renal transplantation, most of which has been established historically without clear evidence of benefit for the patient. Monitoring serum creatinine as an estimate of kidney function for detection of acute rejection is associated with good outcomes for most patients, at least in the short term. The natural history of acute rejection and the favourable features of serum creatinine testing (e.g. speed, low cost, low intra-individual variability) overcome the test's shortcomings (e.g. a poorer signal-to-noise ratio at more normal kidney function).

New monitoring strategies need to be assessed using randomized controlled trials when the spectrum of disease is altered by the use of the new test.

Acknowledgements

We gratefully acknowledge the financial support of the National Health and Medical Research Council of Australia (Program Grant no. 402764 and Postgraduate Research Scholarship no. 402981). With thanks to Rita Horvath, Peter Bunting, Les Irwig and Siobhan Cross for reviewing the manuscript.

References

1 Wolfe RA, Ashby VB, Milford EL, et al. Comparison of mortality in all patients on dialysis, patients on dialysis awaiting transplantation, and recipients of a first cadaveric transplant. *N Engl J Med* 1999; **341**: 1725–30.
2 Overbeck I, Bartels M, Decker O, Harms J, Hauss J, Fangmann J. Changes in quality of life after renal transplantation. *Transplant Proc* 2005; **37**: 1618–21.
3 De Wit GA, Ramsteijn PG, de Charro FT. Economic evaluation of end stage renal disease treatment. *Health Policy* 1998; **44**: 215–32.
4 Chadban S, McDonald SP, Excel LR, Livingston BE, Shtangey V. Transplantation. In: McDonald SP, Excel LR (eds), *ANZDATA Registry Report 2005*. Adelaide: Australia and New Zealand Dialysis and Transplant Registry, 2005, Chapter 8, pp. 103–24.
5 Kasiske BL, Gaston RS, Gourishankar S, et al. Long-term deterioration of kidney allograft function. *Am J Transplant* 2005; **5**: 1405–14.
6 Kasiske BL, Vazquez MA, Harmon WE, et al. Recommendations for the outpatient surveillance of renal transplant recipients. *J Am Soc Nephrol* 2000; **11**(Suppl 15): S1–86.
7 EBPG Expert Group on Renal Transplantation. European best practice guidelines for renal transplantation. Section IV: Long-term management of the transplant recipient. IV.1. Organization of follow-up of transplant patients after the first year. *Nephrol Dial Transplant* 2002; **17**(Suppl 4): 3–4.
8 almer SC, Strippoli GFM, McGregor DO. Interventions for preventing bone disease in kidney transplant recipients: a systematic review of randomized controlled trials. *Am J Kidney Dis* 2005; **45**: 638–49.
9 Cunningham J, Sprague SM, Cannata-Andia J, et al.; Osteoporosis Work Group. Osteoporosis in chronic kidney disease. *Am J Kidney Dis* 2004; **43**: 566–71.

10 Penny MJ, Nankivell BJ, Disney AP, Byth K, Chapman JR. Renal graft thrombosis. A survey of 134 consecutive cases. *Transplantation* 1994; **58**: 565–9.

11 Humar A, Key N, Ramcharan T, Payne WD, Sutherland DE, Matas AJ. Kidney retransplants after initial graft loss to vascular thrombosis. *Clin Transplant* 2001; **15**: 6–10.

12 Meier-Kriesche HU, Li S, Gruessner RW, et al. Immunosuppression: evolution in practice and trends, 1994–2004. *Am J Transplant* 2006; **6** (5 Part 2): 1111–31.

13 Loucaidou M, McLean AG, Cairns TD, et al. Five-year results of kidney transplantation under tacrolimus-based regimes: the persisting significance of vascular rejection. *Transplantation* 2003; **76**: 1120–3.

14 Hariharan S, Johnson CP, Bresnahan BA, Taranto SE, McIntosh MJ, Stablein D. Improved graft survival after renal transplantation in the United States, 1988 to 1996. *N Engl J Med* 2000; **342**: 605–12.

15 Abbott KC, Oliver JD, III, Hypolite I, et al. Hospitalizations for bacterial septicemia after renal transplantation in the United States. *Am J Nephrol* 2001; **21**: 120–7.

16 Miemois-Foley J, Paunio M, Lyytikainen O, Salmela K. Bacteremia among kidney transplant recipients: a case-control study of risk factors and short-term outcomes. *Scand J Infect Dis* 2000; **32**: 69–73.

17 Brennan DC, Agha I, Bohl DL, et al. Incidence of BK with tacrolimus versus cyclosporine and impact of preemptive immunosuppression reduction. *Am J Transplantation* 2005; **5**: 582–94. Erratum 2005; **5** (4 Pt 1): 839.

18 Nankivell BJ, Borrows RJ, Fung CL, O'Connell PJ, Allen RD, Chapman JR. The natural history of chronic allograft nephropathy. *N Engl J Med* 2003; **349**: 2326–33.

19 Rouviere O, Berger P, Beziat C, et al. Acute thrombosis of renal transplant artery: graft salvage by means of intra-arterial fibrinolysis. *Transplantation* 2002; **73**: 403–9.

20 Englesbe MJ, Punch JD, Armstrong DR, Arenas JD, Sung RS, Magee JC. Single-center study of technical graft loss in 714 consecutive renal transplants. *Transplantation* 2004; **78**: 623–6.

21 Cockcroft DW, Gault MH. Prediction of creatinine clearance from serum creatinine. *Nephron* 1976; **16**: 31–41.

22 Levey AS, Bosch JP, Lewis JB, Greene T, Rogers N, Roth D. A more accurate method to estimate glomerular filtration rate from serum creatinine: a new prediction equation. Modification of Diet in Renal Disease Study Group. *Ann Intern Med* 1999; **130**: 461–70.

23 Poggio ED, Wang X, Greene T, Van Lente F, Hall PM. Performance of the modification of diet in renal disease and Cockcroft–Gault equations in the estimation of GFR in health and in chronic kidney disease. *J Am Soc Nephrol* 2005; **16**: 459–66.

24 Myers GL, Miller WG, Coresh J, et al.; National Kidney Disease Education Program Laboratory Working Group. Recommendations for improving serum creatinine measurement: a report from the laboratory working group of the National Kidney Disease Education Program. *Clin Chem* 2006; **52**: 5–18.

25 Coresh J, Astor BC, McQuillan G, et al. Calibration and random variation of the serum creatinine assay as critical elements of using equations to estimate glomerular filtration rate. *Am J Kidney Dis* 2002; **39**: 920–9.

26 Rosano TG, Brown HH. Analytical and biological variability of serum creatinine and creatinine clearance: implications for clinical interpretation. *Clin Chem* 1982; **28**: 2330–1.

27 Keevil BG, Kilpatrick ES, Nichols SP, Maylor PW. Biological variation of cystatin C: implications for the assessment of glomerular filtration rate. *Clin Chem* 1998; **44**: 1535–9.

28 Nickerson P, Jeffery J, Gough J, et al. Identification of clinical and histopathologic risk factors for diminished renal function 2 years posttransplant. *J Am Soc Nephrol* 1998; **9**: 482–7.

29 Nankivell BJ, Fenton-Lee CA, Kuypers DR, et al. Effect of histological damage on long-term kidney transplant outcome. *Transplantation* 2001; **71**: 515–23.

30 Rush D, Nickerson P, Gough J, et al. Beneficial effects of treatment of early subclinical rejection: a randomized study. *J Am Soc Nephrol* 1998; **9**: 2129–34.

31 Ponticelli C, Banfi G. The case against protocol kidney biopsies. *Transplant Proc* 2002; **34**: 1716–8.

32 Levey AS, Greene T, Schluchter MD, et al. Glomerular filtration rate measurements in clinical trials. Modification of Diet in Renal Disease Study Group and the Diabetes Control and Complications Trial Research Group. *J Am Soc Nephrol* 1993; **4**: 1159–71.

33 Gaspari F, Perico N, Remuzzi G. Application of newer clearance techniques for the determination of glomerular filtration rate. *Curr Opin Nephrol Hypertens* 1998; **7**: 675–80.

34 Chapman JR, O'Connell PJ, Nankivell BJ. Chronic renal allograft dysfunction. *J Am Soc Nephrol* 2005; **16**: 3015–26.

35 Gaspari F, Ferrari S, Stucchi N, et al.; MY.S.S. Study Investigators. Performance of different prediction equations for estimating renal function in kidney transplantation. *Am J Transplant* 2004; **4**: 1826–35.

36 Hariharan S. BK virus nephritis after renal transplantation. *Kidney Int* 2006; **69**: 655–62.

37 Lord SJ, Irwig L, Simes RJ. When is measuring sensitivity and specificity sufficient to evaluate a diagnostic test, and when do we need randomized trials? *Ann Intern Med* 2006; **144**: 850–5.

CHAPTER 21
Monitoring in pre-eclampsia

Pisake Lumbiganon, Malinee Laopaiboon

Eclampsia is a potentially fatal complication of pregnancy characterized by convulsions. It is preceded by pre-eclampsia, which is defined as hypertension and proteinuria detected for the first time in the second half of pregnancy (after 20 weeks gestation). Monitoring for pre-eclampsia is a major element of antenatal checks [1].

During normal pregnancy, the blood pressure remains relatively stable in the first trimester, falls by about 5–10 mmHg in the second trimester and returns to pre-pregnancy values by term. Hypertension in pregnancy is usually defined as a systolic blood pressure of at least 140 mmHg and/or a diastolic blood pressure of at least 90 mmHg. It is no longer thought that a *change* in blood pressure is more important than the absolute blood pressure because there is no evidence that it is related to outcomes [2].

Changes in kidney function occur in healthy pregnancy and there is increased protein excretion in the third trimester. In pregnancy, excretion of up to 300 mg protein in the urine in 24 hours is considered normal. Proteinuria during pregnancy is therefore defined as the urinary protein excretion of 300 mg/d or more. In a single midstream urine sample, this usually correlates with a concentration of 30 mg/dl, or 1+ or more on a dipstick, or a spot urine protein/creatinine ratio of at least 30 mg/mmol [2].

Pre-eclampsia is considered severe in the presence of one or more of the following criteria [3]:

1 a systolic blood pressure of 160 mmHg or higher or a diastolic blood pressure of 110 mmHg or higher on two occasions, at least 6 hours apart during bed rest;
2 proteinuria of 5 g or more in a 24-hour urine specimen or 3+ or greater on two random urine samples collected at least 4 hours apart;
3 oliguria, with a urine output of less than 500 ml in 24 hours;
4 cerebral or visual disturbances;
5 pulmonary oedema or cyanosis;
6 epigastric or right upper quadrant pain;
7 impaired liver function;

Evidence-based Medical Monitoring: from Principles to Practice. Edited by Paul Glasziou, Les Irwig and Jeffrey K. Aronson. © 2008 Blackwell Publishing, ISBN: 978-1-4051-5399-7.

8 thrombocytopaenia;
9 foetal growth restriction.

21.1. Pathophysiology of pre-eclampsia

Pre-eclampsia is the result of an initial placental trigger and a maternal systemic reaction that produces the clinical signs and symptoms [4]. It occurs only in the presence of a placenta. It is associated with the failure of the normal invasion of trophoblast cells, leading to maladaptation of maternal spiral arterioles [5]. It can also be associated with hyperplacentation disorders, such as diabetes, hydatidiform mole, hydrops foetalis and multiple pregnancies. Aberration of the interaction between placental and maternal tissue is probably the primary cause, but the exact differences from normal pregnancy are still unclear [6]. Inadequate blood supply to the placenta leads to the release of unknown factors or materials into the maternal circulation, which activate or injure endothelial cells, resulting in endothelial dysfunction [7]. Perfusion to all organs decreases because of intense vasospasm secondary to increased sensitivity of the vasculature to pressor agents. Perfusion is further compromised by activation of the coagulation cascade, and especially platelets, with attendant formation of microthrombi. Plasma volume is reduced by loss of fluid from the intravascular space, further compromising organ blood flow [6]. Epidemiological studies have shown that the cause of pre-eclampsia is at least partly genetic. A single pre-eclampsia gene is unlikely; there are probably several modifier genes along with environmental factors [8].

21.2. Epidemiology of pre-eclampsia

About 2–3% of all pregnant women (5–7% of nulliparae) develop pre-eclampsia, of whom 1.9% develop eclampsia. Thus, 1,500,000–8,000,000 women will develop pre-eclampsia worldwide per year and up to 150,000 of them will have eclampsia [9]. Over 90% of the most serious cases of maternal and foetal morbidity and mortality occur in developing countries [9]. Pre-eclampsia is currently the leading cause of maternal death in Latin America and the Caribbean (26%) and the second leading cause of maternal death (16%) after other direct causes in developed countries [10]. Perinatal mortality is also increased after pre-eclampsia, mainly because of utero-placental insufficiency and pre-term births [11]. Factors that are associated with an increased risk of pre-eclampsia include [12]

- a first pregnancy,
- pre-eclampsia in a previous pregnancy,
- 10 or more years since the previous pregnancy,
- age 40 years or over,
- a body mass index of 35 or more at booking in,
- a family history of pre-eclampsia (especially in the mother or sister),
- a diastolic blood pressure of 80 mmHg or higher at booking in,

- a multiple pregnancy,
- an underlying medical condition (chronic hypertension, renal disease, diabetes and the presence of antiphospholipid antibodies).

21.3. Screening for pre-eclampsia

Current routine screening for pre-eclampsia is based on measurement of blood pressure and urinalysis for proteinuria. However, these are not ideal, as both have considerable within-person variability and hence high false-positive and false-negative rates. Other potential screening and monitoring tests for pre-eclampsia include [13]:

- placental perfusion and vascular resistance dysfunction-related tests, for example mean blood pressure in the second trimester, 24-hour ambulatory blood pressure monitoring, Doppler ultrasound;
- foetoplacental unit endocrinology dysfunction-related tests, for example human chorionic gonadotropin, alpha-fetoprotein, estriol;
- renal dysfunction-related tests, for example serum uric acid, microalbuminuria, urinary calcium excretion;
- endothelial and oxidant stress dysfunction-related tests, for example platelet count, fibronectin, insulin resistance, placental growth factors.

However, a WHO systematic review of screening tests for pre-eclampsia showed that as of 2004 there was no clinically useful screening test that could predict the development of pre-eclampsia [13].

21.4. Treatment of pre-eclampsia

The objectives of management of women with pre-eclampsia are the safety of the mother and then the delivery of a mature neonate. The interventions and timing depend on the severity of the disease, foetal gestational age, and maternal and foetal status. Delivery is the ultimate cure for pre-eclampsia. Management includes monitoring by maternal and foetal assessments and treatments such as antiepileptic drugs, antihypertensive drugs, foetal management, delivery and follow-up [14].

Maternal assessment includes repeated blood pressure measurements, quantitative measurements of protein in urine, platelet counts, serum uric acid and liver function tests [14].

About 30% of patients with pre-eclampsia have placental insufficiency, leading to intrauterine growth restriction. Foetal assessment includes ultrasonographic evaluation of foetal growth and amniotic fluid, umbilical artery Doppler assessment and cardiotocography to evaluate foetal well-being. If gestational age is less than 34 weeks, glucocorticoids should be given to accelerate foetal lung maturity.

Patients with mild pre-eclampsia can be managed expectantly, but they should undergo elective induction of labour at or near term [15]. All patients with severe pre-eclampsia should be hospitalized. For severe pre-eclampsia in patients at gestational age of 34 weeks or over, delivery should be advised after stabilizing with magnesium sulphate with or without antihypertensive therapy as appropriate. The optimal timing for delivery of women with severe pre-eclampsia before 32–34 weeks is still controversial. It involves a balance between protecting the mother by ending the pregnancy versus maximizing foetal maturity by delaying delivery [12]. The management of these patients should be in tertiary care.

Intravenous magnesium sulphate reduces the risk of eclampsia by more than half in women with pre-eclampsia, and probably reduces the risk of maternal death. It does not improve the outcome in the baby in the short term. A quarter of women who receive magnesium sulphate have adverse effects, particularly flushing [16]. Cost-effectiveness analysis suggests that magnesium sulphate for pre-eclampsia costs less and prevents more eclampsia in countries with a low gross national income than those with a high gross national income [17]. The cost-effectiveness substantially improves if magnesium sulphate is used only for severe pre-eclampsia or if the purchase price is reduced in countries with a low gross national income [17].

If the blood pressure is above 170/110 mmHg, most obstetricians would use antihypertensive agents [18]. In mild pre-eclampsia, the role of antihypertensive therapy is less clear. A threshold of 150/100 mmHg should give a reasonable balance between the number of women treated and the benefit achieved [14].

21.5. **Monitoring schedules**

Measurements of blood pressure and urinary protein excretion are non-invasive and are routinely used in antenatal care. They are also commonly used as monitoring for pre-eclampsia in pregnant women of at least 20 weeks' gestation.

21.5.1. **Blood pressure**

For blood pressure measurement, the method should be properly standardized: the woman should be rested and reclining at an angle of 45°. The blood pressure cuff should be of an appropriate size (encircling at least 2/3 of the upper arm diameter) and placed at the level of the heart. The blood pressure should be measured with an auscultatory device, as oscillometric techniques systematically under-record during pregnancy; Korotkoff sound V is recommended for assessment of diastolic blood pressure [2]. Any rise in blood pressure should be confirmed by a second measurement, ideally at least 4–6 hours later. The value of ambulatory blood pressure recording in diagnosing pre-eclampsia has yet to be established [19].

Blood pressure measurement is non-invasive and inexpensive, and should be a good method for monitoring pre-eclampsia. However, there is difficulty in obtaining accurate blood pressure measurements. White coat hypertension is defined as a persistently raised clinic blood pressure with a normal blood pressure at other times [19]. It is more common if the patient is female and young, and may therefore be important in pregnancy [19]. Thus, a single blood pressure measurement may not be a reliable predictor of pre-eclampsia. Some investigators, aware of the random variation in normal blood pressure, have recommended several readings to confirm the diagnosis [14, 20, 21].

Biological and measurement variations are important sources of error in blood pressure determination. However, to date we have not found information on variations in blood pressure in pre-eclampsia. This information is needed for generating control charts in individual subjects and for estimating the number of repeated measurements required to confirm the validity of blood pressure measurement.

The optimal frequency of blood pressure measurement in pregnancy has not been established and is thus left to clinical discretion [22]. However, there is evidence in non-pregnant women that four measurements made at 1-minute intervals are needed to obtain a stable blood pressure [23]. This was confirmed in a later study of the variability in observed blood pressure between two measurements associated with use of the Dinamap PRO 100 in 60 volunteers, 30 aged 23–35 years and 30 aged 54–82 years [24]. The authors used the same interval of 1 minute between measurements. The results suggested that short-term biological variation in blood pressure is small compared with other sources of variability, and that the average of two or more measurements should be used.

Applying the methods described in earlier chapters, we require knowledge of (a) the within-person variability of blood pressure during pregnancy and (b) the rate of progression of increased blood pressure in pre-eclampsia. Currently this information is not available, so we still lack good evidence for recommending intervals for blood pressure measurement in monitoring pre-eclampsia.

21.5.2. Proteinuria

Repeated testing of urinary protein excretion gives differing results because of two major sources of random variation: biological and measurement variation.

The two sources of random variation can be expressed as coefficient of variations (CV). CV_w represents the within-individual biological variation and CV_m represents the measurement variation. The total random variation (CV_t) is calculated as the square root of ($CV_w^2 + CV_m^2$). The coefficients of variation, CV_w and CV_m, of many tests are available in the electronic database of biological variation [25]. CV_t can be used to calculate the dispersion of any test result at a determined probability limit when those results are normally distributed. For example, the dispersion of a test result at 95% probability of that test result is $\pm 1.96 \ [(CV_w^2 + CV_m^2)^{1/2}]$, and this accounts for total random variation in test results. The interval of test results is more useful for clinical decision-making [26].

We can calculate the total random variation in proteinuria. Given a CV_w of 36% and a CV_m of 18% for albumin in the first morning urine specimen, taken from the databases of biological variation values [25], the dispersion of random

Table 21.1 95% dispersion intervals of proteinuria

Protein result (mg/24 h)	Dispersion value (%)	Interval (mg/24 h)
250	198 (79)	52,448
300	237 (79)	63,537
350	277 (79)	73,627

variation for an individual with any degree of proteinuria is $\pm 1.96[(36^2 + 18^2)^{1/2}]$, which is $\pm 79\%$. If, for example, individual proteinuria is 250, 300 and 350 mg/24 h, the 95% dispersion intervals can be estimated as shown in Table 21.1.

Random variation in proteinuria makes the diagnosis of pre-eclampsia problematic. This is because proteinuria has very high values of CV_w (36%) and CV_m (18%). These lead to very wide 95% dispersion intervals. The lower limit, 63 mg/24 h, of the threshold of 300 mg/d is too sensitive and not appropriate to make a diagnosis of proteinuria.

Thus, the technique of accounting for random variation in proteinuria for monitoring pre-eclampsia, although desirable, is not feasible in practice, and more reliable tests are needed. Random variation is usually less for measurement in serum than in the urine. For example, the CV_w (3.1%) and CV_m (1.6%) for serum albumin are much lower than for urine albumin, which are 36% and 18% respectively [25]. The very high random variation in proteinuria measurement makes the use of control charts in individual patients inappropriate. In addition, 24-hour proteinuria measurement is time-consuming and may not be practical.

Theoretically, the number of repeated measurements of proteinuria undertaken to make the dispersion small enough to allow good decision-making in pre-eclampsia can be estimated from the formula [26]

$$n = \left[\frac{Z(CV_w^2 + CV_m^2)^{1/2}}{D} \right]^2$$

where n is the required number of measurements to get $D\%$ precision of estimated mean values of proteinuria and Z represents the standard coefficient of the normal distribution at a determined level of probability. The formula assumes a single analysis of each measurement. If we wanted to achieve 10% precision of estimated means of proteinuria with 95% probability, we should have to repeat about 62 measurements in each pregnant woman. This is unrealistic, and we must therefore work with more measurement variation than is ideal.

The single threshold of proteinuria of 300 mg/24 h is also widely used without scientific evidence. Proteinuria does not satisfy any one of the four criteria for good monitoring tests, as described in Chapter 2. Therefore, current methods for measuring proteinuria might not be useful in monitoring pre-eclampsia. However, we still do not have anything better.

Table 21.2 Intra-individual variability assessed by the median coefficient of variation for urinary albumin measures in samples frozen at -20°C*

| | Median coefficient of variation (%) | | | | | |
| | Albumin concentration $\geq$10 g/l | | Albumin excretion <30 mg/d and albumin concentration $\geq$10 g/l | | Albumin excretion 30–299 mg/d | |
Urinary measures	Men	Women	Men	Women	Men	Women
Albumin concentration	26	28	25	26	42	78
24-h albumin excretion	28	31	28	29	39	78
Albumin:creatinine ratio	28	31	27	30	39	81

Note: *Adapted from Table 3 of [28].

21.5.3. Protein:creatinine ratio and albumin:creatinine ratio

Although 24-hour urinary protein measurement may not be particularly useful in monitoring pre-eclampsia, it is nevertheless looked on as a gold standard. However, 24-hour urine collection is usually difficult in most subjects. A simpler alternative for the patient is to use the protein:creatinine ratio to adjust for hydration status.

In a systematic review in which the protein:creatinine ratio was compared with 24-hour protein excretion, the authors concluded that the protein:creatinine ratio measured in a random urine specimen provides evidence to rule out the presence of significant proteinuria, as defined by 24-hour urinary excretion [27]. A comparison of albumin:creatinine ratio and urinary albumin concentration with 24-hour urinary albumin excretion in 4678 participants from four countries showed that both are acceptable alternatives to measuring the 24-hour urinary albumin excretion and that the simpler urinary albumin concentration may be preferable to the albumin:creatinine ratio because of its simplicity and smaller within-person coefficients of variation, as shown in Table 21.2 [28].

However, this conclusion was not supported by Gansevoort et al. [29], because fresh urine should be used instead of urine stored at -20°C, which increases the variability in albumin concentration. Moreover, specifically collected urine samples and not a portion of a 24-hour urine sample should be used. They therefore proposed that there is still a need for a carefully designed prospective study to clarify this issue. A more recent study showed that a random measurement of the albumin:creatinine ratio is not stable during the day and cannot predict 24-hour urinary protein excretion accurately [30].

In conclusion, we still do not have enough evidence to support the use of the protein:creatinine ratio or albumin:creatinine ratio to detect proteinuria in women with pre-eclampsia. However, since the available information suggests that the protein:creatinine ratio is less variable than 24-hour urinary protein excretion, the protein:creatinine ratio might be a better monitoring test. A well-planned study is urgently needed to answer this very important clinical question.

21.6. Response to treatment and maintenance schedule

If it is decided to continue the pregnancy, maternal and foetal evaluations are required. Frequent blood pressure monitoring is essential. Unfortunately, there is no evidence on which to base guidelines on how often blood pressure should be measured. It has been suggested that platelet count, liver enzymes, renal function and a 24-hour urine collection for protein should be repeated weekly or sooner if disease progression is questionable [3].

The two main goals in managing patients with pre-eclampsia during labour and delivery are prevention of eclampsia and control of hypertension. Blood pressure and proteinuria should be monitored very closely, although there is still insufficient information to recommend how closely.

Patients who received magnesium sulphate should be monitored for adverse effects, including effects on respiratory rate, hourly urine output and deep tendon reflexes.

Although delivery is the definitive treatment for pre-eclampsia, the condition persists for some time after delivery and most maternal deaths occur in the post-partum period [31]. Most post-natal eclampsia occurs within the first 24 hours after delivery. Magnesium sulphate is usually continued for 24 hours after delivery. Patients should also be closely monitored in this period.

21.7. Organization of care

Hospitalization is usually recommended for women with newly diagnosed pre-eclampsia. After maternal and foetal evaluation, subsequent management could be continued in the hospital, at a day-care unit or at home depending on the severity of the disease and patient adherence [3]. Ambulatory management is an option for mild pre-eclampsia in women who are remote from term. If this is selected, it should include frequent maternal and foetal evaluation and access to care providers [3]. Women with severe pre-eclampsia are best managed in tertiary care by experienced obstetricians [3].

21.8. Conclusions

There is a need for well-designed studies to obtain biological and measurement variations in blood pressure in pre-eclampsia. This will allow us to generate control charts for blood pressure monitoring. We also need information about when and how often blood pressure should be taken to diagnose hypertension correctly. Uterine artery blood flow and biochemical markers of oxidative stress and endothelial dysfunction are potentially good candidates for screening [32]. Further studies are also needed to establish accurate screening tests.

References

1 Gifford RW, Jr, August PA, Cunningham G, et al. Report of the National High Blood Pressure Education Program Working Group on High Blood Pressure in Pregnancy. *Am J Obstet Gynecol* 2000; **183**: S1–S22.

2 Brown MA, Lindheimer MD, De Swiet M, Van Assche A, Moutquin JM. The classification and diagnosis of the hypertensive disorders of pregnancy: statement from the International Society for the Study of Hypertension in Pregnancy (ISSHP). *Hypertens Pregnancy* 2001; **20**: ix–xiv.

3 ACOG Practice Bulletin No.33. Diagnosis and management of pre-eclampsia and eclampsia. *Obstet Gynecol* 2002; **99**: 159–67.

4 Redman CW, Sacks GP, Sargent IL. Pre-eclampsia: an excessive maternal inflammatory response to pregnancy. *Am J Obstet Gynecol* 1999; **180**: 499–506.

5 Meekins JW, Pijnenborg R, Hanssens M, McFadyen IR, van Asshe A. A study of placental bed spiral arteries and trophoblast invasion in normal and severe pre-eclamptic pregnancies. *Br J Obstet Gynaecol* 1994; **101**: 669–74.

6 Roberts JM, Cooper DW. Pathogenesis and genetics of pre-eclampsia. *Lancet* 2001; **357**: 53–6.

7 Roberts JM, Lain KY. Recent insights into the pathogenesis of pre-eclampsia. *Placenta* 2002; **23**: 359–72.

8 Broughton Pipkin F. What is the place of genetics in the pathogenesis of pre-eclampsia? *Biol Neonat* 1999; **76**: 325–30.

9 Critchley H, MacLean A, Poston L, Walker J. *Pre-Eclampsia*. London: RCOG Press, 2003.

10 Khan KS, Wojdyla D, Say L, Gulmezoglu AM, Van Look PF. WHO analysis of causes of maternal death: a systematic review. *Lancet* 2006; **367**: 1066–74.

11 Department of Health, Scottish Executive Health Department, and Department of Health, Social Services, Public Safety. Northern Ireland. *Why Mothers Die. The Sixth Report on Confidential Enquiries into Maternal Deaths in the United Kingdom 2000–2002*. London: RCOG Press, 2001.

12 Duley L, Meher S, Abalos E. Management of pre-eclampsia. *BMJ* 2006; **332**: 463–8.

13 Conde-Agudelo A, Villar J, Lindheimer M. World Health Organization systematic review of screening tests for pre-eclampsia. *Obstet Gynecol* 2004; **104**: 1367–91.

14 Walker JJ. Pre-eclampsia. *Lancet* 2000; **356**: 1260–5.

15 Sibai BM. Diagnosis and management of gestational hypertension and pre-eclampsia. *Obstet Gynecol* 2003; **102**: 181–92.

16 Duley L, Gülmezoglu AM, Henderson-Smart DJ. Magnesium sulphate and other anticonvulsants for women with pre-eclampsia. In: *Cochrane Database Syst Rev* 2003; (2): CD000025.

17 Simon J, Gray A, Duley L; on behalf of the Magpie Trial Collaborative Group. Cost-effectiveness of prophylactic magnesium sulphate for 9996 women with pre-eclampsia from 33 countries: economic evaluation of the Magpie Trial. *BJOG* 2006; **113**: 144–51.

18 Brown MA, Whitworth JA. Management of hypertension in pregnancy. *Clin Exp Hypertens* 1999; **21**: 907–16.

19 Higgins JR, de Swiet M. Blood-pressure measurement and classification in pregnancy. *Lancet* 2001; **357**: 131–5.

20 Feldman DM. Blood pressure monitoring during pregnancy. *Blood Press Monit* 2001; **6**: 1–7.

21 Pickering TG. Reflections in hypertension. How should blood pressure be measured during pregnancy? *J Clin Hypertens* 2005; **7**: 46–9.

22 Beaulieu MD. Prevention of preeclampsia. In: *Canadian Task Force on the Periodic Health Examination. Canadian Guide to Clinical Preventive Health Care.* Ottawa: Health Canada, 1994, pp. 136–43.

23 Shimada N. Significance of short-term blood pressure variation in health management. *Nippon Koshu Eisei Zasshi* 1993; **40**: 9–16.

24 Chang JJ, Rabinowitz D, Shea S. Sources of variability in blood pressure measurement using the Dinamap PRO 100 automated oscillometric device. *Am J Epidemiol* 2003; **158**: 1218–26.

25 Ricós C, Vicente J, Lario G, et al. Biological variation database, and quality specifications for imprecision, bias and total error. The 2006 update. Available from http://www.westgard.com/guest32.htm.

26 Fraser CG. Test result variation and the quality of evidence-based clinical guidelines. *Clin Chim Acta* 2004; **346**: 19–24.

27 Price CP, Newall RG, Boyd JC. Use of protein:creatinine ratio measurements on random urine samples for prediction of significant proteinuria: a systematic review. *Clin Chem* 2005; **51**: 1577–86.

28 Dyer AR, Greenland P, Elliott P, et al.; INTERMAP Research Group. Evaluation of measures of urinary albumin excretion in epidemiological studies. *Am J Epidemiol* 2004; **160**: 1122–31.

29 Gansevoort RT, Brinkman J, Bakker SJ, de Jong PE, de Zeeuw D. Evaluation of measures for urinary albumin excretion. *Am J Epidemiol* 2006; **164**(8): 725–7.

30 Wikstrom A-K, Wikstrom J, Larsson A, Olovsson M. Random albumin/creatinine ratio for quantification of proteinuria in manifest pre-eclampsia. *BJOG* 2006; **113**: 930–4.

31 Department of Health. *Why Mothers Die. Report on Confidential Enquiries into Maternal Death in the United Kingdom 1994–96.* London: Stationery Office, 1999.

32 Parra M, Rodrigo R, Barja P, et al. Screening test for pre-eclampsia through assessment of uteroplacental blood flow and biochemical markers of oxidative stress and endothelial dysfunction. *Am J Obstet Gynecol* 2005; **193**: 1486–91.

CHAPTER 22

Monitoring in intensive care

Jan M. Binnekade, Patrick M.M. Bossuyt

In this chapter, we discuss the characteristics of monitoring in the intensive care unit (ICU). In other chapters, monitoring has been discussed in relation to a therapy for a single disease or disorder. By contrast, the majority of monitoring in an ICU focuses on generic physiological consequences (vital functions) and diseases that have precipitated severe illnesses. Monitoring is a large component of the work of an ICU, and clearer evidence about what forms of monitoring improve patient outcomes is of vital importance. An example is monitoring of pulmonary artery pressure using a Swan–Ganz catheter; this was once common, but now several randomized trials have shown that it has no impact on mortality [1].

New therapies, improved techniques and lower costs have caused a transition from occasional measurement to regular monitoring of a number of items. For example, selective decontamination of the digestive tract has altered the frequency of bacteriological culture, from clinical indications only to several times a week to monitor the effectiveness of selective decontamination.

Sometimes this process is reversed. Some accepted tests have no value when used repeatedly for monitoring purposes. An example is the now discarded daily chest x-ray; routine chest x-rays seldom show unexpected clinically relevant abnormalities and they rarely prompt action [2].

We shall briefly discuss the patients who benefit from an ICU admission. We shall then describe some principles of monitoring physiological variables, such as biosignals, blood chemistry, patient–machine interactions, the use of measurement scales, diagnostics and alarms. We shall finish by discussing in more detail monitoring problems during intensive insulin therapy in ICUs.

22.1. Serious illnesses and monitoring—a functional dependency

Intensive care has been defined as a service for patients with potentially recoverable conditions who can benefit from more detailed observation and invasive treatment [3]. Intensive care applies to all medical specialties, but its

Evidence-based Medical Monitoring: from Principles to Practice. Edited by Paul Glasziou, Les Irwig and Jeffrey K. Aronson. © 2008 Blackwell Publishing, ISBN: 978-1-4051-5399-7.

limitations largely define the categories of patients who will be admitted to an ICU. Indications for treatment (with examples) are

1 intensive monitoring while preparing aggressive interventions before surgery (open heart surgery) and after surgery, allowing abnormal physiology to reverse (postoperative cardiac surgery);

2 the need for very intensive nursing care (burns, trauma);

3 the need for control over physiology in order to prevent organ injury (neurosurgical critical care);

4 minimal physiological reserve with a risk of acute potentially reversible injury, requiring life support until abnormalities have been reversed and reserve restored (COPD with pneumonia requiring mechanical ventilation);

5 massive physiological disruption (stress response to injury or inadequate compensation to the response) due to major trauma or sepsis.

A common denominator is sudden deterioration in multiorgan systems' functions, with which an ICU is designed to cope and for which time critical decisions can be made. An ICU is equipped for and proficient in performing detailed observations of vital physiological functions. Derangements that provoke such monitoring can be found in the cardiovascular system, the respiratory system, renal function, the central nervous system, fluid and electrolyte balance, and blood gases.

22.2. What do we monitor in the ICU?

Monitoring activities in the ICU encompass a wide range of techniques. Extensive patient monitoring is necessary to manage life-threatening problems. Serious illnesses can involve single or multiple organ failure that threatens to spread to other organs. Monitoring in the ICU is used both to guide therapy and to keep a careful preventive watch over the functions of other threatened organs. This means that the number of frequently measured variables that are monitored in the ICU can easily add up to a few hundred.

Most conspicuous are the continuous bedside displays of biosignals derived from cardiac, respiratory and neurological variables. Blood samples are often taken and fluid balance is also monitored. Coded (ordinal) observations of consciousness, pain, skin colour and skin condition are all part of these monitoring activities. At the end of the monitoring spectrum are severity of illness scores and therapeutic intensity scores. Monitoring allows daily appraisal of the progress of sequential organ failure and therapeutic intervention scores.

22.2.1. Biosignals

Most monitoring efforts in the ICU are related to biosignals, either electrical signals detected by electrodes or chemicals or mechanical signals that are transformed into electrical form after being detected by sensors. The purpose of processing biosignals is to derive information about the source (the heart, the brain, the circulation, etc.). For this a biosignal has to be acquired, processed, computed and interpreted. The first two of these processes concern the syntax of the signal: maximization of the signal-to-noise ratio or, simply put, obtaining signals with the least possible disturbance. The concern of syntax is to digitize the signal and remove redundant data. This preprocessing stage reshapes the data in such a way that it becomes possible to read it. However, decisions can only be made after other variables have been added. If this signal represents the heart frequency, for example, these parameters will determine when the signal is flagged as a bradycardia or tachycardia.

22.2.2. Blood chemistry

The sampling frequency for whole blood chemistry depends on the timescale of changes, which is strongly influenced both by pathological conditions and by the intensity of treatment. Timescales vary. For example, O_2 and CO_2 can change in seconds, creatinine for evaluating kidney function changes in hours, and cholesterol in days [4]. Although a centralized laboratory that delivers data within hours or days may be satisfactory for most general wards, ICU physicians consider delivery times in excess of small fractions of hours unsatisfactory.

The time needed to process a sample was drastically reduced when point-of-care testing was introduced. In general, point-of-care testing reduces therapeutic turnaround time, the number of errors and blood volume lost for analyses. Point-of-care testing is a prerequisite for early recognition of life-threatening conditions and for titration of commonly used interventions. Point-of-care testing data must be integrated into the patient's medical record and institutional information systems. At present, point-of-care testing is a supplement, not a replacement for conventional laboratory services.

The tests that are most often needed in ICU are P_aO_2, P_aCO_2, pH and bicarbonate in arterial blood. With an additional sample from mixed venous blood, oxygen consumption can be calculated. Sodium, potassium and chloride can also change rapidly, owing to acid-base balance disturbances or when extensive derangements are treated. The effects of blood and plasma transfusions can be monitored much more effectively. Insulin therapy should be carefully monitored—insulin resistance in the critically ill requires frequent blood glucose measurements. Calcium and magnesium concentrations have become more usual in cardiac intensive care. Measures of renal function are obtained through a central laboratory, as are frequently tested coagulation parameters, such as prothrombin time and activated partial thromboplastin time [5].

22.3. Machines in the ICU

22.3.1. The interaction of patients and machines

ICU admissions are most often based on the necessity to support one or more organ systems. Mechanical ventilation is the most commonly used technique. This adds an extra dimension to monitoring: the patient–machine interaction. Adapted synchronized ventilation is a mode of mechanical ventilation that uses a closed-loop algorithm to determine and adjust ventilator settings. This technique can wean the patient from the ventilator by monitoring dynamic compliance and the expiratory time constant. Based on ideal body weight, other ventilator settings are automatically tuned. Since more sophisticated ventilation techniques (sensitive tuning) have become available, patients can comply with ventilation with little or no sedation for most of the time.

22.3.2. Monitoring alarms

Safety concerns in intensive therapy require each device to be equipped with extensive alarm systems, to alert staff to changes in the patient's condition or to equipment malfunction. The complexities of interventions require a different combination of devices for each patient. Each of these devices contributes to the overwhelming total of audio and visual alarms, placing a considerable demand on the alarm user. Many alarms are adjusted too loud ('better safe than sorry'), can become irritating, and lead to sleep deprivation and continuous stress for patients and nurses [6]. As a result, nurses may delay intervention, trying to recognize life-threatening alarms by sound only. Alarm sounds are often difficult to tell apart. The total number of alarms and confusion between devices with similar alarms have been associated with serious adverse events resulting in death of patients [7]. Even experienced nurses can recognize only 38% of vital alarms [8].

It is difficult for users of alarms to learn about and master the large number of alarms in an ICU. Psychological research has shown that our ability to remember pieces of unrelated information is limited to seven, plus or minus two, which includes different sounds [9]. People cannot remember large numbers of different alarm sounds. Standards have therefore been developed to reduce the number of alarms, and in particular alarm signals that are triggered by physiological functions rather than by equipment [10]. There is evidence that suggests that we should develop alarm sounds that are easy to localize, resistant to masking by other sounds and therefore not easily missed, that do not interfere with communication and that are easy to distinguish from other alarm sounds [8].

False-positive alarms are a common problem in the ICU, and only a small proportion of all alarms represent potentially life-threatening risk to the patient [6, 11, 12]. People tend to adjust their behaviour to high false-alarm rates—they do not respond to alarms or simply turn them off. Despite this, they usually set alarm limits conservatively, so that alarms sound without an immediate risk. Although high false-alarm rates reduce the value of monitoring they have become part of normal practice in ICUs.

22.4. Evidence-based monitoring

Evidence-based practice is defined as the conscientious, explicit and judicious use of current best evidence in decision-making. It customizes worker experience with the various forms of evidence to the specific problem under investigation [13].

ICU monitoring practice is seldom questioned. We mention two examples. The first is the use of daily routine chest x-rays. These seldom show unexpected, clinically relevant abnormalities, and rarely prompt action. There is no benefit from daily monitoring by chest radiography in patients on ICU undergoing mechanical ventilation [2].

The second example is continuous monitoring by pulmonary artery catheter, a device used to measure blood flow and pressures in blood vessels in the heart and lungs. These measurements are used to guide treatment of critically ill patients or patients undergoing major surgery. Pulmonary artery catheters were first used in ICUs about 30 years ago. Although, the pulmonary artery catheter allows physicians to describe the patient's clinical and haemodynamic status more accurately, it can also trigger the use of drugs that ultimately worsen outcomes. Several randomized trials have shown that there is no effect on mortality [1]. There is no clear evidence that using pulmonary artery catheters to guide treatment actually allows patients to recover faster, or that more of them survive their illness [14].

Like most other technologies used in ICUs, daily chest radiography and pulmonary artery catheters were widely disseminated without any rigorous evaluation as to whether they reduce mortality or the costs of care in these patients. We feel that one should make an effort to evaluate a specific monitoring practice, especially when there are large variations in practice and lack of evidence. Evaluation is not limited to the monitoring technique itself, but must also include the monitoring strategy (preferable accurately described in a protocol), definitions of action thresholds and the actions to be taken if any of the thresholds is reached (see Chapter 12).

22.5. Costs of monitoring

The provision of intensive care requires highly trained staff, expensive modern equipment and intensive use of diagnostic tests, pharmaceuticals and interventions. An ICU consumes about one-third of all hospital resources [15]. It is important to understand the costs of ICU treatment and its consequences.

A researcher who wants to investigate the cost-effectiveness of an ICU faces large problems. The study object, treatment of the complex ICU patient, involves dealing with multiple concurrent problems, for which often numerous interventions are used at the same time. Measuring the effectiveness of each of these interventions is difficult, because most ICU therapies are supportive and not directly related to outcomes.

Any effort to study cost-effectiveness in the ICU will also be frustrated by ubiquitous variations in care. There are large differences between ICU physicians in the amounts of resources used to manage critically ill patients in a single medical ICU [16]. For example, between ICUs the odds ratio for using pulmonary artery catheters varied by 200–400% across 34 ICUs, according to how the ICU was organized and staffed [17].

One of the rare examples of evaluation of the costs of monitoring in the ICU is a 'before and after' study of intensive glycaemic control in ICU, in which there were substantial savings due to reductions in all major categories of resource utilization [18].

Despite the substantial costs of intensive care, the number of cost-effectiveness analyses is small compared with other types of clinical interventions [15]. The cost-effectiveness of specific monitoring techniques, as well as that of continuous renal replacement therapy, goal-directed therapy for sepsis and 24-hour intensivist coverage, has not yet been evaluated [15]. Most economic studies of ICU costs also lack scientific rigour [19].

22.6. Intensive insulin therapy: glucose monitoring in the ICU

A substantial portion of modern day critical care practice is based on the principle of restoring aberrant respiratory, cardiovascular and other functions to physiological values. This principle creates the necessity to monitor a number of related physiological variables. An extension of this principle can be observed in the use of strict glycaemic control by monitoring and by balanced administration of insulin to prevent hyperglycaemic periods in the largely non-diabetic, critically ill population [20]. This example illustrates some general principles of monitoring in critical care.

22.6.1. Glucose metabolism

In healthy individuals without diabetes mellitus an increase in blood glucose concentration stimulates the release of insulin from the pancreas, which in turn mediates peripheral glucose disposal and suppresses gluconeogenesis to maintain blood glucose homoeostasis. Skeletal muscle is the major site of peripheral insulin-mediated glucose uptake. Key factors that regulate blood glucose concentration in healthy subjects are a combination of hormonal, neural and hepatic autoregulatory mechanisms.

22.6.2. Glucose metabolism in severely ill patients

Hyperglycaemia in critically ill patients without diabetes has traditionally been viewed as a mechanism for delivering enough glucose to the brain and other essential cells during times of stress. As a result, the prevailing practice has been to accept hyperglycaemia in non-diabetic patients as an adaptive response, the rationale being that regulation would not contribute to the overall outcome. However, the persistent hyperglycaemia experienced by patients without diabetes is now thought to be secondary to insulin resistance. It may therefore not be entirely beneficial or adaptive.

Critical illness induces a state of relative insulin resistance. It exists when the metabolic features of insulin deficiency (notably hyperglycaemia, increased lipolysis and protein catabolism) are observed in the presence of normal or raised concentrations of plasma insulin. Effective nutritional support can be compromised by insulin resistance in the critically ill patient because of the associated hyperglycaemia and the failure of feeding regimens to restore lean body mass [21].

22.6.3. Intensive insulin therapy: monitoring blood glucose concentration

Does normalizing physiological variation make an important clinical difference? In a randomized clinical trial in surgical patients in ICU with a blood glucose concentration over 6.1 mmol/l (110 mg/dl), tight regulation of the arterial blood glucose concentration with intensive insulin therapy towards a target of 4.4–6.1 mmol/l (80–110 mg/dl) reduced morbidity and mortality [20].

However, intensive insulin therapy is associated with a high risk of hypoglycaemia, defined as a blood glucose concentration that is insufficient to meet metabolic demands, which has potentially devastating effects on the brain and sometimes causes death [22]. Even moderate hypoglycaemia is associated with a significant stress response, behavioural changes and alterations in cerebral blood flow and metabolism [23]. Although hypoglycaemia is uncommon, in a retrospective ICU study 30 of 156 non-diabetic patients with documented hypoglycaemia were not given insulin [24].

It is difficult to define causal factors for hypoglycaemia in the ICU, and many inter-related factors play a part, including the use of bicarbonate-based substitution fluid during continuous venovenous haemofiltration, reduced nutrition without adjustment for insulin infusion, a prior diagnosis of diabetes mellitus, sepsis and inotropic support [24].

The key to preventing hypoglycaemia is frequent blood glucose testing. Intensive insulin therapy is associated with a sixfold increase in serious hypoglycaemia, and even with a less aggressive approach to glycaemic control and a less stringent glucose target (4.4–8.0 mmol/l; 80–144 mg/dl) rates of hypoglycaemia are comparable [20, 24]. Intensive insulin therapy depends on proper glucose monitoring and timely adjustment of insulin dosages. Considering the many uncontrollable factors, each patient presents a separate individual learning curve in arriving at controlled glucose concentrations.

22.6.4. Alternative options to monitoring blood glucose concentrations in the ICU

As in most other forms of physiological monitoring, there are several options in selecting a monitoring test. Improvements in techniques, device features and performance can now be observed within months. New point-of-care testing devices have a shorter marketing time than the time needed to perform proper evaluation studies. Although not discussed here, the reliability, accuracy and efficiency of these methods should be evaluated before choices are made.

22.6.4.1. Point-of-care-testing

Point-of-care testing can be carried out using a blood glucose meter on capillary blood obtained from a finger prick or on arterial blood obtained from an arterial catheter. However, the performance of bedside point-of-care testing is poor in critically ill patients. In a prospective evaluation of four different glucose meters, 62% of glucose measurements in intensive care wards were more than ±20% different from the laboratory reference [25]. The use of these meters would have resulted in significant errors in insulin dosages. In a comparison of glucose meter analysis of capillary blood, glucose meter analysis of arterial blood, and combined arterial blood gas and blood chemistry analysis, clinical agreement with the central laboratory was significantly better with arterial blood analysis (70% and 77% for glucose meter and blood gas/chemistry analysis respectively) than with capillary blood analysis (57%) [26]. During hypoglycaemia, clinical agreement was only 26% with capillary blood analysis and 56% and 65% for glucose meter and blood gas/chemistry analysis of arterial blood respectively. Glucose meter analysis of both arterial and capillary blood tended to give higher glucose readings, whereas arterial blood gas/chemistry analysis tended to give lower readings. However, despite this poor agreement between these different methods of glucose estimation, there are probably no differences in estimated glucose concentration when a single method is used in patients with different pathologies, clinical signs and/or treatments.

22.6.4.2. Central laboratory testing

In a central laboratory, blood samples are analysed outside the ICU. There is a glucose concentration difference of about 11% between plasma and whole blood, depending on the haematocrit of the sample, and the whole blood glucose concentration is lower than the plasma glucose concentration [27]. Many, but not all, whole blood methods of glucose measurement have their results factored to be in closer agreement with plasma methods.

22.6.4.3. Continuous measurement

Glucose can be measured continuously with a transcutaneous or needle glucose sensor [28], by near-infrared spectroscopy [29] or by microdialysis [30]. Microdialysis is based on sampling soluble molecules from the interstitial fluid by means of a semipermeable membrane at the tip of a probe. The probe's inflowing tubing is constantly perfused with a physiological solution at a rate of 1 μl/min. Samples are continuously collected from the outflow tube. In 20 patients in ICU after cardiac surgery, the mean arterial glucose concentration was 6.7 mmol/l and the absolute glucose concentration in the interstitial fluid measured by microdialysis was 3.55 mmol/l. The mean correlation coefficient between arterial and interstitial concentrations was 0.77 [31]. The usefulness of continuous monitoring techniques remains to be evaluated [32].

22.6.5. The use of a clinical algorithm

Although intensive care is to a great extent provided through routine practice, there is also an excess of information, which may exceed decision-making capabilities. During intensive therapy with insulin several decisions have to be made: the target glucose concentration range, the glucose sampling method, and the frequencies of sampling and of making adjustments to the insulin dosage. All of these steps will affect the results of glucose monitoring, as they interact with one another.

Since glucose control cannot be modelled as a simple cause-and-effect system, a clinical algorithm is necessary to avoid variation in the performance of glucose control by ICU nurses. Despite the fact that physiological variation in blood glucose concentration has been generally assumed to be linear, there appears to be a chaotic, non-linear, unpredictable component in the profiles of people with and without diabetes [33].

In the case of intensive insulin therapy the underlying problem can persist over a long period of time, shifting dynamically in response to complications and therapy, while numerous decisions (which can each turn out to be wrong) have to be made. Glucose monitoring during intensive insulin therapy requires increased mental effort. The interpretation of deviating glucose concentrations, relative to the current insulin dosage and the recent history of insulin dosage adjustments and glucose concentrations, requires a flexible interpretation of rules that are usually abstract. The mental effort required exceeds that of routine problem-solving [34].

Protocols prescribe actions by taking into account both the insulin dosage and the blood glucose concentration. Intensive insulin therapy is guided by the glucose concentration, the current dosage of insulin and the time it took to change from the previous glucose concentration to the current one. Formalization of this process aspires to improve calculability, predictability and overall control of the process [35].

22.6.6. Protocol elements related to glucose monitoring

Elements of intensive insulin therapy that should be covered in nurse-driven protocols include
- the clinical conditions associated with hyperglycaemia;
- the initial glucose concentration that triggered the intensive insulin therapy;
- the type and characteristics of the prescribed insulin;
- the target blood glucose concentration;
- the method of glucose measurement and its characteristics;
- the maximum dosage of insulin per unit time (before consulting the physician);
- the changes in dosage (ml/h) of insulin adapted to the glucose concentration;
- the frequency of glucose measurement as a function of the upward or downward trend of the glucose concentration and the latest absolute quantity;
- risk factors for hypoglycaemia incorporated into daily care (such as feeding patterns, changes in medication, changes in medical condition);

- reduction in the dose of insulin when stability is achieved;
- conditional decision rules for insulin dosage.

Most protocols have formulated additional rules for a number of exceptions, that is, when to notify the physician.

22.6.7. Monitoring ICU performance

Monitoring in the ICU also includes daily classification of patients and processes. Classification implies assigning patients to specific groups according to set criteria. The results are ranked expressions of sequential organ failure scores, severity of illness, probability of survival, therapeutic load and nursing workload. Such monitoring is used to predict mortality and to help allocate resources and staff. Trends can be detected in a timely manner and the quality of care can be monitored.

A summary measure of ICU performance is the standardized mortality ratio (SMR). ICU mortality depends on the severity of the illness. This mortality can be compared with the expected mortality, based on the severity of illness (Apache II) score and the diagnostic category. If the ICU mortality compares favourably with the SMR it performs better than average, but worse if mortality is higher. Other, more patient-oriented monitoring techniques are used to classify the depth of sedation to prevent over-sedation and to predict or recognize delirium.

22.7. Conclusions

A common feature in severely ill patients is the risk of deterioration in organ function. The primary purpose of monitoring physiology is to restore aberrant respiratory, cardiovascular and other functions to functional levels. Monitoring in the ICU relies on a range of techniques that vary from the automated processing of biosignals to the repeated classification of the therapeutic load and the nursing workload. Many of the challenges in monitoring in the ICU are well illustrated by the difficulties in monitoring intensive insulin therapy.

References

1 Shah MR, Hasselblad V, Stevenson LW, et al. Impact of the pulmonary artery catheter in critically ill patients: meta-analysis of randomized clinical trials. *JAMA* 2005; **294**: 1664–70.

2 Graat ME, Choi G, Wolthuis EK, et al. The clinical value of daily routine chest radiographs in a mixed medical-surgical intensive care unit is low. *Crit Care* 2006; **10**: R11.

3 Smith G, Nielsen M. ABC of intensive care. Criteria for admission. *BMJ* 1999; **318** (7197): 1544–7.

4 Tudos AJ, Besselink GA, Schasfoort RBM. Trends in miniaturized total analysis systems for point of care testing in clinical chemistry. *Lab Chip* 2001; **1**: 83–95.

5 Drenck NE. Point of care testing in critical care medicine: the clinician's view. *Clin Chim Acta* 2001; **307**: 3–7.

6 Chambrin MC, Ravaux P, Calvelo-Aros D, Jaborska A, Chopin C, Boniface B. Multicenter study of monitoring alarms in the adult intensive care unit (ICU): a descriptive analysis. *Int Care Med* 1999; **25**: 1360–6.

7 Edworthy J, Hellier E. Alarms and human behaviour: implications for medical alarms. *Br J Anaesth* 2006; **97**: 12–17.

8 Cropp AJ, Woods LA, Raney D, Bredle DL. Name that tone: the proliferation of alarms in the intensive care unit. *Chest* 1994; **105**: 1217–20.

9 Miller GA. The magical number seven, plus or minus two: some limits on our capacity for processing information. *Psychol Rev* 1957; **63**: 81–96.

10 Edworthy J, Hellier E. Fewer but better auditory alarms will improve patient safety. *Qual Saf Health Care* 2005; **14**: 212–5.

11 Tsien CL, Fackler JC. Poor prognosis for existing monitors in the intensive care unit. *Crit Care Med* 1997; **25**: 614–9.

12 Koski EM, Makivirta A, Sukuvaara T, Kari A. Frequency and reliability of alarms in the monitoring of cardiac postoperative patients. *Int J Clin Monit Comput* 1990; **7**: 129–33.

13 Sackett DL, Straus S, Richardson S, Rosenberg W, Haynes RB. Evidence-based medicine. *How to Practice and Teach EBM*, 2nd edn. London: Churchill Livingstone, 2000.

14 Harvey S, Young D, BramptonW, et al. Pulmonary artery catheters for adult patients in intensive care. *Cochrane Database Syst Rev* 2006; **3**: CD003408.

15 Talmor D, Shapiro N, Greenberg D, Stone PW, Neumann PJ. When is critical care medicine cost-effective? A systematic review of the cost-effectiveness literature. *Crit Care Med* 2006; **34**: 2738–47.

16 Garland A, Shaman Z, Baron J, Connors AF. Physician-attributable differences in intensive care unit costs. A single-center study. *Am J Respir Crit Care Med* 2006; **174**: 1206–10.

17 Rapoport J, Teres D, Steingrub J, Higgens T, McGee W, Lemenshow S. Patient characteristics and ICU organizational factors that influence frequency of pulmonary artery catheterization. *JAMA* 2000; **283**: 2559–67.

18 Krinsley JS, Jones RL. Cost analysis of intensive glycemic control in critically ill adult patients. *Chest* 2006; **129**; 644–50.

19 Heyland DK, Kernerman P, Gafni A, Cook DJ. Economic evaluations in the critical care literature: do they help us improve the efficiency of our unit? *Crit Care Med* 1996; **24**: 1591–8.

20 van den Berghe G, Wouters P, Weekers F, et al. Intensive insulin therapy in the critically ill patients. *N Engl J Med* 2001; **345**: 1359–67.

21 Carlson GL. Insulin resistance in sepsis. *Br J Surg* 2003; **90**: 259–60.

22 Cryer PE, Davis SN, Shamoon H. Hypoglycemia in diabetes. *Diabetes Care* 2003; **26**: 1902–11.

23 Sieber FE, Traystman RJ. Special issues: glucose and the brain. *Crit Care Med* 1992; **20**: 104–14.

24 Vriesendorp TM, van Santen S, deVries JH, et al. Predisposing factors for hypoglycemia in the intensive care unit. *Crit Care Med* 2006; **34**: 96–101.

25 Ting C, Nanji AA. Evaluation of the quality of bedside monitoring of the blood glucose level in a teaching hospital. *CMAJ* 1988; **138**: 23–6.

26 Kanji S, Buffie J, Hutton B, et al. Reliability of point of care testing for glucose measurement in critically ill adults. *Crit Care Med* 2005; **33**: 2778–85.

27 Nichols JH. A critical review of blood glucose testing. *Point Care* 2003; **2**: 49–61.

28 Goldberg PA, Siegel MD, Russell RR, et al. Experience with the continuous glucose monitoring system in a medical intensive care unit. *Diabetes Technol Ther* 2004; **6** (3): 339–47.

29 Maruo K, Oota T, Tsurugi M, et al. Noninvasive near-infrared blood glucose monitoring using a calibration model built by a numerical simulation method: trial application to patients in an intensive care unit. *Appl Spectrosc* 2006; **60** (12): 1423–31.

30 Muller M. Clinical review. Microdialysis. *BMJ* 2002; **324**: 588–91.

31 Kremen J, Blaha J, Matias M, et al. Monitoring of glucose concentration in critical patients, comparing arterial blood glucose concentrations and interstitial glucose concentration measured by microdialysis technique. *Vnitr Lek* 2006; **52** (9): 777–81.

32 Vogelzang M, Ligtenberg JJ. Practical aspects of implementing tight glucose control in the ICU. *Curr Opin Clin Nutr Metab Care* 2007; **10** (2): 178–80.

33 Kroll MH. Biological variation of glucose and insulin includes a deterministic chaotic component. *Biosystems* 1999; **50** (3): 189–201.

34 Reason J. *Human Error*. Cambridge: Cambridge University Press, 1994.

35 Eitel F, Kanz KG, Hortig E, Tesche A. Do we face a fourth paradigm shift in medicine—algorithms in education? *J Eval Clin Pract* 1999; **6**: 321–33.

CHAPTER 23

Monitoring intraocular pressure in glaucoma

Les Irwig, Paul R. Healey, Jefferson D'Assunção, Petra Macaskill

Glaucoma is a common chronic neurodegenerative disease [1]. It takes the form of a slowly progressive optic neuropathy, which causes visual field loss and eventually blindness. The most important modifiable risk factor for glaucoma is intraocular pressure: the prevalence, incidence, severity and progression rate of the disease all increase with increasing intraocular pressure [2, 3]. There is evidence from randomized trials that reducing intraocular pressure delays progression of visual field loss when the initial intraocular pressure is raised above the 95th percentile for the population, as well as when it is within the range considered normal, the so-called normal-tension glaucoma [4–7]. Therefore, the major focus of glaucoma management is reduction of intraocular pressure.

23.1. Potential measures, a causal schema and choosing measures

The pathway from intraocular pressure to visual field loss is shown in Figure 23.1. There are non-modifiable risk factors for glaucoma, such as age, family history and myopia [8–10]. The major modifiable risk factor is intraocular pressure, which can be lowered by drugs, laser trabeculoplasty or surgical drainage procedures. Methods of monitoring include late outcome measures of functional loss (visual fields) and structural loss (optic nerve head topography and retinal nerve fibre layer thickness) and measurement of the risk factor itself, intraocular pressure. It is important that there is currently no intermediate monitoring test between the early responsive changes in intraocular pressure and the late outcomes of structural and functional changes. The characteristics of these tests are summarized in Table 23.1 and described below.

Evidence-based Medical Monitoring: from Principles to Practice. Edited by Paul Glasziou, Les Irwig and Jeffrey K. Aronson. © 2008 Blackwell Publishing, ISBN: 978-1-4051-5399-7.

Table 23.1 Characteristics of possible monitoring tests in glaucoma

Measure	Clinical validity	Responsiveness	Signal-to-noise ratio	Practicality
Functional tests: visual field testing	**High: outcome of interest**	Low	Low	Moderate: subjective test—difficult for some patients
Structural tests: optic nerve and retinal nerve lplp thickness	Moderate: mechanism of visual field loss	Low	Low	High: objective and easy
Early biomarker: intraocular pressure	Moderate	**High**	**High**	**High: objective and easy**

Note: Bold entries mark the preferred choice in each column.

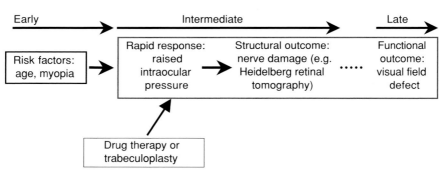

Figure 23.1 The pathophysiological pathway from intraocular pressure to visual field loss.

23.2. Visual field tests

Visual field loss is usually quantified using automated static perimetry, with statistical analysis of visual sensitivities for comparison with both the normal population and the patient's previous field test results. Visual field testing is essentially subjective, relying on the patient's ability to detect flashes of light of varying intensity throughout the visual fields. Although good algorithms have been developed to improve repeatability (e.g. the Humphrey Field Analyzer 24-2 SITA standard algorithm), from a monitoring perspective the test is intended to detect small changes that occur over a long period of time. Monitoring the outcome of treatment involves determining whether the rate of change differs from that which would have occurred in the absence of treatment, as discussed in Chapter 5 in relation to Figure 5.3. Because of the slow time-course of progression of visual field loss, the monitoring interval is set at 6–12 months in most countries. There is little research on the most appropriate monitoring schedule, given the relatively small expected change over time (the signal) and the measurement variability (the noise) [11]. As monitoring after the commencement of treatment relies heavily on the stability of the estimate of the pre-treatment value, it is best established using several measurements, which can be made over a few weeks or months [12, 13].

23.3. Tests of optic nerve head topography and retinal nerve fibre layer thickness

Several tests have been developed to assess the topography of the optic nerve head, such as Heidelberg retinal tomography (HRT) and retinal nerve fibre layer thickness, including scanning laser polarimetry (SLP) and optical coherence tomography (OCT). They are easier for patients and quicker to perform than visual field testing and provide good summary estimates of changes and the extent to which they may be due to measurement variability. However, structural change does not correlate well with functional change, making its clinical significance for vision loss unclear [14].

23.4. Intraocular pressure

Although measurement of intraocular pressure is the mainstay of the management of glaucoma, and although considerable reductions in intraocular pressure can be achieved in trials, the target intraocular pressure may not be reached during usual practice. Even using liberal criteria for adequate control, intraocular pressure has been reported to be controlled in only 66% of follow-up visits in patients with mild glaucoma and 52% of visits in patients with moderate to severe glaucoma [15].

Intraocular pressure changes rapidly in response to drugs. Immediate effects can be measured in hours and the effect of continuing treatment within days. However, there is considerable measurement variability. Sources of systematic variability include the instrument used, the operator, diurnal variation and the time elapsed since the last dose of medication. These can be minimized by standardization. The remaining random measurement variability (noise) is small in relation to the changes in intraocular pressure when treatment is first started (signal), but the noise may be large in relation to the signal of change in intraocular pressure in response to a change in treatment. Therefore, long-term management of the intraocular pressure is ideally suited to the use of control charts, which is the topic of the rest of this chapter.

In attempting to implement ideal practice, one of the difficulties faced by practitioners is identifying real deviations of intraocular pressure away from the target (the signal) against the background measurement variability in intraocular pressure (noise). Some measurement variability can be explained by diurnal variation or the time that has elapsed since the last dose of a drug. However, most of the variation is unexplained: even on a single occasion, measurements of intraocular pressure have a 50% chance of differing by as much as 2 mmHg and a 30% chance of differing by at least 3 mmHg [16].

   To help identify which test results are important and which reflect no more than measurement variability, we now demonstrate the use of one type of control chart for intraocular pressure (see Chapter 7).

23.4.1. A statistical process control chart for intraocular pressure

Statistical process control charts are usually constructed to determine whether measurements deviate from pre-existing values (see Chapter 7). However, an alternative way of constructing charts has been proposed for medical monitoring [17]. To illustrate the latter approach, intraocular pressure data from a man with normal-tension glaucoma at age 57 were used. Intraocular pressure measured at annual visits to an optometrist over the previous 12 years had been 15–17 mmHg in the right eye and 15–18 mmHg in the left eye. Later measurements tended to be higher. A control chart was constructed as follows:

- *Choosing a target.*   Based on randomized trial evidence and guidelines [6, 7, 18, 19], the target was set at 12 mmHg in both eyes.
- *Setting control limits.*   To reflect measurement variability, control limits are commonly set at 1 and 2 standard deviations (SDs) from the target. Few normative data are available, so we set control limits using Reichert (non-contact) tonometry repeated several times during office hours over 2 weeks of stable treatment. These data were asymmetrical (Figure 23.2), with a skew to the right. An Altman–Bland plot [20] showed that within-eye measurement variability increased as the mean intraocular pressure increased (Figure 23.3). We therefore set control limits based on percentiles rather than symmetrical SD-based limits.
- *Detecting real deviations from target.*   We identified deviations from target that were likely to be real rather than measurement variability broadly based on guides derived from statistical process control, that is, eight successive measurements on one side of the target, four successive measurements beyond the 16th or 84th percentile (equivalent to ±1 SD), and two successive measurements beyond the 2nd or 98th percentile (equivalent to ±2 SD) (see Chapter 7 for a discussion of these guides).

A similar sequence of steps was taken to develop a control chart for differences between the left and right eyes. The target pressure was replaced by the mean inter-eye difference on stable treatment (0.61 mmHg) and control limits reflected measurement variability between the eyes, based on SDs, as inter-eye differences were symmetrically distributed.

   The control charts shown in Figure 23.4 show the target or mean difference (solid straight lines), the control limit percentiles (dashed and dotted lines) and the pressure-lowering interventions used (noted at the top of the chart).

Percentage of patients

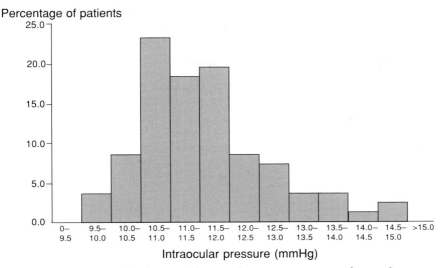

Intraocular pressure (mmHg)

Figure 23.2 Frequency distribution of intraocular pressures measured every few hours, between 0800 hours and 1800 hours over 2 weeks using non-contact tonometry (82 measurements pooled across both eyes).

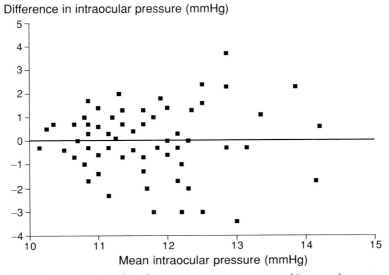

Mean intraocular pressure (mmHg)

Figure 23.3 Altman–Bland plot of successive measurements of intraocular pressure every few hours, between 0800 hours and 1800 hours over 2 weeks measured using non-contact (Reichert) tonometry; data for both eyes.

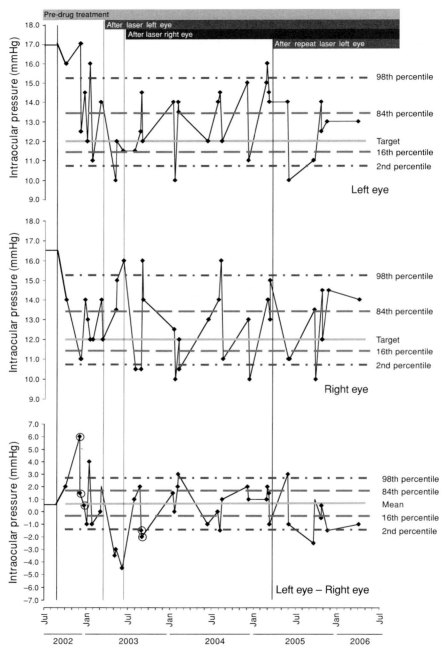

Figure 23.4 Control charts for intraocular pressure. Top panel: right eye; middle panel: left eye; bottom panel: inter-eye difference (left eye minus right eye); pre-treatment value based on the four most recent measurements before treatment.

Although the monitoring interval was never more than a few months, the exact interval was not fixed. Measurement was more frequent if previous results suggested that a change in management might be considered. Often, two measurements were taken within 1 week of each other to reduce measurement variability before a consultation at which a change in treatment was being considered. During treatment with latanoprost for the initial 6 months, most of the measurements were above target. After left selective laser trabeculoplasty, one intraocular pressure measurement was on target and two were below target, one of which was below the 16th percentile, suggesting a beneficial effect. The chart of inter-eye differences confirmed this, with three differences below the 16th percentile. After right selective laser trabeculoplasty, two successive measurements were below the 16th percentile. During the following year, the intraocular pressure in the right eye was reasonable, with five measurements above target, one on target and four below. In the left eye control was not as good, with six measurements above target, two on target and two below.

Over the next 6 months, the intraocular pressure increased, with four consecutive measurements above the 84th percentile in the left eye, and three of four measurements in the right eye. Selective laser trabeculoplasty was repeated on the left eye; three of the four subsequent measurements were below the 16th percentile and one was below the 2nd percentile. Measurements over the next 6 months were all above target, suggesting that this effect was not sustained. However, the inter-eye difference chart suggested some beneficial effect—six of the eight measurements were below the mean, of which five were below the 16th percentile.

The encircled points in the inter-eye display (Figure 23.4, bottom panel) show one-eyed masked trials of additional drugs, in the left eye in both cases. The first set of encircled points shows the ineffectiveness of adding dorzolamide: intraocular pressure was actually higher than in the untreated right eye, with one measurement above the 98th percentile. The second set of encircled points shows the benefit of adding brimonidine, with two successive measurements below the 2nd percentile.

23.4.2. Signal, noise and construction of control charts

There is considerable measurement variability in intraocular pressure. Against this background of measurement variability (noise), control charts provide a means to identifying true changes (signal). The data from this patient demonstrate their value in ensuring appropriate long-term reduction in intraocular pressure in the management of glaucoma. Control charts help avoid over- and under-interpretation. Over-interpretation occurs, for example, when a change in measurement is attributed to a change in treatment rather than to measurement variability. Under-interpretation occurs, for example, when a patient is assumed to be on target because recent measurements are all close to target, when in fact charting shows that several sequential measurements are above target, suggesting that the target has not been reached. Control charts also offer a framework for the conduct of one-eyed therapeutic trials, using the other eye as a control when there is limited systemic absorption of the drug.

It is possible that measurement variability differs between patients, making it desirable to construct control limits based on an individual patient's measurement variability, as has been done in this patient. Although obtaining these data may sound onerous, it is a relatively small effort to improve the management of a condition that requires lifelong treatment. Obtaining such data would be facilitated by the development of reliable easy-to-use tonometers for home use.

When it is not feasible to use individual patient data to construct control limits, it may be possible to use estimates of measurement variability from the published literature. Unfortunately, studies are not usually designed and analysed in a way that allows them to be used in constructing control charts. Studies should follow the approach we have used in our study of short-term intraocular pressure variability:

1 They should be in patients with glaucoma using treatment; the measurement variability may be different to that in unaffected people or untreated patients.
2 They should include biological variability, not just technical variability: technical variability is concerned with how intraocular pressure varies on one occasion; biological variability is concerned with how intraocular pressure varies over hours, days or weeks without any changes in treatment.
3 They should show the distribution of within-person variability, not just SDs, to assess asymmetry.
4 They should provide Altman–Bland plots [20] to see if measurement variability changes with intraocular pressure.

The usefulness of control charts will be enhanced if measurement variability is reduced. This can be achieved in several ways. Firstly, known causes of variability can be dealt with, for example by taking measurements at set times to avoid diurnal variation and at set time after the last dose of ocular drug. Secondly, if several tonometers are used, they should be calibrated against each other. Thirdly, the number of measurements can be increased at critical times for decision-making.

23.4.3. Using control charts

The wider use of control charts will require them to be easy to use. In the case of intraocular pressure, individualized control charts will need to be created to ensure that the target is correct for the patient and the control limits appropriate for the target. This will require the development of accessible software allowing easy input of the data and generating clinician- and consumer-friendly graphs.

A control chart can be useful in communicating between doctor and patient, as shown here. In addition to joint treatment decisions, the timing of additional measurements can be arranged according to needs. For example, if measurements suggest that the intraocular pressure may be off-target, discussion can centre on the need for multiple measurements to be taken over the next few days or weeks to finalize a decision.

Plotting intraocular pressure, setting a target, displaying control limits and annotating interventions are several beneficial features that control charts contribute to monitoring intraocular pressure and making management decisions. The impact on quality of care of wider adoption of control charts should be assessed.

Acknowledgements

This work was funded by program grants (211205 and 402764) from the National Health and Medical Research Council of Australia. We are grateful to Christine Craigie for taking some of the intraocular pressure measurements; Siew Chan for help with data management; Paul Glasziou, Ronald Ingle, Christine Craigie, Carl Heneghan and Sumit Dhingra for helpful comments; and Miranda Cheung for assistance in preparing the manuscript.

References

1 Quigley HA, Broman AT. The number of people with glaucoma worldwide in 2010 and 2020. *Br J Ophthalmol* 2006; **90**: 262–7.
2 Leske MC, Heijl A, Hyman L, Bengtsson B, Komaroff, E. Factors for progression and glaucoma treatment: the Early Manifest Glaucoma Trial. *Curr Opin Ophthalmol* 2004; **15**: 102–6.
3 Sommer A, Tielsch JM, Katz J, et al. Relationship between intraocular pressure and primary open angle glaucoma among white and black Americans. The Baltimore Eye Survey. *Arch Ophthalmol* 1991; **109**: 1090.
4 Maier PC, Funk J, Schwarzer G, Antes G, Falck-Ytter YT. Treatment of ocular hypertension and open angle glaucoma: meta-analysis of randomised controlled trials. *BMJ* 2005; **331**: 134–6.
5 Heijl A, Leske MC, Bengtsson B, Hyman L, Bengtsson B, Hussein M; Early Manifest Glaucoma Trial Group. Reduction of intraocular pressure and glaucoma progression: results from the Early Manifest Glaucoma Trial. *Arch Ophthalmol* 2002; **120**: 1268–79.
6 Collaborative Normal-Tension Glaucoma Study Group. The effectiveness of intraocular pressure reduction in the treatment of normal-tension glaucoma. *Am J Ophthalmol* 1998; **126**: 498–505.
7 Collaborative Normal-Tension Glaucoma Study Group. Comparison of glaucomatous progression between untreated patients with normal-tension glaucoma and patients with therapeutically reduced intraocular pressures. *Am J Ophthalmol* 1998; **126**: 487–97.
8 Drance S. Chronic open angle glaucoma: risk factors in addition to intraocular pressure. *Acta Ophthalmol Scand* 2001; **79**: 545.
9 Leske MC, Connell AM, Wu SY, et al. Incidence of open-angle glaucoma: the Barbados Eye Studies. The Barbados Eye Studies Group. *Arch Ophthalmol* 2001; **119**: 89–95.

10 Mitchell P, Smith W, Attebo K, Healey PR. Prevalence of open-angle glaucoma in Australia. The Blue Mountains Eye Study. *Ophthalmol* 1996; **103**: 1661–9.

11 Schulzer M. The Normal-Tension Glaucoma Study Group. Errors in the diagnosis of visual field progression in normal-tension glaucoma. *Ophthalmol* 1994; **101**: 1589–95.

12 Heijl A, Bengtsson B. The effect of perimetric experience in patients with glaucoma. *Arch Ophthalmol* 1996; **114**: 19–22.

13 Irwig L. This added to my myopia. *BMJ* 2003; **326**: 1336.

14 Strouthidis NG, Scott A, Peter NM, Garway-Heath DF. Optic disc and visual field progression in ocular hypertensive subjects: detection rates, specificity, and agreement. *Invest Ophthalmol Vis Sci* 2006; **47**: 2904–10.

15 Fremont AM, Lee PP, Mangione CM, et al. Patterns of care for open-angle glaucoma in managed care. *Arch Ophthalmol* 2003; **121**: 777–83.

16 Phelps CD, Phelps GK. Measurement of intraocular pressure: a study of its reproducibility. *Albrecht Von Graefes Arch Klin Exp Ophthalmol* 1976; **198**: 39–43.

17 Glasziou P, Irwig L, Mant D. Monitoring in chronic disease: a rational approach. *BMJ* 2005; **330**: 644–8.

18 American Academy of Ophthalmology. Primary Open-Angle Glaucoma Preferred Practice Pattern™. September 2005. Available from http://www.aao.org/education/library/ppp/poag_new.cfm (last accessed 5 April 2007).

19 Damji KF, Behki R, Wang L; for the Target Intraocular Pressure Workshop participants. Canadian perspectives in glaucoma management: setting target intraocular pressure range. *Can J Ophthalmol* 2003; **38**: 189–97.

20 Bland JM, Altman DG. Statistical methods for assessing agreement between two methods of clinical measurement. *Lancet* 1986; **327**: 307–10.

CHAPTER 24

Monitoring in osteoarthritis

George Peat, Mark Porcheret, John Bedson, Alison M. Ward

Osteoarthritis is a significant part of the workload of primary-care clinicians. About 2 million adults in the UK [1] and 7.1 million in the USA [2] consult a clinician in ambulatory care with symptoms attributed to osteoarthritis each year. In Canada about 40 per 1000 adults visit their doctor for osteoarthritis each year [3] and visit an average of twice a year.

General practice consultations for osteoarthritis occur in only a very small proportion of patients aged 35 years and under, but are significantly more common in middle and later life (Figure 24.1) [4]. This reflects the strong age-related patterns of osteoarthritis incidence and prevalence.

Figures based on recorded physician-diagnosed cases probably underestimate how often patients with osteoarthritis are seen in primary care. The diagnosis of knee osteoarthritis is conservatively used by clinicians, often invoked several years after the symptoms first occur, and recorded under non-specific labels.

Patients who present to primary care represent only a minority of those affected. For instance, in the second Dutch survey of General Practice, of the 149 per 1000 adults aged 25 years and over with self-reported osteoarthritis of the hip or knee, 23 had presented to the general practitioner and received a diagnosis of osteoarthritis [5]. Non-consulters may have less severe problems, but as many as 50% of those with severe knee pain and disability have not consulted their general practitioner within the past year [6].

Ageing populations and the increased prevalence of major determinants such as obesity mean that osteoarthritis is projected to increase further over the next 15 years [7]. Care for individuals with osteoarthritis extends over many years. Serial re-evaluation of patients with osteoarthritis already happens in primary care and the community. However, the processes (whether clinician-dependent or patient self-monitoring) appear to be largely unmeasured and undocumented.

Evidence-based Medical Monitoring: from Principles to Practice. Edited by Paul Glasziou, Les Irwig and Jeffrey K. Aronson. © 2008 Blackwell Publishing, ISBN: 978-1-4051-5399-7.

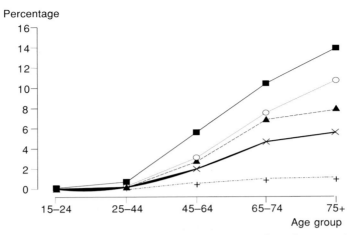

Figure 24.1 Age-specific consulting prevalence rates by people with osteoarthritis aged 15 and over in the UK, using different databases. (Adapted from [4].)

24.1. The condition

Perceptions remain that osteoarthritis (and the accompanying pain) is benign, a part of normal ageing, a disease primarily of cartilage, 'just a bit of wear and tear', inevitably progressive, for which nothing can be done. Perhaps these attitudes contribute to the relatively low profile of osteoarthritis. But research evidence paints a different picture.

- Osteoarthritis is projected to be in the top 10 leading causes of years lived with disability in developed regions of the world.
- It is not an inevitable consequence or intrinsic part of ageing.
- Osteoarthritic disease can evolve in subchondral bone, synovium, capsule, periarticular muscles, sensory nerve endings, meniscus and supporting ligaments.
- Osteoarthritis involves aberrant repair, not just tissue destruction.
- The typical course of structural disease and symptoms is gradual deterioration, but not invariably so; only a minority progress to the stage of requiring joint replacement.
- Many effective conservative treatments are available, although their average effect in reducing symptoms and disability is often relatively modest.

Osteoarthritis is not a simple disease entity [8] but a group of overlapping distinct diseases that can be characterized by clinical, pathological, biomechanical and biochemical features. The joints most commonly affected are the knees, hips and hands [9]. The diagnosis of spinal osteoarthritis, once popular, has now almost completely disappeared [10].

The pathological features incorporate the whole of the joint and include focal hyaline cartilage loss, changes in subchondral bone (marginal outgrowth, osteophyte formation, sclerosis) and changes in surrounding soft tissues (e.g.

inflammation of the synovium, ligamentous laxity, muscle inhibition and weakness). Plain radiography has traditionally been the method by which the structural pathology of osteoarthritis is assessed, although more sophisticated imaging (e.g. MRI) is increasingly being used in research.

The clinical effects of osteoarthritis are joint pain (particularly use-related), affecting one or a few regions only (often bilaterally), stiffness after inactivity ('gelling') and in the early morning (<30 minutes), joint line and/or periarticular tenderness, reduced joint movement and function, bony enlargement, coarse crepitus, a mild to modest effusion (if at all) and Heberden's and/or Bouchard's nodes [11]. Signs such as bony enlargement, used in existing classification criteria, may represent relatively late signs of advanced disease [12].

24.2. Why might we monitor osteoarthritis?

Monitoring can help decide whether treatment should be started, adjusted or stopped, and to establish what the response to treatment has been (including detecting adverse effects).

The goals of management are to reduce symptoms, maintain or improve joint mobility, limit the progression of joint damage and reduce functional disability, while avoiding or reducing the use of drugs when possible [11]. Effective pharmacological, non-pharmacological and surgical interventions are available [13, 14]. These can be arranged in a stepped-care model (Figure 24.2), with failure to respond to treatments at one level leading to the next step up [15].

Monitoring might be expected to inform management in primary care, but also when to refer to a specialist (e.g. a rheumatologist or orthopaedic surgeon).

There is no clearly established system for monitoring osteoarthritis. Here we consider what can be monitored and take the example of pain severity as a subjective marker for monitoring osteoarthritis to illustrate some of the problems involved. We return to the question 'should osteoarthritis be monitored?' at the end of the chapter.

24.3. What can we monitor?

24.3.1. Potential measures and a causal schema

Osteoarthritis may not be a single disease entity but a collection of heterogeneous diseases that share a similar endpoint, joint failure [9]. Hence, multiple causal pathways are thought to cause symptomatic osteoarthritis (Figure 24.3) [16].

24.3.2. Choosing domains for monitoring

The range of possible candidate variables for monitoring osteoarthritis is vast (Table 24.1). The challenge of selecting a monitoring test includes the substantial discordance between pathological features and the clinical syndrome

Step 4 To be considered if persisting pain or disability[4]	Surgical referral	
Step 3 Further interventions to be considered if persisting pain or disability[4]	Cognitive behavioural therapy Intra-articular hyaluronan Intra-articular glucocorticoids Occupational therapy TENS[3] Topical NSAIDs[2]	
Step 2 Interventions to be considered if persisting pain ordisability[4]	Physiotherapy Group education Wedged insoles Walking aids Appliances	Non-selective NSAIDs[2] Selective NSAIDs[2] Opioid analgesics Capsaicin Acupuncture
Step 1 Interventions to be offered to all knee pain sufferers	Written information Exercise Weight loss Restorative sleep advice	Thermotherapy Paracetamol SYSADOA[1] (glucosamine, chondroitin, diacerein, avocado–soya unsaponifiables)

Figure 24.2 A stepped model of care for the treatment of knee pain and osteoarthritis. (1) Symptomatic slow-acting drugs for osteoarthritis.(2) Non-steroidal anti-inflammatory drug (NSAID). (3) Transcutaneous Electrical Nerve Stimulation. (4) Despite the use of interventions from lower steps. (Reproduced from [15] with permission.)

of joint pain and disability. This discordance is also evident as the disease progresses—changes in structural disease are weakly related to changes in pain and disability.

The progression of structural disease, any single disease pathway and any one conservative treatment are all likely to have only a relatively small causal effect on pain and disability. Monitoring symptoms are not synonymous with monitoring disease activity nor are they likely to reflect a simple direct effect of interventions. Pain severity will also reflect the influence of co-morbidities, psychological factors, sociocultural determinants and individual responses in the form of accommodative and assimilative coping [17–19].

In the rest of this chapter we focus on one domain for monitoring: pain severity, a term we use for the combination of pain intensity and interference with daily activities [20]. The reasons for choosing to focus on pain severity for monitoring osteoarthritis are as follows:

1 Most treatment decisions are driven by symptoms. There is currently no model of preventive action for asymptomatic osteoarthritis. Even decisions such as referral to hospital specialists and the need for joint replacement are likely to be strongly influenced by pain severity [21, 22].

Table 24.1 Options for monitoring osteoarthritis

Type	Examples
Pathological	Plain radiography
	Magnetic resonance imaging
	Ultrasound
Biochemical	Urinary CTXII
	Serum COMP
Clinical	Self-reported
	Pain, disability, participation
	Physician-assessed impairment
	Effusion, limited range of movement, muscle strength, mal-alignment
	Observed physical performance
	Timed walking test, time step test, timed chair stand, standing balance
Risk indicators	Body mass index, physical inactivity
Treatment	Exercise/physical activity, long-term NSAID therapy
Adverse events	Gastrointestinal toxicity, gastrointestinal bleeding

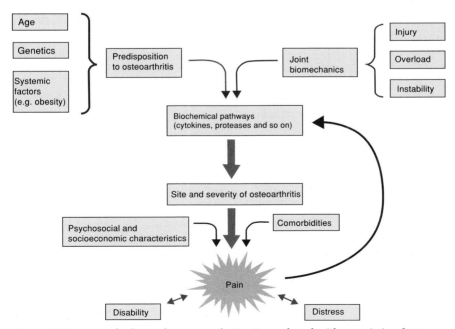

Figure 24.3 A causal schema for osteoarthritis (Reproduced with permission from [16]).

2 Pain control and minimizing disability are commonly cited as the principal goals in the management of osteoarthritis. Pain and disability are important domains for evaluating upper and lower limb osteoarthritis [8] and for evaluating chronic pain [23, 24] and the effectiveness of its treatment [25].

3 Pain intensity, interference with activities and the fear that these will escalate are likely to be principal reasons for seeking the advice of health-care professionals.

4 Pain severity is generally perceived to be under-assessed, under-estimated and under-managed, particularly in older adults [26–28]. Several professional bodies have already recommended that pain measurement form part of routine assessment [29, 30].

5 There is considerable evidence about available measures and their psychometric properties, as well as some consensus on which measures are preferred and how they may be interpreted.

There are no good monitoring alternatives to pain severity. Plain radiography is a relatively crude measure of the disease process, and alternative imaging techniques (MRI, ultrasonography) are still being investigated for their diagnostic value. The scientific and clinical value of biomarkers has yet to be established.

Certain important arguments are sacrificed by a focus on pain severity. Other markers may be more appropriate for specific purposes. A combination of markers may provide a better overview of progress over time (e.g. self-reported measures could be supplemented by observed physical function tests to obtain a fuller impression of disability). There are likely to be trade-offs between different outcomes or targets for monitoring (e.g. achieving satisfactory pain control but at the risk of adverse effects from long-term drug therapy). As yet, there is no established basis for combining different targets for monitoring osteoarthritis [31].

24.3.3. Choosing measures of pain severity for monitoring

There is a wide range of available self-completed or interviewer-administered measures of pain severity. Measures that include pain intensity and interference with daily activities may be generic, disease-specific or condition-specific, region-specific or site-specific, unidimensional or multidimensional, patient-specific, or simple summary measures [32]. Table 24.2 lists some of the more commonly used and extensively investigated measures that can be considered for monitoring pain severity in patients with osteoarthritis [33–44].

Making a recommendation based on a review of their relative merits is not our purpose, but we encourage the reader to consult relevant review articles [45–48]. Instead we take two measures that have a track record of use in research and clinical practice, have been recommended by expert panels for use in clinical trials and clinical settings [8, 24, 25] and have empirical evidence that can be used to illustrate how they might be used and interpreted.

The first is the Western Ontario and McMaster Universities Osteoarthritis Index (WOMAC), specific for osteoarthritis of the hips and knees, which

Table 24.2 Examples of self-completed measures of pain severity used in populations with osteoarthritis

Measure	Recall period	Items	Scales
Generic			
SF-36 [32]	4 wk	36	General health; physical function; role – physical; role – emotional; bodily pain; mental health; social functioning; vitality
AIMS2 [33]	4 wk	56	Mobility; physical activity; dexterity; activities of daily living; social role; social activity; anxiety; depression; pain
WONCA-COOP [34]	4 wk	9	Physical fitness; feelings; daily activities; social activities; change in health; overall health; social support; quality of life; pain
Brief pain inventory [35]	24 h	10	Pain, impact of pain on mood; impact of pain on activities
Site- or disease-specific			
Any chronic pain grade [36]	3 or 6 mo	7	Characteristic pain intensity; disability points; single index: grade I–IV
Lower extremity			
WOMAC [37]	48 h	24	Pain; stiffness; physical functioning
HOOS [38]	7 d	40	Symptoms; pain; activities of daily living; sports and recreation; quality of life
KOOS [39]	7 d	42	Symptoms; pain; activities of daily living; sports and recreation; quality of life
Oxford Hip Score [40]	4 wk	12	Single index
Oxford Knee Score [41]	4 wk	12	Single index
Upper extremity			
AUSCAN [42]	48 h	15	Pain; stiffness; physical functioning
DASH [43]	7 d	30	Disability/symptoms

consists of 24 questions providing a summative score for subscales on pain (five items), stiffness (two items) and physical functioning (17 items) [38]. Responses are recorded either on a visual analogue scale or a five-point ordinal scale (none/mild/moderate/severe/extreme) giving subscale scores of 0–100 on the visual analogue scale or 0–20 (pain), 0–8 (stiffness), 0–68 (physical functioning) on the ordinal scale. Completion time is about 5 minutes. The second is a single-item measure of pain intensity, the 11-point numerical rating scale, which provides a score of 0–10. Different periods of recall are possible, including current pain intensity, pain intensity within the past week and average and worst pain intensity in the previous 3 or 6 months [20, 37]. Completion time is less than 1 minute.

24.4. Has this individual responded sufficiently?

24.4.1. Clinically relevant changes

There has been much effort in recent years to understand how best to design and analyse studies of clinical relevant changes in patient-reported outcomes and to derive estimates for commonly used measures (reviews of progress and current expert opinion in this field are provided in the proceedings of meetings of OMERACT [49, 50] and IMMPACT IV [51].

Clinically relevant changes as they relate to individual patient monitoring concern between- and within-person minimal clinically important differences (MCID) [52] over time. One of the most frequently used methods for deriving an estimate of MCID is the anchor-based transition method. This relies on patients' judgements of whether, during a specified period, they are unchanged, better or worse. Change scores observed during this period are then related to this transition rating. This approach has been applied to both the WOMAC and the 11-point numerical rating scale to derive estimates of the MCID. A summary of sample studies is provided in Table 24.3 [53–56].

Minimally clinically important improvements for WOMAC pain scores of 41% have been reported in 603 rheumatology out-patients with knee osteoarthritis [57]. There was a reduction of 41% or more in WOMAC pain scores at 4 weeks after oral non-steroidal treatment in 75% of those who rated their response to treatment as 'good' or 'excellent' (sensitivity 75%). Only 25% of the patients who rated their response to the same treatment as 'fair', 'poor' or 'none' experienced this degree of pain reduction (specificity 75%). Others have used a more lenient anchor of being 'slightly improved' and estimated minimally clinically important worsening, which has been less frequently studied but is nevertheless useful in the context of monitoring [53].

On the basis of other studies [54, 55], a reduction of 30% is now recommended as the minimal clinically important improvement for the 0–10 numerical rating scale for pain intensity [24]. Single-item measures need not be inferior to longer multiple-item measures (Table 24.4).

Evidence is mixed on whether the value of MCID varies between patient groups. In most studies, however, MCID has varied depending on patient

Table 24.3 Examples of MCID estimates for WOMAC and PI-NRS from anchor-based transition method studies involving osteoarthritis patients

Setting, intervention, population	Anchor	Pain severity measure	MCID (%)	Sensitivity, specificity (%)	Reference
2724 patients with chronic pain in clinical trials of pregabalin (10% osteoarthritis).	Patient reports minimally, much or very much improved at 5–12 wk	PI-NRS (0–10)*	−15	77, 77	[53]
	Patient reports much or very much improved at 5–12 wk	PI-NRS (0–10)*	−28	78, 78	
	Patient reports very much improved at 5–12 wk	PI-NRS (0–10)*	−47	82, 82	
814 rheumatology out-patients with knee osteoarthritis (n = 603) or hip osteoarthritis (n = 211)	Response to treatment rated by patient as good or excellent at 4 wk	WOMAC pain (0–100)	−41 (knee)	75, 75	[54]
		WOMAC function (0–100)	−32 (hip)	75, 75	
			−26 (knee)	75, 75	
			−21 (hip)	75, 75	
Rehabilitation in-patients with knee osteoarthritis (n = 113) or hip osteoarthritis (n = 79)	Patient reports 'slightly better' at 3 mo	WOMAC pain (0–10)	−18	—	[55]
		WOMAC function (0–10)	−17	—	
	Patient reports 'slightly worse' at 3 mo	WOMAC pain (0–10)	+14	—	
		WOMAC function (0–10)	+22	—	
825 rheumatology out-patients with knee osteoarthritis (n = 233), hip osteoarthritis (n = 89), hand osteoarthritis (n = 133), rheumatoid arthritis (n = 290) or ankylosing spondylitis (n = 83)	Patient reports slightly better, much better at 3 mo	PI-NRS (0–100)	−15	90, 80	[56]
	Patient reports much better at 3 mo	PI-NRS (0–100)	−33	84, 93	

Note: *Mean of seven daily measurements at baseline and at follow-up.
MCID, minimum clinically important difference; WOMAC, Western Ontario and McMaster Universities Osteoarthritis Index; PI-NRS, pain intensity–numerical rating scale.

Table 24.4 Comparison of estimates of percentage changes in different pain severity measures for detecting patient-rated improvement or deterioration at 18 months of follow-up

	Pain severity measure (area under the curve)						
	WOMAC subscales			Chronic pain grade single items			
	Pain	Stiffness	Functioning	Current pain	Average pain	Pain interference	
*Definition of improvement**							
Completely recovered or much better	0.85	0.74	0.95	0.93	0.95	0.79	
Completely recovered, much better or better	0.79	0.65	0.77	0.84	0.88	0.68	
Definition of deterioration							
Much worse or worse	0.74	0.66	0.69	0.74	0.76	0.70	
Much worse	0.69	0.65	0.70	0.79	0.83	0.71	

Note: *Based on responses to the question 'Compared to when you came for your assessment 18 months ago, how do you think your knee pain has changed?'.

baseline scores—the higher the baseline score, the greater the reduction needed before the patient recognizes it as being important. This applies particularly to raw scores, but also to percentage changes.

24.4.2. Clinically relevant state

An alternative to measuring the size of change is to define a clinically relevant state, such as the 'patient acceptable symptom state' (PASS) [56]. Patients value improvements principally if their symptoms become tolerable [58]. Clinically relevant changes are secondary to achieving a clinically relevant state. This suggests concentrating on maintaining patients within a target range of pain severity, similar to a target blood pressure in hypertension or international normalized ratio in anticoagulation.

The PASS values for WOMAC pain and physical function scores (0–100) are estimated at 32 and 35 for knee osteoarthritis and 31 and 34 for hip osteoarthritis [56]. Of patients who felt that their overall state was satisfactory 75% had scores below the PASS; 75% of those who felt that their state was not satisfactory had scores above the PASS.

Similar arguments have been developing for the 0–10 numerical rating scale item on pain intensity. There appears to be a fairly consistent interpretation of values across different types of chronic pain, including osteoarthritis. Values of 1–4 are generally interpreted as 'mild', 5–6 or 5–7 as 'moderate' and 7–10 or 8–10 as 'severe' [59]. Significant disability begins to emerge at 'moderate' degrees of pain [60]. Scores of less than 5 on the 0–10 numerical rating scale may form part of a concept of 'manageable pain control'.

24.4.3. Problems in estimating clinical relevant changes and states

Despite much progress and the appeal of single universal values for MCID or clinically relevant states, it is unlikely that such a simple solution exists. Different stakeholders may have different definitions of what constitutes an important change or state. To date, studies have principally been from patients' perspectives. The anchor-based methods used to date are somewhat circular: why not just ask patients if they are better? [61] Values may be context-specific and time-dependent. Without standardization, different estimates will result from studies using different designs and instruments [62]. Considering MCID and clinically relevant states without also being aware of the costs required to produce them is just 'plain wrong' [63].

These arguments illustrate the current 'state of the science' of measuring and interpreting pain severity. Interpreting outcome data in clinical trials has been a major driving force behind such evidence. The application and usefulness of monitoring pain severity for osteoarthritis care in routine clinical settings are still developing.

24.5. Monitoring pain severity

24.5.1. How and when can we monitor pain severity?

It is conceptually useful to distinguish short-term and long-term monitoring of pain severity.

Short-term monitoring is the initial evaluation of pain severity and its re-evaluation in response to the introduction of a new intervention, the withdrawal of an existing treatment or an alteration in the dose of an existing treatment within an episode of care lasting anywhere from several days to 3 months. This short-term evaluation is probably made relatively informally by asking patients to return to the clinician in the event of continuing problems and to describe them.

Long-term monitoring need not be tied to an episode of care, but could instead involve retaining an overview of the course of the illness by repeated assessments at fixed intervals. Re-evaluating pain severity at annual intervals is suggested as a quality indicator for the care of older adults with osteoarthritis [64]. Monitoring in this way may reduce the likelihood that severe pain and disability will go unnoticed and avoid some of the inherent difficulties in relying on patient recall for comparative estimates of changes over such long periods of time. Currently, there is no established process for routine long-term monitoring of osteoarthritis.

24.5.2. How can we evaluate the effect of monitoring pain severity?

Simply introducing patient-reported measures into routine practice has little effect on management decisions or patient outcomes [65, 66]. Any effects of monitoring on patient outcomes rely on a chain of events that connects formal eliciting of the degree of pain severity through to changes in a patient's current health status and the prevention of future adverse events and illness progression. Unless we seriously scrutinize this causal chain, further clinical trials of monitoring osteoarthritis are likely to be uninformative.

24.5.3. Should we monitor pain severity in osteoarthritis?

Continued management of osteoarthritis generally occurs outside the remit of chronic disease clinics. Such clinics have developed over many years and deliver high-quality care, but in the UK, for example, they are also driven by financial rewards for achieving targets. However, for osteoarthritis there are no such financial incentives. Primary health-care practitioners currently rely on a combination of patient-initiated consultations and opportunistic checks to monitor osteoarthritis. Formal measurement is seldom involved.

Monitoring pain severity in osteoarthritis is different in several ways from monitoring biological markers. Patients can self-monitor their pain and disability constantly. Furthermore, they have direct access to many of the effective options for managing osteoarthritis (over-the-counter medications, weight loss, exercise and physical activity) without needing to consult health-care professionals.

However, there are several reasons why monitoring pain severity could be beneficial for osteoarthritis sufferers. It is important to include the patient's perceptions of treatment efficacy in the management of osteoarthritis—not only do patients and clinicians judge treatment efficacy differently but patients may also alter their efficacy criteria to stay with their preferred treatment [67]. Monitoring pain severity may be a useful way to inform this process and target acceptable degrees of treatment efficacy for each patient.

For example, in 116 single n-of-1 trials using a within-patient randomized, double-blind, crossover comparison of treatments for osteoarthritis, in which patient-completed daily diaries of pain and stiffness were used to evaluate treatment response, the results supported the recommendation to use parac-etamol as the first-line pharmacological treatment in preference to NSAIDs [68].

A potential adverse effect of monitoring pain severity in osteoarthritis is that drawing attention to the pain and disability that sufferers experience may increase their awareness of the pain and reduce their coping ability [19]. However, to date there is no evidence that this is the case in osteoarthritis. However, the problem is made more complex by the fact that perception of pain severity and physical functioning is influenced by socioeconomic status and psychosocial factors such as self-efficacy, pessimism, coping style, depression and anxiety [17].

Finally, from the doctor's perspective, monitoring the progress of pain and disability is an important process that is integral to treatment strategies throughout the patient's illness. It helps define specific management options, gives both doctor and patient expectations of the outcomes of treatments, and establishes their long-term success. It can help determine when treatment can be safely stopped, and thereafter acts as a trigger to further intervention. It seems that without monitoring, osteoarthritic patients would not be in a position to receive optimal care.

24.6. Scheduled follow-up

Each year a significant minority of older adults with severe joint pain and disability do not appear to consult primary-care doctors [6, 60], although many are 'very dissatisfied' with the prospect of living the rest of their lives with their symptoms (Figure 24.4) [69]. Those with depression are less likely to consult [70]. This may be indirect evidence of disillusionment with formal health-care services. A more proactive approach to monitoring would provide opportunities to identify clinically important deterioration or persisting unmanageable pain.

Oral NSAIDs are commonly used by patients to manage osteoarthritis. This usage can often be reduced or eliminated without rebound effects on pain or function, either by organizing a review by a community pharmacist or by

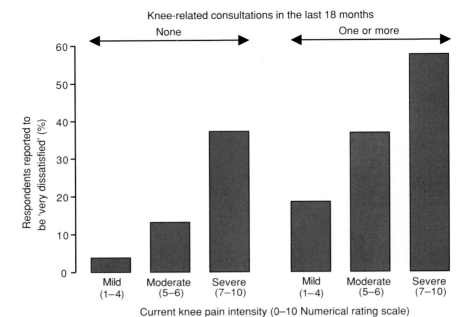

Figure 24.4 Percentages of individuals with symptomatic knee osteoarthritis who would be 'very dissatisfied' if they had to spend the rest of their lives with their current knee symptoms (data from 212 community-dwelling adults aged 50 years and over reporting knee pain within the previous 6 months, symptoms on most days in the past month and definite radiographic osteoarthritis on plain x-rays) (Adapted from [69]).

offering alternative non-pharmacological treatment [71]. Given the risks and costs of adverse effects from using long-term NSAIDs, scheduled monitoring of patients with osteoarthritis may help reduce the length of time during which the patients are at risk of adverse effects from unnecessary treatment.

Since osteoarthritis is a common condition, a small improvement in care would have large population benefits, but clinicians are also wary of 'opening the floodgates' by encouraging more frequent consultations. For every scheduled visit that is instrumental in preventing unnecessary pain or disability, or reducing unnecessary use of NSAIDs, how many more will be uninformative or result in unnecessary 'tinkering' with treatment? Selecting and targeting the groups that are most likely to benefit from monitoring is a logical solution. However, if we draw an analogy with disease prevention, in which many people need to engage in preventive action to prevent disease in a few, it may still be necessary to monitor many individuals with osteoarthritis to tackle a few cases of significant preventable suffering [72].

By separating the monitoring of osteoarthritis from the management of other chronic conditions, we also neglect some of the important collateral benefits that patients with osteoarthritis experience when their co-morbidities are better controlled. For example, effective management of depression reduces perceived arthritis-related disability [73]. Annual medication reviews, now a standard requirement for all registered patients, may be sufficient to identify problems with long-term use of NSAIDs by patients with osteoarthritis. Monitoring obesity is likely to be a population-wide concern, but presumably any benefit will also accrue for patients with osteoarthritis. For some patients with osteoarthritis the most effective intervention will be one aimed at reducing the burden of co-morbidities [74]. Under these circumstances, an approach to monitoring that focuses solely on osteoarthritis will miss opportunities for such collateral benefit.

Rather than alter the pattern of follow-up for patients with osteoarthritis, would introducing formal quantitative measurement of pain severity into the existing arrangements be worthwhile? These have, after all, been widely accepted and applied in clinical trials of the effectiveness of treatments for osteoarthritis.

24.7. Formal quantitative measurement

Recognizing pain appears to be the first challenge in primary-care consultations. In a study of 105 primary-care physicians in the USA, physicians recorded information about pain in 47% of patients who consulted them with moderate degrees of pain and 70% of patients who consulted them with severe pain [75]. This clearly leaves a significant minority of cases potentially unrecognized.

Even when pain is recognized, clinicians generally underestimate patients' pain, particularly if the patient rates it as severe [26, 76–80]. Assessing change over time is also problematic. It is likely that over longer periods, the ability of patients and clinicians to report improvement retrospectively or deterioration accurately may decline [81]. This has two implications: simple global ratings of change ('are you better?') may provide misleading responses if a long period has elapsed and current anchor-based calculations of MCID need to be supplemented by other approaches [82].

The use of repeated quantitative measurement may help clinicians recognize pain and disability, obtain accurate estimates of pain severity and provide a common language for communicating about pain. The benefits of shared decision-making are now widely accepted [83, 84]. Owing to the large number of possible treatments and the wide range of non-treatment factors that influence pain and disability [17], the selection and titration of treatment for osteoarthritis is unlikely to be done purely on the basis of pain severity. A patient's preference for different treatments is likely to be an important determinant of treatment selection, and may itself influence the effectiveness of treatment. But recognition and accurate assessment of pain severity would be an important component of effective communication and decision-making.

Nevertheless, there are several potential difficulties and unresolved matters that relate to the use of formal quantitative measurements to monitor pain severity. Although less likely to recall bias, response shift is a feature of self-reported quality-of-life measures [85, 86]. This is likely to affect self-reported measures of pain and disability in those with osteoarthritis as they become older and their condition and their general health change. Other potential adverse effects of introducing repeated quantitative measurement of pain severity into osteoarthritis consultations include disrupting doctor–patient communication (measures designed for research are often too long), unduly focusing attention on pain (medicalization, creating worried well), the risk of conscious manipulation of self-reporting, and the relative lack of appropriate measures in certain groups of individuals who may be particularly vulnerable to under-recognized and under-treated pain (e.g. severe cognitive impairment). Each of these deserves attention, although some concerns may have been overstated. For example, brief measures may be just as responsive to perceived changes over time (Table 24.4). Studies in other chronic pain conditions have shown little reactivity from repeated pain measurement, even intensive electronic diary completion [87]. Greater involvement of other members of the primary-care multidisciplinary team (and perhaps even community-based individuals) could remove some of the burden of monitoring from general practitioners.

24.8. Conclusions

Osteoarthritis is a common and increasingly prevalent condition responsible for a large number of primary-care consultations. Small improvements in care would bring major population benefits. However, the role of monitoring in bringing about such improvements is unclear. Current arrangements for monitoring osteoarthritis rely on a combination of patient-initiated consultations and opportunistic evaluations during consultations for other illness. Formal measurement is seldom involved. The heterogeneity of the disease and the degree of discordance between this and subjective status mean that a single obvious target for monitoring osteoarthritis is not currently available.

By considering pain severity as the target of osteoarthritis monitoring, we have raised a broader question: do (should) the concepts and practice of monitoring chronic disease extend to monitoring common chronic symptoms and subjective states? We need more research before being able to decide whether and how to monitor osteoarthritis more formally than at present. In the meantime, greater recognition and more accurate assessment of pain severity in the consultation would be a step in the right direction.

24.8.1. Research agenda
The following is a suggested research agenda for monitoring in osteoarthritis:
• Basic descriptive epidemiology on the course of joint pain and osteoarthritis over time.

- Selective monitoring: identifying which individuals with osteoarthritis would most benefit from formal monitoring.
- The role of disease monitoring and the effectiveness of treatment guided by such markers.
- The association between symptom control and disability management and the progression of disease and risk of future significant events and outcomes (e.g. joint replacement, hospitalization, dependency, social isolation).
- The development of psychometrically robust brief measures of pain assessment for use in the primary-care consultation and for self-monitoring.
- The effectiveness and cost-effectiveness of multiple-episode, longer term care plans.
- The conceptual basis and practical value of monitoring states of 'subjective significance'.

Acknowledgements

Peter Croft for his initial ideas and encouragement. Nadine Foster for advice on patient preferences, members of the research team for CAS(K). Workshop participants at the Primary Care Rheumatology Society's Annual Meeting in 2006, whose ideas and suggestions on monitoring osteoarthritis we drew on for this chapter.

References

1 Arthritis Research Campaign. Arthritis: the big picture. 1. Statistics from the ARC Epidemiology Unit, 2002. Available from
http://www.arc.org.uk/about_arth/bigpic.htm (last accessed 18 September 2006).

2 Hootman JM, Helmick CG, Schappert SM. Magnitude and characteristics of arthritis and other rheumatic conditions on ambulatory medical care visits, United States, 1997. *Arthritis Rheum* 2002; **47**: 571–81.

3 Health Canada. Arthritis in Canada. *An Ongoing Challenge*. Ottawa: Health Canada, 2003. Available from http: //www.acreu.ca/pdf/Arthritis_in_Canada.pdf (last accessed 26 July 2006).

4 Jordan K, Clarke AM, Symmons DPM, et al. Measuring disease prevalence: a comparison of musculoskeletal disease using four general practice consultation databases. *Br J Gen Pract* 2007; **57**: 7–14.

5 Westert GP, Schellevis FG, de Bakker DH, Groenewegen PP, Bensing JM, van der Zee J. Monitoring health inequalities through general practice: The Second Dutch National Survey of General Practice. *Eur J Public Health* 2005; **15**: 59–65.

6 Jinks C, Jordan K, Ong N, Croft P. A brief screening tool for knee pain in primary care (KNEST). 2. Results from a survey in the general population aged 50 and over. *Rheumatology* 2004; **43**: 55–61.

7 Perruccio AV, Power JD, Badley EM. Revisiting arthritis prevalence projections—it's more than just the aging of the population. *J Rheumatol* 2006; **33**: 1856–62.

8 World Health Organization. The burden of musculoskeletal conditions at the start of the new millennium. Report of a WHO Scientific Group. *WHO Technical Report*

Series No. 919. Geneva: WHO, 2003. Available from http://whqlibdoc.who.int/trs/WHO_TRS_919.pdf (last accessed 26 July 2006).

9 Felson DT, Lawrence RC, Dieppe PA, Hirsch R, Helmick CG. Osteoarthritis: the disease and its prevalence and impact. In: Felson DT (conference chair), *Osteoarthritis: New Insights. Part 1: The Disease and Its Risk Factors. Ann Intern Med* 2000; **133**: 635–6.

10 Croft P. Diagnosing regional pain: the view from primary care. *Baillieres Best Pract Res Clin Rheumatol* 1999; **13**: 231–42.

11 Prodigy. Guidance. Osteoarthritis, 2005. Available from http://www.prodigy.nhs.uk/osteoarthritis (last accessed 12 September 2006).

12 Peat G, Thomas E, Duncan R, Wood L, Hay E, Croft P. Clinical classification criteria for knee osteoarthritis: performance in the general population and primary care. *Ann Rheum Dis* 2006; **65**: 1363–7.

13 Jordan KM, Arden NK, Doherty M, et al.; Standing Committee for International Clinical Studies Including Therapeutic Trials ESCISIT. EULAR Recommendations 2003. An evidence based approach to the management of knee osteoarthritis. Report of a Task Force of the Standing Committee for International Clinical Studies Including Therapeutic Trials (ESCISIT). *Ann Rheum Dis* 2003; **62**: 1145–55.

14 Zhang W, Doherty M, Arden N, et al.; EULAR Standing Committee for International Clinical Studies Including Therapeutics (ESCISIT). EULAR evidence based recommendations for the management of hip osteoarthritis: report of a task force of the EULAR Standing Committee for International Clinical Studies Including Therapeutics (ESCISIT). *Ann Rheum Dis* 2005; **64**: 669–81.

15 Porcheret M, Jordan K, Croft P; Primary Care Rheumatology Society. Treatment of knee pain in older adults in primary care: development of an evidence-based model of care. *Rheumatol (Oxford)* 2007; **46**: 638–48.

16 Dieppe PA, Lohmander LS. Pathogenesis and management of pain in osteoarthritis. *Lancet* 2005; **365**: 965–73.

17 Keefe FJ, Smith SJ, Buffington AL, Gibson J, Studts JL, Caldwell DS. Recent advances and future directions in the biopsychosocial assessment and treatment of arthritis. *J Consult Clin Psychol* 2002; **70**: 640–55.

18 Stang PE, Brandenburg NA, Lane MC, Merikangas KR, von Korff MR, Kessler RC. Mental and physical comorbid conditions and days in role among persons with arthritis. *Psychosom Med* 2006; **68**: 152–8.

19 De Vlieger P, Bussche EV, Eccleston C, Crombez G. Finding a solution to the problem of pain: conceptual formulation and the development of the Pain Solutions Questionnaire (PaSol). *Pain* 2006; **123**: 285–93.

20 Von Korff M, Jensen MP, Karoly P. Assessing global pain severity by self-report in clinical and health services research. *Spine* 2000; **25**: 3140–51.

21 Hadorn DC, Holmes AC. The New Zealand priority criteria project. Part 1: Overview. *BMJ* 1997; **31**: 131–4.

22 Woolhead GM, Donovan JL, Chard JA, Dieppe PA. Who should have priority for a knee joint replacement? *Rheumatology (Oxford)* 2002; **41**: 390–4.

23 Turk DC, Dworkin RH, Allen RR, et al. Core outcome domains for chronic pain clinical trials: IMMPACT recommendations. *Pain* 2003; **106**: 337–45.

24 Dworkin RH, Turk DC, Farrar JT, et al; IMMPACT. Core outcome measures for chronic pain clinical trials: IMMPACT recommendations. *Pain* 2005; **113**: 9–19.

25 Bellamy N, Kirwan J, Boers M, et al. Recommendations for a core set of outcome measures for future phase III clinical trials in knee, hip, and hand osteoarthritis. Consensus development at OMERACT III. *J Rheumatol* 1997; **24**: 799–802.

26 Mantyselka P, Kumpusalo E, Ahonen R, Takala J. Patients' versus general practitioners' assessments of pain intensity in primary care patients with non-cancer pain. *Br J Gen Pract* 2001; **51**: 995–7.

27 Rosemann T, Wensing M, Joest K, Backenstrass M, Mahler C, Szecsenyi J. Problems and needs for improving primary care of osteoarthritis patients: the views of patients, general practitioners and practice nurses. *BMC Musculoskelet Disord* 2006; **7**: 48.

28 Breivik H, Collett B, Ventafridda V, Cohen R, Gallacher D. Survey of chronic pain in Europe: prevalence, impact on daily life, and treatment. *Eur J Pain* 2006; **10**: 287–333.

29 Wenger NS, Shekelle PG; the ACOVE Investigators. ACOVE quality indicators. *Ann Intern Med* 2001; **135**: 652–67.

30 AGS Panel on Persistent Pain in Older Persons. The management of persistent pain in older persons. *JAGS* 2002; **50** (Suppl 6): S205–S224.

31 Dougados M. Monitoring osteoarthritis progression and therapy. *Osteoarthritis Cartilage* 2004; **12** (Suppl 1): 55–60.

32 Fitzpatrick R, Davey C, Buxton MJ, Jones DR. Evaluating patient-based outcome measures for use in clinical trials. *Health Technol Assess* 1998; **2**: 14.

33 Ware JE, Jr, Sherbourne CD. The MOS 36-item short-form health survey (SF-36). I. Conceptual framework and item selection. *Med Care* 1992; **30**: 473–83.

34 Ren XS, Kazis L, Meenan RF. Short-form arthritis impact measurement scales. 2: Tests of reliability and validity among patients with osteoarthritis. *Arthritis Care Res* 1999; **12**: 163–71.

35 Nelson E, Wasson J, Kirk J, et al. Assessment of function in routine clinical practice: description of the COOP Chart method and preliminary findings. *J Chronic Dis* 1987; **40** (Suppl 1): 55S–69S.

36 Mendoza T, Mayne T, Rublee D, Cleeland C. Reliability and validity of a modified Brief Pain Inventory short form in patients with osteoarthritis. *Eur J Pain* 2006; **10**: 353–61.

37 Von Korff M, Ormel J, Keefe FJ, Dworkin SF. Grading the severity of chronic pain. *Pain* 1992; **50**: 133–49.

38 Bellamy N. *WOMAC Osteoarthritis Index. A User's Guide*. Ontario: London Health Services Centre, McMaster University, 1996.

39 Nilsdotter AK, Lohmander LS, Klassbo M, Roos EM. Hip disability and osteoarthritis outcome score (HOOS)—validity and responsiveness in total hip replacement. *BMC Musculoskelet Disord* 2003; **4**: 10.

40 Roos EM, Roos HP, Lohmander LS, Ekdahl C, Beynnon BD. Knee Injury and Osteoarthritis Outcome Score (KOOS)—development of a self-administered outcome measure. *J Orthop Sports Phys Ther* 1998; **28**: 88–96.

41 Dawson J, Fitzpatrick R, Carr A, Murray D. Questionnaire on the perceptions of patients about total hip replacement. *J Bone Joint Surg Br* 1996; **78**: 185–90.

42 Dawson J, Fitzpatrick R, Murray D, Carr A. Questionnaire on the perception of patients about total knee replacement. *J Bone Joint Surg Br* 1998; **80**: 63–9.

43 Bellamy N, Campbell J, Haraoui B, et al. Dimensionality and clinical importance of pain and disability in hand osteoarthritis: development of the Australian/Canadian (AUSCAN) Osteoarthritis Hand Index. *Osteoarthritis Cartilage* 2002; **10**: 855–62.

44 Hudak PL, Amadio PC, Bombardier C. Development of an upper extremity outcome measure: the DASH (disabilities of the arm, shoulder and hand). The Upper Extremity Collaborative Group (UECG). *Am J Ind Med* 1996; **29**: 602–8.

45 Sun Y, Sturmer T, Gunther KP, Brenner H. Reliability and validity of clinical outcome measurements of osteoarthritis of the hip and knee—a review of the literature. *Clin Rheumatol* 1997; **16**: 185–98.

46 Ortiz Z, Shea B, Garcia Dieguez M, et al. The responsiveness of generic quality of life instruments in rheumatic diseases. A systematic review of randomized controlled trials. *J Rheumatol* 1999; **26**: 210–6.

47 Garratt AM, Brealey S, Gillespie WJ, DAMASK Trial Team. Patient-assessed health instruments for the knee: a structured review. *Rheumatol (Oxford)* 2004; **43**: 1414–23.

48 Dziedzic KS, Thomas E, Hay EM. A systematic search and critical review of measures of disability for use in a population survey of hand osteoarthritis (osteoarthritis). *Osteoarthritis Cartilage* 2005; **13**: 1–12.

49 OMERACT 5. *International Consensus Conference on Outcome Measures in Rheumatology, Toulouse, France, 4–8 May 2000. J Rheumatol* 2001; **28** (2): 394.

50 OMERACT 6. *International Consensus Conference on Outcome Measures in Rheumatology, Gold Coast, Australia, 11–14 April 2002. J Rheumatol* 2003; **30** (5): 1101.

51 IMMPACT-IV, 11–12 June 2004, Washington, DC. http://www.immpact.org/meetings.html (last accessed 17 May 2007).

52 Beaton DE, Bombardier C, Katz JN, et al. Looking for important change/differences in studies of responsiveness. OMERACT MCID Working Group. Outcome measures in rheumatology. Minimal clinically important difference. *J Rheumatol* 2001; **28** (2): 400–5.

53 Angst F, Aeschlimann A, Michel BA, Stucki G. Minimal clinically important rehabilitation effects in patients with osteoarthritis of the lower extremities. *J Rheumatol* 2002; **29**: 131–8.

54 Farrar JT, Young JP, Jr, LaMoreaux L, Werth JL, Poole RM. Clinical importance of changes in chronic pain intensity measured on an 11-point numerical pain rating scale. *Pain* 2001; **94**: 149–58.

55 Salaffi F, Stancati A, Silvestri CA, Ciapetti A, Grassi W. Minimal clinically important changes in chronic musculoskeletal pain intensity measured on a numerical rating scale. *Eur J Pain* 2004; **8**: 283–91.

56 Tubach F, Ravaud P, Baron G, et al. Evaluation of clinically relevant states in patient reported outcomes in knee and hip osteoarthritis: the patient acceptable symptom state. *Ann Rheum Dis* 2005; **64**: 34–7.

57 Tubach F, Ravaud P, Baron G, et al. Evaluation of clinically relevant changes in patient reported outcomes in knee and hip osteoarthritis: the minimal clinically important improvement. *Ann Rheum Dis* 2005; **64**: 29–33.

58 Tubach F, Dougados M, Falissard B, Baron G, Logeart I, Ravaud P. Feeling good rather than feeling better matters more to patients. *Arthritis Rheum* 2006; **55**: 526–30.

59 Palos GR, Mendoza TR, Mobley GM, Cantor SB, Cleeland CS. Asking the community about cutpoints used to describe mild, moderate, and severe pain. *J Pain* 2006; **7**: 49–56.

60 Peat G, Thomas E, Croft P. Staging joint pain and disability: a brief method using persistence and global severity. *Arthritis Care Res* 2006; **55**: 411–9.

61 Wright JG. Evaluating the outcome of treatment: shouldn't we asking patients if they are better? *J Clin Epidemiol* 2000; **53**: 549–53.

62 Tubach F, Wells GA, Ravaud P, Dougados M. Minimal clinically important difference, low disease activity state, and patient acceptable symptom state: methodological issues. *J Rheumatol* 2005; **32**: 2025–9.

63 Hays RD, Woolley JM. The concept of clinically meaningful difference in health-related quality-of-life research. How meaningful is it? *Pharmacoeconomics* 2000; **18**: 419–23.

64 Ganz DA, Chang JT, Roth CP, et al. Quality of osteoarthritis care for community-dwelling older adults. *Arthritis Rheum* 2006; **55**: 241–7.

65 Greenhalgh J, Meadows K. The effectiveness of the use of patient-based measures of health in routine practice in improving the process and outcomes of care: a literature review. *J Eval Clin Pract* 1999; **5**: 401–16.

66 Huas D, Pouchain D, Gay B, Avouac B, Bouvenot G; The French College Of Teachers In General Practice. Assessing chronic pain in general practice: are guidelines relevant? A cluster randomized controlled trial. *Eur J Gen Pract* 2006; **12**: 52–7.

67 Bellamy N, Carr A, Dougados M, Shea B, Wells G. Towards a definition of 'difference' in osteoarthritis. *J Rheumatol* 2001; **28**: 427–30.

68 Nikles CJ, Yelland M, Glasziou PP, Del Mar C. Do individualized medication effectiveness tests (n-of-1 trials) change clinical decisions about which drugs to use for osteoarthritis and chronic pain? *Am J Ther* 2005; **12**: 92–7.

69 Peat G, Thomas E, Handy J, et al. The Knee Clinical Assessment Study—CAS(K). A prospective study of knee pain and knee osteoarthritis in the general population. *BMC Musculoskelet Disord* 2004; **5**: 4.

70 Jordan K, Jinks C, Croft P. A prospective study of the consulting behaviour of older people with knee pain. *Br J Gen Pract* 2006; **56**: 269–76.

71 Hay EM, Foster NE, Peat G, et al. Pragmatic randomised clinical trial of the effectiveness of community physiotherapy and enhanced pharmacy review for knee pain in older people presenting to primary care. *BMJ* 2006; **333**: 995–1003.

72 Rockhill B, Kawachi I, Colditz GA. Individual risk prediction and population-wide disease prevention. *Epidemiol Rev* 2000; **22**: 176–80.

73 Lin EH, Katon W, Von Korff M, et al.; IMPACT Investigators. Effect of improving depression care on pain and functional outcomes among older adults with arthritis: a randomized controlled trial. *JAMA* 2003; **290**: 2428–9.

74 Dieppe P, Brandt KD. What is important in treating osteoarthritis? Whom should we treat and how should we treat them? *Rheum Dis Clin North Am* 2003; **29**: 687–716.

75 Bertakis KD, Azari R, Callahan EJ. Patient pain in primary care: factors that influence physician diagnosis. *Ann Fam Med* 2004; **2**: 224–30.

76 Tait RC, Chibnall JT. Physician judgments of chronic pain patients. *Soc Sci Med* 1997; **45**: 1199–205.

77 Suarez-Almazor ME, Conner-Spady B, Kendall CJ, Russell AS, Skeith K. Lack of congruence in the ratings of patients' health status by patients and physicians. *Med Decis Making* 2001; **21**: 113–21.

78 Marquie L, Raufaste E, Lauque D, Marine C, Ecoiffier M, Sorum P. Pain rating by patients and physicians: evidence of systematic pain miscalibration. *Pain* 2003; **102**: 289–96.

79 Kappesser J, Williams AC, Prkachin KM. Testing two accounts of pain underestimation. *Pain* 2006; **124**: 109–16.

80 Panda M, Staton LJ, Chen I, et al. The influence of discordance in pain assessment on the functional status of patients with chronic nonmalignant pain. *Am J Med Sci* 2006; **332**: 18–23.

81 Norman GR, Stratford P, Regehr G. Methodological problems in the retrospective computation of responsiveness to change: the lesson of Cronbach. *J Clin Epidemiol* 1997; **50**: 869–79.

82 Guyatt GH, Osoba D, Wu AW, Wyrwich KW, Norman GR; The Clinical Significance Consensus Meeting Group. Methods to explain the clinical significance of health status measures. *Mayo Clin Proc* 2002; **77**: 371–83.

83 Haynes RB, Devereaux PJ, Guyatt GH. Physicians' and patients' choices in evidence based practice. *BMJ* 2002; **342**: 1350.

84 Straus SE, Richardson WS, Glasziou P, Haynes RB. Evidence-based medicine. *How to Practice and Teach EBM*. London: Elsevier, 2005.

85 Sprangers MAG, Schwartz CE. Integrating response shift into health-related quality of life research: a theoretical model. *Soc Sci Med* 1999; **48**: 1507–15.

86 Rapkin BD, Schwartz CE. Towards a theoretical model of quality-of-life appraisal: implications of findings from studies of response shift. *Health Qual Life Outcomes* 2004; **2**: 14.

87 Aaron LA, Turner JA, Mancl L, Brister H, Sawchuk CN. Electronic diary assessment of pain-related variables: is reactivity a problem? *J Pain* 2005; **6**: 107–15.

Index